Pharmacotherapy Principles & Practice Study Guide: A Case-Based Care Plan Approach

Pharmacotherapy Principles & Practice Study Guide: A Case-Based Care Plan Approach

FOURTH EDITION

Editors

Michael D. Katz, PharmD
Professor and Director of International Programs
Director of Residency Programs
Department of Pharmacy Practice and Science
College of Pharmacy
University of Arizona
Tucson, Arizona

Kathryn R. Matthias, PharmD, BCPS (AQ-ID)
Assistant Professor
Department of Pharmacy Practice and Science
College of Pharmacy
University of Arizona
Tucson, Arizona

Marie A. Chisholm-Burns, PharmD, MPH, FCCP, FASHP
Dean and Professor
College of Pharmacy
University of Tennessee
Memphis, Knoxville, and Nashville, Tennessee

New York   Chicago   San Francisco   Athens   London   Madrid   Mexico City
Milan   New Delhi   Singapore   Sydney   Toronto

Pharmacotherapy Principles & Practice Study Guide: A Case-Based Care Plan Approach, Fourth Edition

1 2 3 4 5 6 7 8 9 LMN 21 20 19 18 17 16

ISBN 978-0-07-184396-6
MHID 0-07-184396-5

This book was set in Minion Pro by Cenveo® Publisher Services.
The editors were Michael Weitz and Peter J. Boyle.
The production supervisor was Catherine Saggese.
Project management was provided by Srishti Malasi, Cenveo Publisher Services.
The designer was Alan Barnett; the cover designer was Dreamit, Inc.
LSC Communications was printer and binder.

This book is printed on acid-free paper.

Library of Congress Cataloging-in-Publication Data

Names: Katz, Michael D., editor. | Matthias, Kathryn R., editor. | Chisholm-Burns, Marie A., editor.
Title: Pharmacotherapy principles & practice study guide : a case-based care plan approach / editors,
    Michael D. Katz, Kathryn R. Matthias, Marie A. Chisholm-Burns.
Other titles: Pharmacotherapy principles and practice study guide | Complemented by (expression):
    Pharmacotherapy principles & practice. 4th edition.
Description: Fourth edition. | New York : McGraw-Hill Education, [2017] |
    Complemented by: Pharmacotherapy principles & practice / editors, Marie A. Chisholm-Burns,
    Terry L. Schwinghammer, Barbara G. Wells, Patrick M. Malone, Jill M. Kolesar, Joseph T. DiPiro.
    Fourth edition. [2016]. | Includes bibliographical references and index.
Identifiers: LCCN 2016044870| ISBN 9780071843966 (pbk. : alk. paper) | ISBN 0071843965
    (pbk. : alk. paper)
Subjects: | MESH: Drug Therapy | Case Reports | Problems and Exercises
Classification: LCC RM262 | NLM WB 18.2 | DDC 615.5/8—dc23 LC record available at
    https://lccn.loc.gov/2016044870

McGraw-Hill books are available at special quantity discounts to use as premiums and sales promotions, or for use in corporate training programs. To contact a representative please visit the Contact Us pages at www.mhprofessional.com.

CONTENTS

CONTRIBUTORS

Shirley M. Abraham, MD
Assistant Professor, Department of Pediatrics, University of New Mexico, Albuquerque, New Mexico
Chapter 100

Sarah M. Adriance, PharmD, BCPS
Specialty Practice Pharmacist, Critical Care, The Ohio State University Wexner Medical Center, Columbus, Ohio
Chapter 85

Ronda L. Akins, PharmD
Infectious Diseases Clinical Specialist, Methodist Charlton Medical Center; Adjunct Associate Professor, University of Texas at Dallas, Department of Biological Sciences, Richardson, Texas
Chapter 82

Rita Alloway, PharmD, BCPS, FCCP
Research Professor of Medicine, Director, Transplant Clinical Research, Director, Transplant Pharmacy Residency and Fellowship, University of Cincinnati, Cincinnati, Ohio
Chapter 61

Samah Alsherhi, PharmD
Postdoctoral Fellow, Department of Pharmacy Practice and Science, College of Pharmacy, University of Arizona, Tucson, Arizona
Chapter 26

Emily Anastasia, PharmD
Clinical Pharmacy Specialist, Cardiology, Durham Veterans Affairs Medical Center, Durham, North Carolina
Chapter 3

David A. Apgar, PharmD
Assistant Professor (retired), University of Arizona College of Pharmacy, Tucson, Arizona
Chapter 67

Katie E. Barber, PharmD
Assistant Professor, Department of Pharmacy Practice, University of Mississippi School of Pharmacy, Mississippi
Chapter 82

Kim W. Benner, PharmD, BCPS, FASHP, FPPAG
Professor of Pharmacy Practice, Director, Post-graduate Programs in Pharmacy Practice, Samford University McWhorter School of Pharmacy; Pediatric Clinical Pharmacy Specialist, Children's of Alabama, Birmingham, Alabama
Chapter 71

Emily B. Borders, PharmD, BCOP
Assistant Professor, University of Oklahoma, Oklahoma City, Oklahoma
Chapter 99

Sheila R. Botts, PharmD, FCCP, BCCP
Chief, Clinical Pharmacy Research and Academic Affairs, Kaiser Permanente Colorado, Aurora, Colorado
Chapter 43

Adam Bress, PharmD, MS-CTS
Research Assistant Professor, Pharmacotherapy Outcomes Research Center, Department of Pharmacotherapy, College of Pharmacy, University of Utah, Salt Lake City, Utah
Chapter 5

Gretchen M. Brophy, PharmD, BCPS, FCCP, FCCM, FNCS
Professor of Pharmacotherapy and Outcomes Science and Neurosurgery, Virginia Commonwealth University, Medical College of Virginia, Richmond, Virginia
Chapter 33

Susan P. Bruce, PharmD, BCPS
Associate Dean of Pharmacy Education and Interprofessional Studies, College of Pharmacy, Chair and Professor, Pharmacy Practice, Northeast Ohio Medical University, Rootstown, Ohio
Chapter 63

Diana Cao, PharmD, BCPS (AQ Cardiology)
Vice Chair of Clinical and Administrative Sciences Department, Assistant Professor of Clinical and Administrative Sciences, College of Pharmacy, California Northstate University, Elk Grove, California

Diana Cao, PharmD, BCPS
Assistant Professor, School of Pharmacy, Loma Linda University, Loma Linda, California
Chapter 4

Diane M. Cappelletty, PharmD
Professor, University of Toledo College of Pharmacy, Toledo, Ohio
Chapter 77

Joshua C. Caraccio, PharmD, BCPS
Antimicrobial Stewardship and Infectious Diseases Pharmacist, Utah Valley Regional Medical Center, Provo, Utah
Chapter 96

Larisa H. Cavallari, PharmD, BCPS, FCCP
Associate Professor and Associate Chair, Department of Pharmacotherapy and Translational Research, Director, Center for Pharmacogenomics, Associate Director, Personalized Medicine Program, University of Florida, Gainesville, Florida
Chapter 5

Kevin W. Chamberlin, PharmD
Associate Clinical Professor, Assistant Head, Department of Pharmacy Practice, School of Pharmacy, University of Connecticut, Farmington, Connecticut
Chapter 38

Juliana Chan, PharmD, FCCP, BCACP
Clinical Associate Professor, Gastroenterology and Hepatology, Clinical Pharmacist, Ambulatory Pharmacy Services, Clinical Associate Professor, Pharmacy Practice, Colleges of Pharmacy and Medicine, University of Illinois, Chicago, Illinois
Chapters 23 & 24

Jack J. Chen, PharmD, FCCP, BCPS, CGP
Professor and Department Chair, Department of Pharmacy Practice, College of Pharmacy, Marshall B. Ketchum University, Fullerton, California
Chapter 34

Aimee B. Chevalier, PharmD
Clinical Assistant Professor, Pharmacy Practice, Clinical Pharmacist, Ambulatory Pharmacy Services, College of Pharmacy, University of Illinois, Chicago, Illinois
Chapter 8

Marie A. Chisholm-Burns, PharmD, MPH, MBA, FCCP, FASHP
Dean and Professor, College of Pharmacy, University of Tennessee, Memphis, Knoxville, and Nashville, Tennessee
Chapter 1

Amanda H. Corbett, PharmD, BCPS, FCCP
Clinical Associate Professor, Infectious Diseases, University of North Carolina, Eshelman School of Pharmacy, Chapel Hill, North Carolina
Chapter 97

Susan Cornell, BS, PharmD, CDE, FAPhA, FAADE
Associate Director of Experiential Education, Associate Professor of Pharmacy Practice, Midwestern University Chicago College of Pharmacy, Clinical Pharmacist/Diabetes Educator, Access DuPage Community Clinic, Downers Grove, Illinois
Chapter 48

Brian L. Crabtree, PharmD, BCPP
Interim Associate Dean and Professor, Department of Pharmacy Practice, Eugene Applebaum College of Pharmacy and Health Sciences, Wayne State University, Detroit, Michigan
Chapter 42

Jean E. Cunningham, PharmD, BCPS
Senior Clinical Content Specialist, Truven Health Analytics Findaly, Ohio
Chapter 70

Clarence E. Curry, Jr, PharmD
Associate Professor Emeritus of Pharmacy Practice, College of Pharmacy, Howard University, Washington, DC
Chapters 20 & 21

Dawne Cylwik, PharmD
Advanced Practice Pharmacist, El Rio Community Health Center, Tucson, Arizona
Chapter 72

Devra K. Dang, PharmD, BCPS, CDE
Associate Clinical Professor of Pharmacy Practice, University of Connecticut School of Pharmacy; Clinical Faculty, Burgdorf Primary Care Clinic, Storrs, Connecticut
Chapter 52

Stephanie Davis, PharmD, BCACP
Program Manager, Education and Clinical Services, Southern Arizona VA Healthcare System, Clinical Assistant Professor, University of Arizona College of Pharmacy, Tucson, Arizona
Chapter 16

Kristina De Los Santos, PharmD, BCPS
Chief, Pharmacy Service Line, Southern Arizona VA Healthcare System, Adjunct Clinical Assistant Professor, Pharmacy, Practice and Science, University of Arizona College of Pharmacy, Tucson, Arizona
Chapter 10

Robert J. DiDomenico, PharmD, BCPS (AQ Cardiology), FCCP
Clinical Professor, Department of Pharmacy Practice, College of Pharmacy, University of Illinois at Chicago, Chicago, Illinois
Chapter 5

Eric Dietrich, PharmD, BCPS
Assistant Professor of Pharmacy and Medicine, Departments of Pharmacotherapy and Translational Research and Community Health and Family Medicine, Colleges of Pharmacy and Medicine, University of Florida, Gainesville, Florida
Chapter 64

Monica A. Donnelley, PharmD, BCPS
Infectious Diseases Pharmacist, University of California Davis Medical Center, Stockton, California
Chapter 84

Jeremiah J. Duby, PharmD, BCPS
Senior Critical Care Pharmacist, Specialty Critical Care Residency Program Director, University of California Davis Medical Center; Assistant Clinical Professor, University of California Davis School of Pharmacy; Assistant Clinical Professor, University of California San Francisco School of Pharmacy; Adjunct Associate Professor, Touro University, Sacramento, California
Chapter 84

Christopher J. Edwards, PharmD, BCPS
Clinical Assistant Professor, Department of Pharmacy Practice and Science, Department of Emergency Medicine, Colleges of Pharmacy and Medicine, University of Arizona; Senior Pharmacy Manager, Clinical Pharmacy Services, Banner - University Medical Center Tucson, Tucson, Arizona
Chapter 47

Megan J. Ehret, PharmD, MS, BCPP
Associate Professor, Pharmacy Practice (Affiliate), Institute for Collaboration on Health, Intervention, and Policy, University of Connecticut, Storrs, Connecticut
Chapter 38

Shareen Y. El-Ibiary, PharmD, FCCP, BCPS
Professor of Pharmacy Practice, Department of Pharmacy Practice, Midwestern University College of Pharmacy-Glendale, Glendale, Arizona
Chapter 54

Kirsten E. Ellis, PharmD
Assistant Clinical Instructor, International Programs, College of Pharmacy, University of Arizona; Clinical Pharmacist, Infectious Diseases and HIV/AIDS, Banner - University Medical Center Tucson, Tucson, Arizona
Chapter 44

John Erramouspe, PharmD, MS
Professor, Pharmacy Practice and Administrative Sciences, College of Pharmacy, Idaho State University, Pocatello, Idaho
Chapter 45

Brian L. Erstad, BCPS, MCCM
Professor and Head, University of Arizona College of Pharmacy, Tucson, Arizona
Chapters 85 & 91

Echo Fallon, PharmD
Clinical Pharmacist, Banner - University Medical Center Tucson, Tucson, Arizona
Chapter 36

William Travis Foxx-Lupo, PharmD
Oncology Clinical Pharmacist, Seattle Cancer Care Alliance at Northwest Hospital, Seattle, Washington
Chapter 98

Andrea S. Franks, PharmD, BCPS
Associate Professor of Clinical Pharmacy, University of Tennessee Health Science Center, Knoxville, Tennessee
Chapter 59

Wendy Gabriel, PharmD, BCPS
Assistant Professor, South College School of Pharmacy, Knoxville, Tennessee
Chapter 27

Ronak Gandhi, PharmD, BCPS
Clinical Pharmacist-Infectious Diseases, Massachusetts General Hospital, Boston, Massachusetts
Chapter 86

Heather L. Girand, PharmD
Professor of Pharmacy Practice, Ferris State University College of Pharmacy, Bronson Methodist Hospital, Kalamazoo, Michigan
Chapters 78 & 79

Lisa W. Goldstone, MS, PharmD, BCPS
Assistant Professor, University of Arizona College of Pharmacy, Clinical Specialty Pharmacist, Psychiatry, Banner - University Medical Center South, Tucson, Arizona
Chapter 46

Maqual R. Graham, PharmD
Professor of Pharmacy Practice, University of Missouri, Clinical Pharmacy Specialist, Veterans Affairs Medical Center, Kansas City, Missouri
Chapter 102

William Joshua Guffey, PharmD, BCACP, BC-ADM, BCPS
Director, Pharmacy Education Center for Advanced Practice and Charlotte AHEC, Carolinas HealthCare System; Assistant Professor of Clinical Education, Eshelman School of Pharmacy, University of North Carolina, Chapel Hill, North Carolina
Chapter 65

Tracy M. Hagemann, PharmD, FCCP, FPPAG
Associate Dean, Nashville and Professor of Clinical Pharmacy, University of Tennessee College of Pharmacy, Nashville, Tennessee
Chapters 56 & 75

Keri D. Hager, PharmD, BCACP
Assistant Professor, Pharmacy Practice and Pharmaceutical
Sciences Department, College of Pharmacy, University of
Minnesota, Duluth, Minnesota
Chapters 2 & 3

Nancy H. Heideman, PharmD, BCPS
Clinical Pharmacy Specialist, Pediatrics, University of
New Mexico Hospital, Albuquerque, New Mexico
Chapter 100

Richard L. Heideman, MD
Emeritus Professor of Pediatrics, Hematology/Oncology
Program, University of New Mexico, Albuquerque,
New Mexico
Chapter 100

Emily L. Heil, PharmD, BCPS-AQ ID, AAHIVP
Assistant Professor - Infectious Diseases, Department of
Pharmacy Practice and Science, University of Maryland
School of Pharmacy, Baltimore, Maryland

Brett H. Heintz, PharmD, BCPS-ID, AAHIVE
Associate Clinical Professor, University of Iowa College of
Pharmacy, Pharmacy Specialist, Internal Medicine and
Infectious Diseases, Iowa City VA Medical Center,
Iowa City, Iowa
Chapter 84

Brian A. Hemstreet, PharmD, FCCP, BCPS
Professor and Assistant Dean for Student Affairs, Regis
University School of Pharmacy, Denver, Colorado
Chapter 18

Daniel Hershberger, PharmD or MD
Pulmonary and Critical Care Fellow, Omaha, Nebrasska
Chapters 30 & 31

Michelle L. Hilaire, PharmD, CDE, BCPS, BCACP, FCCP
Clinical Professor of Pharmacy Practice, University of
Wyoming School of Pharmacy, Laramie, Wyoming
Chapter 68

Marcella Honkonen, PharmD, BCPS
Clinical Assistant Professor, Department of Pharmacy
Practice and Science, University of Arizona, Tucson,
Arizona
Chapters 26 & 27

Rebecca Hoover, PharmD
Clinical Assistant Professor, Pharmacy Practice and
Administrative Sciences, College of Pharmacy, Idaho State
University, Pocatello, Idaho
Chapter 45

Alexis E. Horace, PharmD, BCACP
Assistant Professor, School of Pharmacy, University of
Louisiana at Monroe; Clinical Pharmacist, University of
Louisiana Mid-City Clinic, Baton Rouge, Louisiana
Chapter 12

Jaime R. Hornecker, PharmD, BCPS
Clinical Assistant Professor, University of Wyoming School
of Pharmacy, Casper, Wyoming
Chapter 68

Cherry W. Jackson, PharmD, BCPP, FASHP, FCCP
Professor, Department of Pharmacy Practice, Auburn
University; Clinical Professor, Department of Psychiatric
and Behavioral Neurobiology, School of Medicine,
University of Alabama, Birmingham, Alabama
Chapter 41

Michael P. Kane, PharmD, FCCP, BCPS, BCACP
Professor, Department of Pharmacy Practice, Albany College
of Pharmacy and Health Sciences, Clinical Pharmacy
Specialist, The Endocrine Group, LLP, Albany, New York
Chapter 50

Michael D. Katz, PharmD
Professor and Director of International Programs, Director
of Residency Programs, Department of Pharmacy Practice
and Science, College of Pharmacy, University of Arizona,
Tucson, Arizona
Chapters 1, 17, 36 & 51

Deanna L. Kelly, PharmD, BCPP
Professor of Psychiatry, Director and Chief, Treatment
Research Program, Maryland Psychiatric Research Center,
University of Maryland School of Medicine, Baltimore,
Maryland
Chapter 40

Amy K. Kennedy, PharmD, BCACP
Assistant Professor, University of Arizona College of
Pharmacy, Clinical Pharmacist, El Rio Health Center,
Tucson, Arizona
Chapter 49

Michael D. Kraft, PharmD
Clinical Associate Professor, University of Michigan, College
of Pharmacy, Assistant Director of Pharmacy-Education
and Research and Clinical Pharmacist, Department
of Pharmacy Services, University of Michigan Health
System, Ann Arbor, Michigan
Chapter 101

Jeannie Kim Lee, PharmD, BCPS, CGP, FASHP
Assistant Head, Department of Pharmacy Practice and
Science, Associate Professor, Colleges of Pharmacy and
Medicine, University of Arizona, Tucson, Arizona
Chapters 10, 16

Mary Lee, PharmD, BCPS, FCCP
Vice President and Chief Academic Officer, Midwestern University, Professor of Pharmacy Practice, Chicago College of Pharmacy, Downers Grove, Illinois
Chapters 57 & 58

Russell E. Lewis, PharmD, FCCP, BCPS
Professore Associato, Malattie Infettive (MED/17), Dipartimento di Scienze Mediche e Chirurgiche, Alma Mater Studiorum Università di Bologna, Bologna, Italy
Chapter 94

Jacqueline M. Lucey, PharmD, BCPS, BCACP
Clinical Pharmacy Specialist - Diabetes Specialty Center, Diabetes and Endocrine Health, Health and Wellness Pavilion - Wexford, Wexford, Pennsylvania
Chapter 55

Alex C. Lopilato, PharmD, BCPPS
Clinical Specialist, Neonatal Intensive Care Unit, Florida Hospital for Children, Orlando, Florida
Chapter 47

Mark Malesker, PharmD, FCCP, FCCP, FASHP, BCPS
Professor of Pharmacy Practice and Medicine, Creighton University, Omaha, Nebraska
Chapters 28, 29, 30 & 31

Kathryn R. Matthias, PharmD, BCPS (AQ-ID)
Assistant Professor, Department of Pharmacy Practice and Science, College of Pharmacy, University of Arizona, Tucson, Arizona
Chapters 1, 86, 88 & 96

Lena M. Maynor, PharmD, BCPS
Clinical Associate Professor, West Virginia University School of Pharmacy, Morgantown, West Virginia
Chapter 25

Yolanda McKoy-Beach, PharmD, CDE
Assistant Professor, Howard University College of Pharmacy, Clinical Pharmacist, La Clinica del Pueblo, Washington, DC
Chapter 20

Patrick J. Medina, PharmD, BCOP
Associate Professor, University of Oklahoma College of Pharmacy, OU Cancer Institute, Oklahoma City, Oklahoma
Chapter 99

Charlie Michaudet, MD, CAQSM
Assistant Professor, Family Medicine Residency Program, Community Health and Family Medicine, University of Florida, Gainesville, Florida
Chapter 64

Vanessa E. Millisor, PharmD
Assistant Professor (Clinical), Pharmacy Practice, Eugene Applebaum College of Pharmacy and Health Sciences, Wayne State University, Detroit, Michigan
Chapter 19

Beverly C. Mims, PharmD
Professor of Pharmacy Practice, Howard University, College of Pharmacy, Clinical Pharmacist, Howard University Hospital, Washington, DC
Chapter 21

Phillip L. Mohorn, PharmD, BCPS, BCCCP
Clinical Pharmacy Specialist-Critical Care, Department of Pharmacy, Spartanburg Medical Center, Spartanburg, South Carolina
Chapter 76

Lee Morrow, MD, MSc
Professor, Division of Pulmonary, Critical Care, and Sleep Medicine, Creighton University School of Medicine, Omaha, Nebraska
Chapters 28, 29, 30 & 31

Allison Mruk, PharmD
Clinical Pharmacy Lead, Pediatric Cardiology, Phoenix Children's Hospital, Phoenix, Arizona
Chapter 13

Melinda M. Neuhauser, PharmD, MPH
Clinical Pharmacy Specialist, Infectious Diseases, VA Pharmacy Benefits Management Services, Hines, Illinois
Chapter 90

Tien M.H. Ng, PharmD
Associate Professor of Clinical Pharmacy and Medicine, University of Southern California School of Pharmacy, Los Angeles, California
Chapter 4

Mantiwee Nimworapan, PharmD
Clinical Assistant, Pharmacy Practice and Science, Banner - University Medical Center Tucson, Tucson, Arizona
Chapter 51

David E. Nix, PharmD, BCPS (AQ-ID)
Professor, University of Arizona College of Pharmacy, University of Arizona College of Medicine; Banner-University Medical Center Tucson, Tucson, Arizona
Chapter 89

Chioma Obih, PharmD
Clinical Pharmacy Specialist, Internal Medicine, Ochsner Medical Center, New Orleans, Louisiana
Chapter 26

David Parra, PharmD, FCCP, BCPS
Clinical Pharmacy Program Manager in Cardiology,
Veterans Integrated Service Network 8, Pharmacy Benefits
Management, Bay Pines, Florida; Clinical Associate
Professor, Department of Experimental and Clinical
Pharmacology, College of Pharmacy, University of
Minnesota, Minneapolis, Minnesota
Chapter 3

Asad E. Patanwala, PharmD, BCPS, FCCP, FASHP
Associate Professor, Department of Pharmacy Practice and
Science, University of Arizona College of Pharmacy,
Clinical Pharmacy Specialist, Emergency Medicine,
Banner - University Medical Center Tucson, Tucson,
Arizona
Chapter 35

Krina H. Patel, PharmD
Adjunct Faculty, Department of Pharmacy Practice and
Administration, Philadelphia College of Pharmacy,
University of the Sciences, Philadelphia, Pennsylvania
Chapter 39

Susan L. Pendland, PharmD, MS
Adjunct Associate Professor, University of Illinois at
Chicago; Clinical Staff Pharmacist, St Joseph Berea
Hospital, Berea, Kentucky
Chapter 90

Hanna Phan, PharmD
Associate Professor, Department of Pharmacy Practice and
Science, Department of Pediatrics, Colleges of Pharmacy
and Medicine, University of Arizona, Tucson, Arizona
Chapters 13, 15, 47 & 95

Beth Bryles Phillips, PharmD, FASHP, FCCP, BCPS
Rite Aid Professor, Director, PGY2 Ambulatory Care
Residency, University of Georgia College of Pharmacy,
Athens, Georgia
Chapter 62

James J. Pitcock, PharmD
Clinical Assistant Professor of Pharmacy Practice, School
of Pharmacy, University of Mississippi, University,
Mississippi
Chapter 37

Melissa R. Pleva, PharmD, BCPS, BCNSP
Adjunct Clinical Assistant Professor, Department of Clinical,
Social, and Administrative Sciences, University of
Michigan College of Pharmacy, Ann Arbor, Michigan
Chapter 101

John Leander Po, MD
Department of Medicine, University of Arizona,
Tucson, Arizona
Chapter 83

Allison Ann Presnell, PharmD
Clinical Pharmacy Specialist, St Joseph's/Candler Centers for
Medication Management, Savannah, Georgia
Chapter 62

April Miller Quidley, PharmD, BCPS, FCCM
Critical Care Pharmacist, Clinical Assistant Professor,
Vidant Medical Center, Greenville, North Carolina
Chapter 76

John J. Radosevich, PharmD, BCCCP, BCPS
Clinical Pharmacist - Critical Care, St. Joseph's Hospital and
Medical Center, Barrow Neurological Institute, Phoenix,
Arizona
Chapter 87

P. David Rogers, PharmD, PhD
First Tennessee Chair of Excellence in Clinical Pharmacy,
Vice-chair for Research, Director, Clinical and
Translational Therapeutics, Professor of Clinical
Pharmacy and Pediatrics, University of Tennessee,
Memphis, Tennessee
Chapter 94

Youssef M. Roman, PharmD
Clinical Support Specialist, OneOme, PhD Candidate
Research Assistant, University of Minnesota, Minneapolis,
Minnesota
Chapter 2

Leigh Ann Ross, PharmD, BCPS, FCCP, FASHP
Associate Dean for Clinical Affairs, Professor and Chair,
Department of Pharmacy Practice, School of Pharmacy,
The University of Mississippi, Jackson, Mississippi
Chapter 37

Laurajo Ryan, PharmD, MSc, BCPS, CDE
Clinical Associate Professor, University of Texas at Austin
College of Pharmacy, University of Texas Health Science
Center, Department of Medicine, Pharmacotherapy
Education Research Center, Austin, Texas
Chapter 22

Lauren S. Schlesselman, PharmD
Assistant Clinical Professor, Director of Assessment and
Accreditation, University of Connecticut School of
Pharmacy, Storrs, Connecticut
Chapters 60, 92 & 93

Roohollah Sharifi, MD, FACS
Director, Surgery Clinic, Professor of Surgery, University of
Illinois at Chicago, College of Medicine, Chicago, Illinois
Chapters 57 & 58

Kayce M. Shealy, PharmD, BCPS, BCACP, CDE
Interim Chair and Associate Professor, Department of Pharmacy Practice, Director, Innovation and Entrepreneurship, Department of Pharmacy Practice, Presbyterian College School of Pharmacy, Clinton, South Carolina
Chapter 53

Colin I. Sheffield, PharmD
Coordinator, Cancer Center Specialty Pharmacy, Duke University Hospital, Durham, North Carolina
Chapter 97

Susan M. Sirmans, PharmD, BCPS
Associate Professor, School of Pharmacy, University of Louisiana at Monroe, Monroe, Louisiana
Chapter 12

Nicole Slater, PharmD
Assistant Clinical Professor, Department of Pharmacy Practice, Harrison School of Pharmacy, Auburn University, Mobile, Alabama
Chapter 41

Steven M. Smith, PharmD, MPH, BCPS
Assistant Professor of Pharmacy and Medicine, Departments of Pharmacotherapy and Translational Research and Community Health and Family Medicine, Colleges of Pharmacy and Medicine, University of Florida, Gainesville, Florida
Chapter 64

Sarah A. Spinler, PharmD, BCPS (AQ-Cardiology), FCCP, FCPP, FAHA, FASHP, AACC
Professor of Clinical Pharmacy, Philadelphia College of Pharmacy, University of the Sciences in Philadelphia, Philadelphia, Pennsylvania
Chapter 6

Sara A. Stahle, PharmD, BCPS
Clinical Pharmacy Coordinator, University of Chicago Medicine, Chicago, Illinois
Chapter 91

Robert J. Straka, PharmD, FCCP
Department Head and Professor, Department of Experimental and Clinical Pharmacology, College of Pharmacy, University of Minnesota, Minneapolis, Minnesota
Chapter 2

Janice L. Stumpf, PharmD
Clinical Associate Professor, University of Michigan College of Pharmacy, Ann Arbor, Michigan
Chapters 73 & 74

Meghan K. Sullivan, PharmD, BCAPC
Director, Center for Medication Therapy Management at Creighton University, Omaha, Nebraska
Chapter 69

Brittany Suzuki, PharmD
Pharmacy Resident, Queen's Medical Center, Honolulu, Hawaii
Chapter 28

Joseph M. Swanson, PharmD, BCPS
Associate Professor of Clinical Pharmacy and Pharmacology, University of Tennessee, Colleges of Pharmacy and Medicine, Clinical Specialist, Regional Medical Center at Memphis, Memphis, Tennessee
Chapter 11

Eljim P. Tesoro, PharmD, BCPS
Clinical Associate Professor, College of Pharmacy, Clinical Pharmacist, Neurosciences, Director, PGY2 Critical Care Residency, University of Illinois Hospital and Health Sciences System, Chicago, Illinois
Chapter 33

Kimberly A. Trobaugh, PharmD, BCPS
Adjunct Assistant Professor, University of Kentucky College of Pharmacy, Transplant Clinical Pharmacist, University of Kentucky HealthCare, Lexington, Kentucky
Chapter 61

Toby C. Trujillo, PharmD, BCPS (AQ-Cardiology)
Associate Professor, University of Colorado Skaggs School of Pharmacy and Pharmaceutical Sciences, Clinical Specialist, Cardiology/Anticoagulation, University of Colorado Hospital, Aurora, Colorado
Chapter 7

Nicole M. Varner, PharmD, BCPS
Clinical Pharmacy Specialist, Pediatrics, Banner - University Medical Center Tucson, Diamond Children's; Clinical Assistant Professor, Department of Pharmacy Practice and Science, College of Pharmacy, University of Arizona, Tucson, Arizona
Chapter 15

Daniel J. Ventricelli, PharmD
Assistant Professor, Clinical Pharmacy, Philadelphia College of Pharmacy, University of the Sciences, Philadelphia, Pennsylvania
Chapters 60 & 92

Nicole D. Verkleeren, PharmD, BCPS
Clinical Pharmacist, Critical Care, Forbes Regional Hospital, Monroeville, Pennsylvania
Chapter 14

John Kelly Wachira, MD
Pulmonary and Critical Care Fellow, Creighton University
    School of Medicine, Omaha, Nebraska
Chapter 29

Lynn C. Wardlow, PharmD, MBA, BCPS (AQ ID)
Specialty Practice Pharmacist, Infectious Diseases, Ohio
    State University Wexner Medical Center, Columbus, Ohio
Chapter 95

Heidi J. Wehring, PharmD, BCPP
Assistant Professor of Psychiatry, Maryland Psychiatric,
    Research Center, University of Maryland Baltimore
    School of Medicine, Baltimore, Maryland
Chapter 40

Christy M. Weiland, PharmD, BCPS
Clinical Assistant Professor, University of Wyoming,
    Laramie, Wyoming
Chapters 80 & 81

Timothy Welty, PharmD
Clinical Assistant Professor and Clinical Specialist in
    Internal Medicine, University of West Virginia, Cabell
    Huntington Hospital, Huntington, West Virginia
Chapter 32

Jon P. Wietholter, PharmD, BCPS
Clinical Associate Professor, West Virginia University
    School of Pharmacy; Internal Medicine Clinical
    Pharmacist, WVU-Medicine Ruby Memorial Hospital,
    Morgantown, West Virginia
Chapter 66

Sheila M. Wilhelm, PharmD, FCCP, BCPS
Clinical Associate Professor, Department of Pharmacy
    Practice, Eugene Applebaum College of Pharmacy
    and Health Sciences, Wayne State University; Clinical
    Pharmacy Specialist, Internal Medicine, Harper University
    Hospital, Detroit, Michigan
Chapter 19

Susan R. Winkler, PharmD, BCPS, FCCP
Professor and Chair, Department of Pharmacy Practice,
    Midwestern University Chicago College of Pharmacy,
    Downers Grove, Illinois
Chapter 9

G. Christopher Wood, PharmD, FCCP
Associate Professor, Department of Clinical Pharmacy,
    College of Pharmacy, University of Tennessee,
    Memphis, Tennessee
Chapter 11

Lawrence David York, PharmD
Clinical Pharmacist, Infectious Diseases and HIV/AIDS,
    University of Arizona College of Medicine, Tucson,
    Arizona
Chapter 88

PREFACE

Determining and providing organized patient-specific pharmacotherapy recommendations involves a thorough evaluation of the patient's medical problems and medication issues. *Pharmacotherapy Principles and Practice Study Guide: A Case-Based Care Plan Approach,* fourth edition, contains 102 patient cases that correspond to chapters published in the fourth edition of *Pharmacotherapy Principles and Practice.* Our goal for this companion textbook is to be a study guide for today's learners of the clinical application of pharmacotherapy through either self-study or during patient case discussion sessions with other health care professionals. The aim of this study guide is to help students navigate the process of applying their knowledge of pharmacotherapy to a specific patient case by organizing patient data to logically assess a patient's medication issues and formulate a rational pharmacotherapy care plan.

Using a patient database form as an organized guide, students in the health care profession should learn how to apply their knowledge to evaluate the following key aspects of a patient case:

- *Medical Problem List:* Prioritize and organize each patient's medical problems and corresponding medications

- *Laboratory Values:* Evaluate provided and missing laboratory values for issues related to each patient's medication and medical problem list

- *Drug Therapy Problem Worksheet:* Assess each patient for drug therapy problems and their causes by specifically focusing on drug dosing, missing medications, medications without an obvious indication, drug interactions, and the social and economic impact of certain pharmacotherapy recommendations

- *Pharmacotherapy Care Plan:* Formulate a comprehensive, rational, and practical patient care plan with pharmacotherapy recommendations that are organized by the prioritized medical problem list

- *Patient Education Summary:* Based on a patient's medical problem list and pharmacotherapy recommendations, summarize brief patient education points that are individualized to the patient case

A guide for reviewing and evaluating patient cases and preparing patient database forms is provided in greater detail in Chapter 1. The cases are written in a realistic fashion, using terms and abbreviations that would be seen in a real patient's medical record. Definitions of abbreviations can be found in the fourth edition of *Pharmacotherapy Principles and Practice.* The Online Learning Center at www.PPPstudyguide.com has blank patient database forms that may be downloaded.

We, along with patient case authors, used published literature and our experiences as educators and clinicians to determine the focus of each patient case to be included in this textbook. If upon using this study guide you feel that anything important has been left out, please let us know your thoughts for future editions.

We acknowledge the commitment of more than 150 patient case authors who dedicated their time and knowledge in the preparation of this fourth edition study guide. We also thank all of the editors and authors of *Pharmacotherapy Principles and Practice*, who provided the pharmacotherapy background as reference material for this study guide's patient cases and question hints, and for their thoughts and suggestions as we developed the book.

We are grateful to everyone at McGraw-Hill who advised us and helped prepare this study guide. We specifically thank Michael Weitz for all of his suggestions and insight. In addition, we thank Peter Boyle, Srishti Malasi, Sandhya Joshi, and Laura Libretti for guiding us through the publication process and for the hard work related to the copyediting and formatting of each patient case.

At the University of Tennessee, we thank Dr. Christina Spivey for her suggestions to provide more consistency between this study guide and the companion *Pharmacotherapy Principles and Practice*, fourth edition, textbook.

Lastly, we sincerely thank Dr. Edward W. Randell for conscientiously checking laboratory values for SI unit conversion.

Michael D. Katz, PharmD
Kathryn R. Matthias, PharmD, BCPS (AQ-ID)
Marie A. Chisholm-Burns, PharmD, MPH, FCCP, FASHP

1 Applying Pharmacotherapy Principles and Practice: How to Use This Study Guide

Michael D. Katz   Kathryn R. Matthias
Marie A. Chisholm-Burns

As health care becomes more complex in the 21st century, the health professional student increasingly is challenged to learn a rapidly expanding amount of information as well as necessary skills to apply that knowledge in a patient care setting. Students of pharmacotherapy quickly learn that the field is rapidly changing as our knowledge of human disease evolves and new drugs are developed to improve patient outcomes. Students also learn that while drug therapy can have tremendous beneficial effects on patient outcomes, such therapy also has the potential to cause harm. The "art" of pharmacotherapy is in applying knowledge and making therapeutic decisions that are most likely to have maximum positive benefit *for a specific patient*. As a companion book to *Pharmacotherapy Principles and Practice*, 4th ed. (*PPP*), this study guide is designed to assist the student in learning to apply didactic knowledge to specific patient situations. Such application requires skills that cannot be learned in lectures or in other passive learning situations, but must be learned by practice and repetition. The more students practice applying their knowledge, using their patient assessment skills, and making therapeutic decisions in their preclinical courses, the more prepared they will be to apply these skills to real patients in their clinical rotations.

This study guide is more than a book of patient cases, but it uses patient cases to help students learn to apply pharmacotherapeutic knowledge and skills. Case-based learning is not a new concept in health sciences curricula. As a form of active learning, case-based learning allows the student to practice the skills necessary to provide patient care. The focus of the cases in this study guide is, of course, pharmacotherapeutics. A unique feature of this study guide is the expectation that the student will develop a pharmacotherapy care plan as the "output" for each case. What follows is a general discussion

of the patient care process and then specific information regarding the use of the study guide and development of the pharmacotherapy care plan.

PHARMACEUTICAL CARE AND THE PATIENT CARE PROCESS

Most pharmacy students are taught about pharmaceutical care early in their pharmacy curriculum. Pharmaceutical care, first described in the late 1980s and early 1990s,[1] can be summarized as "… patient-centered practice in which the practitioner assumes responsibility for a patient's drug-related needs and is held accountable for this commitment."[2] Although the definition of pharmaceutical care does not explicitly state that pharmacists are to perform these tasks, many feel that pharmaceutical care is the central mission of the pharmacy profession.

Although it may seem obvious that health professionals practice in a patient-centered way, all too often, practitioners become distracted by technical or administrative tasks. Pharmacy students, upon graduation, commit to patient-centered practice in the Oath of a Pharmacist:[3]

I promise to devote myself to a lifetime of service to others through the profession of pharmacy. In fulfilling this vow:

- I will consider the welfare of humanity and relief of suffering my primary concerns.
- I will apply my knowledge, experience, and skills to the best of my ability to assure optimal outcomes for my patients.
- I will respect and protect all personal and health information entrusted to me.

- I will accept the lifelong obligation to improve my professional knowledge and competence.
- I will hold myself and my colleagues to the highest principles of our profession's moral, ethical, and legal conduct.
- I will embrace and advocate changes that improve patient care.
- I will utilize my knowledge, skills, experiences, and values to prepare the next generation of pharmacists. I take these vows voluntarily with the full realization of the responsibility with which I am entrusted by the public.

A central tenet underlying pharmaceutical care and our desire to improve drug therapy outcomes is the recognition that patients have drug therapy needs. Although sometimes these needs are obvious ("What can I take for my headache?"), in many cases the patient's drug therapy needs are unrecognized. For the practitioner committed to responsibility for a patient's drug-related needs, identifying such needs in an accurate and timely way is paramount. During any pharmaceutical care encounter, the patient must be assessed to determine whether the following drug therapy needs are being met:[2]

1. The medication is appropriate

2. The medication is effective

3. The medication is safe

4. The patient is adherent

The challenge for the beginning pharmacotherapeutic practitioner is in application. How does a student learn to take the scientific and factual information learned in the classroom and in readings and then apply it to patients so that drug therapy outcomes are maximized? This study guide is designed for this purpose, to teach the student the patient care process: how to organize patient information, assess patients in a systematic way, and develop a pharmacotherapy care plan.[4]

All clinicians need a structured rational thought process for making clinical decisions. What sets each profession and professional apart is the application of a unique knowledge base and set of clinical skills to identify and solve problems and to prevent problems from occurring. In the context of drug therapy, Cipolle et al. termed this structured process the "Pharmacotherapy Workup."[2]

There are five steps that comprise the patient care process and constitute the Pharmacotherapy Workup (see Fig. 1-1): Collect, Assess, Plan, Implement and Follow-up. As Figure 1-1 indicates, each stage of the process is connected to and continuous with the other stages, and the process is ongoing as the patient's situation changes.

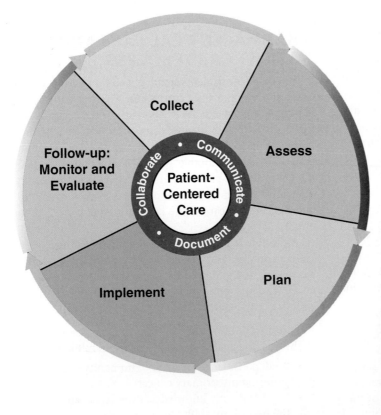

Pharmacists' patient care process
Pharmacists use a patient-centered approach in collaboration with other providers on the health care team to optimize patient health and medication outcomes.

Using principles of evidence-based practice, pharmacists:

Collect
The pharmacist assures the collection of the necessary subjective and objective information about the patient in order to understand the relevant medical/medication history and clinical status of the patient.

Assess
The pharmacist assesses the information collected and analyzes the clinical effects of the patient's therapy in the context of the patient's overall health goals in order to identify and prioritize problems and achieve optimal care.

Plan
The pharmacist develops an individualized patient-centered care plan, in collaboration with other health care professionals and the patient or caregiver that is evidence-based and cost-effective.

Implement
The pharmacist implements the care plan in collaboration with other health care professionals and the patient or caregiver.

Follow-up: Monitor and evaluate
The pharmacist monitors and evaluates the effectiveness of the care plan and modifies the plan in collaboration with other health care professionals and the patient or caregiver as needed.

FIGURE 1-1. The Patient Care Process. (Adapted with permission from the Joint Commission of Pharmacy Practitioners. Pharmacists' Patient Care Process. May 29, 2014. https://www.pharmacist.com/sites/default/files/files/PatientCareProcess.pdf, accessed January 26, 2016.)

Collect

The purpose of the collection stage is to gather patient-specific information and then determine if the patient's drug therapy needs are being met.[5] To develop the best possible pharmacotherapy plan for the patient, the information gathered must be as accurate and complete as possible. Inaccurate or incomplete information may result in bad therapeutic decisions. There are a variety of sources from which such information is gathered. Although the specific sources may differ on the basis of the patient's situation, the clinician must strive to obtain information from all available sources. The patient is a crucial source of information, as are family members, caregivers, and other health professionals. In a health-system setting (hospitals, ambulatory care clinics, etc.), the clinician also will have access to subjective and objective information recorded in the patient's medical record and other institutional databases. For the pharmacotherapy workup, particular attention must be given to obtaining a complete and accurate medication history. Remember that since the patient care process is continuous, the gathering of patient-specific information also must be ongoing. Such information must be documented in an organized and easily retrievable way that maintains patient confidentiality. Since there may be a large volume of patient-specific information generated, particularly in a hospitalized patient, the use of a standardized patient data form facilitates the organization and retrievability of patient-specific information. Despite the clinician's best effort, in most cases there will be information that is inaccurate and/or incomplete. Never assume that you have all the information you need or that the information you have is correct. The clinician must be mindful of this and seek to "fill in the blanks" by asking appropriate follow-up questions or seeking additional information from other sources.

Assess

After all available information is collected, the next step is to develop a problem list.[6] The concept of problem list development is well established in the context of the problem-oriented medical record and the use of the SOAP (Subjective, Objective, Assessment, Plan) method of charting progress notes. The development of an accurate and complete problem list based on the patient's drug therapy needs is crucial in that the development of the pharmacotherapy care plan is derived from the patient's problem list. If a problem is not listed or is not accurate, then the plan will be incomplete or suboptimal. The problem list must be prioritized to ensure that the most important problems are addressed in a timely fashion. For the student learning pharmacotherapy, developing an accurate and complete list of problems is challenging since many pieces of subjective and objective information (findings) have to be interpreted before something can be labeled as a problem. In many cases, problems are medical diagnoses (hypertension, type 2 diabetes, etc.), and in some cases the problem may be a symptom (headache, nausea, pain, etc.). Keep in mind that the definition of a problem may change as more information is gathered. For example, a patient may present with fatigue and, in the absence of other information, that is how the patient's problem is defined at that specific time. However, if the patient is referred to a physician and is found to have hypothyroidism, then the patient's problem list is changed to hypothyroidism, with fatigue as a symptom of the patient's hypothyroidism. A common trap for the beginning student is listing every finding as a problem. With thought and, ultimately, experience, the student will begin to see that the patient's signs and symptoms may be "lumped" into broader problems. If the above-mentioned patient also has cold intolerance, cognitive impairment, weight gain, elevated TSH, and slightly elevated LDL cholesterol, the patient's problem is still hypothyroidism, since each of those findings is a common sign/symptom of hypothyroidism. Although the pharmacotherapy problem list may be very similar to the problem list generated by other clinicians or the problem list present in the patient's medical record, remember that the pharmacist, having a unique body of knowledge, should have a different way of looking at the patient, and the problem list may not be entirely the same. The pharmacotherapy workup must be focused on drug therapy issues, particularly on the presence or risk of drug therapy problems (DTPs). During the entire process, always ask yourself:

- Could the patient's problem(s) be caused by drug therapy?
- Could the patient's problem(s) be managed by a change in drug therapy?

Assessment for Drug Therapy Problems

The primary focus of the pharmacotherapy workup is the identification and management (treatment and prevention) of DTPs. A DTP is defined as any undesirable event or risk experienced by the patient that involves or is suspected to involve drug therapy and that actually or potentially interferes with a desired patient outcome.[7] Strand et al.'s original list of DTP categories has been expanded to 14 categories:

- Correlation between drug therapy and medical problems
- Need for additional drug therapy
- Unnecessary drug therapy
- Appropriate drug selection
- Wrong drug
- Drug regimen
- Dose too low
- Dose too high
- Therapeutic duplication
- Drug allergy/adverse drug event
- Interactions
- Failure to receive therapy
- Financial impact
- Patient knowledge of drug therapy

Since there are so many categories and specific types of DTPs, and since patients often receive multiple medications, it is important to use an organized, systematic approach to identify actual and potential DTPs. Once a DTP is identified and categorized, it is then necessary to identify the cause of the problem, thereby leading to potential solutions. When multiple DTPs are identified, they need to be prioritized to determine which problems should be addressed first. The patient's concerns must be considered in determining the problems that have the highest priority. Remember that the process of DTP identification is connected to the basic tenets of assessing the patient's drug therapy needs—appropriateness, effectiveness and safety of medications, and the patient's adherence.

Plan

The pharmacotherapy care plan[8,9] is the roadmap to achieving improved pharmacotherapy outcomes. It is the action plan developed on the basis of the assessment components described above. Care plans have been an integral component of nursing care, and other professionals or certain health care settings may utilize components of a care plan. However, there is no standard or widely accepted method of care plan development in pharmacy. Standard 2.1 of the 2016 accreditation standards for pharmacy education in the United States[10] requires that "…The graduate is able to provide patient-centered care as the medication expert (collect and interpret evidence, prioritize, formulate assessments and recommendations, implement, monitor and adjust plans, and document activities)." Ideally, the patient's care plan should be constructed with the patient's involvement and, in a multidisciplinary fashion, developed and altered in a cooperative way by all who are involved with the patient's care. Further, pharmacotherapy care planning should be a component of the patient's overall care plan. Care plans developed in isolation or not shared with the patient or other professionals are less likely to have the desired effect on patient outcomes. A pharmacotherapy care plan must be generated as part of the systematic patient care process and should be a dynamic document that reflects changes in the patient's conditions and drug therapy needs. The care plan is developed in a problem-oriented fashion. Each item in the patient's problem list must be addressed in the care plan, and the care plan should be prioritized in the same way as the problem list.

The pharmacotherapy care plan has several key components for each problem:

- Current drug regimen
- Drug therapy problems
- Therapy goals, desired endpoints
- Therapeutic recommendations
- Rationale
- Therapeutic alternatives
- Monitoring and follow-up
- Patient education

In patients who have multiple problems, there likely will be some redundancy in the pharmacotherapy care plan in that some problems may be related, and some medications may be used for multiple indications. As the care plan is developed, it is important for the student to see and understand the connections among multiple problems and the pharmacotherapy plan. For example, a patient with hypertension, type 2 diabetes, and chronic kidney disease may be treated with an ACE-I to lower blood pressure (BP), slow progression of renal disease, and reduce risk of cardiovascular events. The student must understand not only that the one drug may be used for several reasons but that the drug could affect the patient's problems in a variety of ways, such as improving BP control while causing an increase in serum potassium or an acute rise in serum creatinine. The risk and significance of these effects must be considered on the basis of the overall clinical picture. In some patients, unintended effects, at least to a defined point, may be acceptable.

Defining therapy goals and endpoints is crucial. You cannot determine whether the patient's desired outcomes are being achieved if you do not know what those desired outcomes are. Think of goals as broad or general outcomes, whereas endpoints are more specific parameters often used as indicators or surrogate markers to indicate that our goals are being achieved. The goals of therapy must be achievable and realistic for the patient. Drug therapy may aim to (1) cure a disease; (2) reduce or eliminate signs and/or symptoms; (3) slow or halt the progression of a disease; (4) prevent a disease; (5) normalize laboratory values; and/or (6) assist in the diagnostic process. Goals and endpoints must be observable, measurable, and describable using specific parameters.

Going back to our diabetic, hypertensive patient mentioned above, the goals of treating those disorders are to prevent cardiovascular disease (stroke, coronary artery disease, peripheral vascular disease), kidney disease, other microvascular complications of diabetes (retinopathy, neuropathy), etc. We also want the patient to feel better and have improved quality of life (QOL). An important goal of any pharmacotherapy care plan is the avoidance of adverse events. We do not want the patient to have side effects or a worsened QOL due to our recommended drug therapy. What would be endpoints for our patient? In our hypertensive diabetic patient, some endpoints would include BP <130/80 mm Hg, glycated hemoglobin <6.5-7% (0.065-0.07; 48-53 mmol/mol Hb), LDL cholesterol <130 mg/dL (<3.36 mmol/L), and weight loss of 22 lb (10 kg). Goals and endpoints should be associated with a time frame, describing, if possible and realistically, when the goal or endpoint is to be achieved (BP <130/80 mm Hg in 1 month; 22 lb (10 kg) weight loss in 6 months, etc.). The goals and endpoints part of the plan will be directly tied to the monitoring part of the plan, since monitoring is the way we will know if our goals and endpoints have been achieved.

Implement

Therapeutic recommendations are the interventions made to meet the patient's drug therapy needs. The recommendations must be specific and individualized to the patient's condition and drug therapy problems. For most problems, there are several ways to intervene to achieve the desired goals and endpoints. The clinician must consider all the possibilities and recommend a therapeutic course that is best for that patient, based on scientific evidence, patient history, cultural and health beliefs, psychosocial issues, health literacy, and cost. Remember that therapeutic recommendations for one problem may have an impact on other problems, so do not lose sight of the big picture.

Although it is important for the clinician to make appropriate therapeutic recommendations, providing a rationale for those recommendations is necessary. The rationale is *why* you are recommending what you are recommending. From an educational standpoint, providing a well-reasoned rationale shows that the student is thinking and understanding, rather than repeating what is in a book, guideline, or said by others. In the clinical practice setting, it is common for pharmacists to be asked to provide their rationale to physicians as part of a discussion about a patient's therapy. Pharmacists need to be adept at providing such a rationale in a succinct way. The rationale should be stated in a way that clearly describes why the recommendation was made for this patient, including why it was chosen over other alternatives, and any evidence available to support the recommendation should be provided.

In determining your therapeutic recommendations, several reasonable alternative regimens typically are available. Even after you have recommended your primary plan, the best alternatives must be kept in mind. The patient or prescriber may not agree with your primary recommendation and request an alternative. Your primary plan may not be effective, or an intolerable adverse event may occur, thereby requiring implementation of an alternative plan. As with your therapeutic recommendations, be specific with your alternative recommendations and base your alternative choices on relative effectiveness and safety based on the best evidence available.

Follow-up: Monitor and Evaluate

Monitoring and follow-up are important components of the pharmacotherapy care plan and the overall patient care process.[11] Monitoring is how we determine whether our goals and endpoints (achieving positive goals and avoiding negative endpoints) are being reached. An effective monitoring plan must be realistic for the patient setting and include specific monitoring parameters (clinical and laboratory/diagnostic tests), frequency of monitoring, and when the patient needs to be seen again for follow-up. Students often struggle with developing a monitoring plan since references often provide only general recommendations for what to monitor and how often. In most patients, the intensity and frequency of monitoring are dynamic. In a critically ill hospitalized patient, some pharmacotherapy monitoring parameters may be assessed multiple times daily. As the patient becomes more stable, leaves the ICU, and is, hopefully, discharged home, monitoring becomes less frequent. A patient initiated on warfarin in the hospital may have an INR measured daily.

After discharge with a therapeutic international normalized ratio (INR), monitoring may be done weekly, and as the patient's INR and clinical status remain stable, the frequency is slowly reduced until the INR is measured on a monthly basis. If the INR or the clinical picture changes, the frequency of INR monitoring likely will be temporarily increased. Regardless of the setting, the frequency of monitoring, particularly for those parameters involving blood collection or other invasive tests, must be realistic and based on how often the information truly is needed, what the patient can or is willing to allow, availability of vascular access, and, in the outpatient setting, the ability of the patient to travel to a laboratory or the availability of home care services. In the home setting, some of the monitoring may be done by the patient, such as assessing presence and severity of signs and symptoms, basic physical assessment parameters (e.g., weight, presence of edema), and certain diagnostic or laboratory tests (e.g., BP, blood glucose). The monitoring plan must be specific—what parameters, frequency of monitoring, who will monitor, and when and with whom the patient will follow-up. The results of monitoring naturally will influence the pharmacotherapy care plan, and in many cases, there should be an upfront determination of what action will be taken based on the results of the monitoring plan (e.g., "the patient's INR is <2, the warfarin dose will be increased from 4 to 5 mg daily").

Patient education is a crucial piece of the pharmacotherapy care plan. Patient adherence to drug therapy can be improved with effective and ongoing patient education, and ideally, such education should be provided with verbal communication and written materials. Pharmacy students should utilize skills learned in their communications courses and information available in books[12,13] and begin applying those skills in case-based learning, small group discussions, and internship experience in preparation for their pharmacy practice experience rotations and, ultimately, pharmacy practice. The pharmacotherapy care plan must include a summary of what you will tell and provide the patient regarding their drug therapy.

Remember that our model for the patient care process involves continuous follow-up. As the pharmacotherapy care plan is implemented, the patient's response to therapy is monitored, and changes in therapy may be necessary. Changes in previous problems or the development of new signs and symptoms will require the assessment process and changes in the pharmacotherapy care plan. Although the patient care process and the application of your didactic knowledge to the patient care setting may seem daunting, by working through the cases in the Study Guide, your skills can only get better and better. Although this book can be used for self-study, ideally, some of the cases in this Study Guide will be used in a small group discussion setting under the guidance of a group facilitator, so you can see how other students think. Group settings also provide the opportunity to discuss and defend your therapeutic recommendations and practice your verbal communication skills. As you work through the patient cases, you will make mistakes and perhaps choose suboptimal therapy that even could cause harm.

Beginners always make mistakes, and you should use these mistakes as powerful learning opportunities. Here are some tips for success in patient care:

- CARE about the patient!
- Know your stuff—be prepared
- Realize that every patient is different
- Review and assess *all* available information
- Be organized and consistent in your approach
- Do not make snap judgments—is your assessment and approach supported by the evidence?
- NEVER make assumptions
- Be skeptical
- Think ahead, and think it through ("… then what?")

HOW THE CASES ARE ORGANIZED

Each patient case in the study guide has been prepared in a standard format, similar to how you will see cases presented in a clinical setting. The use of an organized case format will assist you in learning where to find information about the patient and help you get accustomed to the format for when you will be presenting patients yourself in case discussions or rotations. The patient cases in the study guide are meant to be realistic. Patients usually will have multiple, sometimes related, problems, though each case will focus on one primary topic or problem. Patients will have DTPs requiring identification and management. The components of each case in the study guide include:

1. *Patient Identification*—name, age, etc.
2. *Chief Complaint*—why the patient is seeking help, in the patient's own words.
3. *History of Present Illness* (HPI)—the patient's story about why they are seeking help.
4. *Past Medical History* (PMH)—including all significant illnesses, surgical procedures, injuries.
5. *Family History*—age and health of immediate family (parents, siblings, children); for deceased relatives, the age and cause of death are included; any hereditary diseases should be noted.
6. *Social History*—may include where the patient is from or lives, ethnicity/race, marital status, number of children, educational background, occupation, diet.
7. *Tobacco/Alcohol/Substance Use.*
8. *Allergy/Intolerances/Adverse Drug Events* (ADEs)—a common area where information from the patient is missing or incomplete.
9. *Medication History*—should include current (or medications prior to admission if hospitalized) and previous medications; the list should include what the patient *actually* is taking, not just what is prescribed, and must include OTC drugs and dietary supplements (including herbal and complementary/alternative products).

10. *Review of Systems* (ROS)—systematic, head-to-toe questions asked to elicit symptoms and potential problems not noted by the patient in the HPI. Positive findings and pertinent negatives (significant absence of a symptom) are included.
11. *Physical Examination* (PE)—nature and completeness of the examination will depend on the patient's history and overall clinical picture. Rarely will a complete PE be done; rather, the examination will be targeted to the situation. Positive and pertinent negative findings will be included in the PE. If you are not familiar with the meaning or significance of some of the examination findings, make sure you look those up. Components of the PE may include:
    - General
    - Vital Signs (include pain as fifth vital sign)
    - Skin
    - HEENT
    - Neck and Lymph Nodes
    - Chest
    - Breasts (in women)
    - Cardiovascular
    - Abdomen
    - Neurology
    - Extremities
    - Genitourinary
    - Rectal
12. *Laboratory and Other Diagnostic Tests*—only data that are common and/or directly relevant to the case will be included. A list of normal laboratory values is included as Appendix B of this study guide. All laboratory results will be presented in conventional units typically used in the United States and in Systéme Internationale (SI) units for students using the book in other countries. If you are not familiar with the meaning or significance of some of the laboratory findings, make sure you look those up.
13. *Assessment*—the clinician's impression and/or diagnosis.
14. *Student Workup*—for each case, you will be asked if there is missing information and to evaluate and develop a Patient Database, Drug Therapy Problem Worksheet, and Pharmacotherapy Care Plan. When you are working with actual patients, you will find that the patient's history and information from other sources will be incomplete and/or inaccurate. Patient cases in the study guide will have missing information, and it is important that, as you evaluate each case, you recognize what needed information is missing so that you can make an accurate assesment of the patient. One way to remember to assess for missing information is to always create as one of your patient's problems "Inadequate Database," and then list the missing information elements under that problem in your Care Plan. A more detailed description of the Patient Database, Drug Therapy Problem Worksheet, and Pharmacotherapy Care Plan forms will follow.
15. *Targeted Questions*—each case will include a series of questions targeted toward helping you better understand

the key elements of the case and the patient's primary problems. A unique feature of this study guide is each question will be followed by a hint, guiding you to the pages in *Pharmacotherapy Principles and Practice*, 4th ed. (PPP) where you can find the information to answer the question.

16. *Follow-up*—some cases will provide a brief clinical follow-up that may include some outcomes of your initial Care Plan. The Follow-up section may include additional Targeted Questions, with hints to further assist your studies.

17. *Global Perspective*—another unique feature of this study guide is the inclusion of a Global Perspective section that highlights an issue related to the case that is important to countries outside North America or involves different ethnic groups or races. Global Perspectives may highlight differences in disease incidence or manifestations, pharmacokinetics or pharmacodynamics, treatment standards, culturally based beliefs and/or treatments, and drug response.

18. *Case Summary*—a short summary of the key points addressed by the case.

19. *References*—will be included in the patient case only if a key reference has been published that is not included in *PPP*. For most cases, the references included in the relevant *PPP* chapters are excellent sources for you to obtain additional information.

STUDENT CASE WORKUP

The desired student workup of each case in this study guide is the development of a Pharmacotherapy Care Plan. The principles of the pharmacotherapy workup, patient assessment, and development of a care plan were reviewed earlier in this chapter. Your workup of the study guide cases will apply these principles. To facilitate your accomplishing these tasks in a thoughtful, organized and systematic way, you are provided three forms—Patient Database, Drug Therapy Problem Worksheet (DTPW), and Pharmacotherapy Care Plan. The forms used in this study guide are adapted with permission from those originally developed by the American Society of Health-System Pharmacists (ASHP) in the early 1990s as part of its Clinical Skills program,[5,6,8,11] and these forms are currently used by particpants in the ASHP Clinical Skills Competition (www.ashp.org/Import/ABOUTUS/Awards/ClinicalSkillsCompetition.aspx).

Different clinicans and institutions use many different types of patient-monitoring forms. Think of the forms used in this study guide as a tool to help you learn to provide the best patient care. The forms are designed to help you organize information and your thinking. Although you will find the use of such forms helpful, do not obsess about the forms or using them the "right" way. Again, the forms are a tool to help you achieve what you *should* obsess about—making the patient's drug therapy the best it can be.

To help you understand how to best utilize these forms as you workup the study guide cases, we have prepared a practice case presented in the same format as other cases in the study guide and a completed student workup. Before you embark on your first study guide patient case, look over the practice case and the completed forms. We added some tips in certain places in the practice case forms to help you better understand their application. Learning to effectively assess patients and develop a care plan involves skills that require practice and repetition. As you begin learning pharmacotherapeutics, applying your didactic knowledge to patient situations may seem difficult, and it is likely you will make mistakes. That's okay! The point of this study guide is to help you learn and to develop your skills. Through your coursework, reading, and use of this guide, you will see your knowledge and skills increase and you will become a great practitioner who will improve patient drug therapy outcomes.

REFERENCES

1. Hepler CD, Strand LM. Opportunities and responsibilities in pharmaceutical care. Am J Hosp Pharm 1990 47: 533-543.

2. Cipolle RJ, Strand L, Morley P. Pharmaceutical Care Practice. The Patient-Centered Approach to Medication Management, 3rd ed. New York, McGraw-Hill, 2012.

3. American Association of Colleges of Pharmacy. www.aacp.org/resources/academicpolicies/studentaffairspolicies/Documents/OATHOFAPHARMACIST2008-09.pdf. Accessed January 10, 2016.

4. American Society of Health System Pharmacists. ASHP guidelines on a standardized method for pharmaceutical care. Am J Health Syst Pharm 1996 53:1713-1716.

5. Mason NA, Shimp LA. Module 2: Building a pharmacist's patient database. In: ASHP Clinical Skills Program—Advancing Pharmaceutical Care. Bethesda, MD, American Society of Health-System Pharmacists, 1993.

6. Shimp LA, Mason NA. Module 3: Constructing a patient's drug therapy problem list. In: ASHP Clinical Skills Program—Advancing Pharmaceutical Care. Bethesda, MD, American Society of Health-System Pharmacists, 1993.

7. Strand LM, Morley PC, Cipolle RJ, et al. Drug-related problems: Their structure and function. DICP 1990 24: 1093-1097.

8. Jones W, Campbell S. Module 4: Designing and recommending a pharmacist's care plan. In: ASHP Clinical Skills Program—Advancing Pharmaceutical Care. Bethesda, MD, American Society of Health-System Pharmacists, 1993.

9. Galt K. Developing Clinical Practice Skills for Pharmacists. Bethesda, MD, American Society of Health-System Pharmacists, 2006.

10. American Council for Pharmacy Education. Accreditation Standards and Key Elements for the Professional Program in Pharmacy Leading to the Doctor of Pharmacy Degree, Standards 2016. https://www.acpe-accredit.org/pdf/Standards2016FINAL.pdf. Accessed January 18, 2016.

11. Frye CB. Module 5: Monitoring the pharmacist's care plan. In: ASHP Clinical Skills Program—Advancing Pharmaceutical Care. Bethesda, MD, American Society of Health-System Pharmacists, 1993.

12. Beardsley RS, Kimberlin CL, Tindall WN. Communication Skills in Pharmacy Practice, 6th ed. Philadelphia, PA, Lippincott Williams & Wilkins, 2012.

13. Rantucci ML. Pharmacists Talking with Patients: A Guide to Patient Counseling, 2nd ed. Philadelphia, PA, Lippincott Williams & Wilkins, 2007.

PRACTICE CASE

Learning Objectives

- Recognize the signs, symptoms, and risk factors for hypovolemia, hypokalemia, and metabolic alkalosis
- Develop an appropriate treatment and monitoring plan for hypovolemia, hypokalemia, and metabolic alkalosis
- Recognize the impact of pregnancy on medication choice and disease management

PATIENT PRESENTATION

Chief Complaint

"I feel so tired and dizzy, and I can't stop throwing up."

History of Present Illness

Susan Jones is a 23-year-old woman brought to an urgent care center c/o severe weakness and dizziness. She states it started 3 days ago when she began to have frequent vomiting. She thinks that "maybe I ate something bad." She also says that her bowel movements have been "a little looser than normal." She states that before she got sick 3 days ago, she felt fine.

Past Medical History

Bulimia with two psychiatric hospitalizations

Depression, s/p suicide attempt × 1 (slashed wrists)

Pelvic inflammatory disease

Family History

Mother died from drug overdose at age 34; she does not know her father.

Social History

Single community college student; no children; works part-time in restaurant.

Tobacco/Alcohol/Substance Abuse

(+) cigarettes half ppd; admits to occasional marijuana use, denies current other illicit or unprescribed drug or alcohol use; used IV heroin until 1 year ago.

Medications

Fluoxetine 20 mg bid po

Trazodone 50 mg q hs po

Potassium chloride 40 mEq q AM po

Methadone 120 mg q AM po

Omeprazole 20 mg q day po

Ethinyl estradiol/norethindrone 1 q AM po

Review of Systems

(+) Weakness, dizziness, fatigue, nausea, and diarrhea; denies headache, chest pain, or abdominal pain; (+) dysuria; (−) vaginal pain or discharge.

Physical Examination

▶ *General*

Very thin, chronically ill–appearing young woman who fainted when sitting up.

▶ *Vital signs*

BP 105/75 mm Hg lying, 70/0 mm Hg sitting; P 110 lying, 160 sitting; RR 12, T 37.1°C

Weight 47 kg (103.4 lb.), height 5′4″ (163 cm)

▶ *Skin*

Dry, poor skin turgor; no rashes or lesions noted

▶ *HEENT*

PERRLA; mouth very dry; poor dentition

▶ *Neck and Lymph Nodes*

JVD 0 (neck veins flat); thyroid gland normal; no lymphadenopathy

▶ *Chest*

Clear to auscultation and percussion

▶ *Breasts*

Examination deferred

▶ *Cardiovascular*

Tachycardic; normal S_1, S_2; no murmurs, rubs, or gallops

▶ *Abdomen*

No tenderness or organomegaly; bowel sounds slightly hyperactive

▶ *Extremities*

Very thin; trace pedal edema; multiple "tracks" both arms

▶ *Genitourinary*

Normal vaginal discharge; uterus appears to contain approximately 12-week pregnancy

▶ *Rectal*

Mild hemorrhoids; Hemoccult (−)

Laboratory Tests

Fasting, Obtained upon Admission

	Conventional Units	SI Units
Na	126 mEq/L	126 mmol/L
K	2.1 mEq/L	2.1 mmol/L
Cl	87 mEq/L	87 mmol/L
CO_2	32 mEq/L	32 mmol/L
BUN	8 mg/dL	2.9 mmol/L
SCr	0.5 mg/dL	44 μmol/L
Glu	110 mg/dL	6.1 mmol/L
Ca	8.7 mg/dL	2.18 mmol/L
Mg	1.8 mEq/L	0.90 mmol/L
Phosphate	3.6 mg/dL	1.16 mmol/L
WBC	$7.4 \times 10^3/mm^3$	$7.4 \times 10^9/L$
Hgb	11.6 g/dL	116 g/L; 7.2 mmol/L
Hct	34.6%	0.346
Albumin	3.2 g/dL	32 g/L
PT	17 s	
INR	1.3	

Urine pregnancy test (+)

ABG: pH 7.56, pO_2 98 mm Hg (13.0 kPa), O_2 sat 99% (0.99), pCO_2 44 mm Hg (5.9 kPa), HCO_3 31 mEq/L (31 mmol/L)

Urine toxicology screen: (+) cocaine, THC, methamphetamine, nicotine, HCTZ

ECG: flat T waves; (+) U wave

Assessment

Twenty-three-year-old pregnant woman with ECF volume depletion, vomiting and diarrhea, significant hypokalemia with ECG changes, hyponatremia, and metabolic alkalosis. Urine tox screen indicates active illicit drug use.

Student Workup

Missing Information?

Evaluate: Patient Database

Drug Therapy Problems

Care Plan (by Problem)

TARGETED QUESTIONS

1. What signs and symptoms of ECF volume depletion, hypokalemia, and metabolic alkalosis does the patient have?

   Hint: See pp. 391, 417, and 442 in PPP

2. What are the causes of this patient's alkalosis?

   Hint: See p. 448 in PPP

3. What are the risks of administering potassium intravenously?

   Hint: See p. 435 in PPP

4. What are the signs and symptoms of opioid withdrawal, and what drug interactions may occur with methadone?

   Hint: See pp. 554 and 558 in PPP

5. What medications have proven to have teratogenic effects in humans?

   Hint: See p. 732 in PPP

FOLLOW-UP

Three months later, the patient calls you after being discharged from an inpatient substance abuse program. She says she feels great, is staying clean, and her baby is doing well ("Look how fat I am!"). Her obstetrician recently told her that she has low thyroid and wants her to take levothyroxine. She is afraid that it will hurt her baby and she wants your advice. You look up her laboratory tests in the computer and note that her TSH is 10.1 μIU/mL (10.1 mIU/L). What is your advice to her?

Hint: See pp. 741-742 in PPP

⊙ GLOBAL PERSPECTIVE

Depression is a common mental disorder that presents with depressed mood, loss of interest or pleasure, feelings of guilt or low self-worth, disturbed sleep or appetite, low energy, and poor concentration. These problems can become chronic or recurrent and may lead to substantial impairments in an individual's ability to take care of his or her everyday responsibilities. At its worst, depression can lead to suicide, with the loss of about 850,000 lives every year.

In 2008, depression was the leading cause of disability worldwide as measured by years lived with disability (YLD) and the fourth-leading contributor to the global burden of disease based on disability-adjusted life-years (DALYs). By the year 2020, depression is projected to reach second place in the ranking of DALYs calculated for all ages and in both sexes. Today, depression already is the second cause of DALYs worldwide in the age category 15-44 years for both sexes combined. According to the World Health Organization, fewer than 25% of depressed patients have access to care, and, in some countries, fewer than 10% have access to care. Barriers to effective care include the lack of resources, lack of trained providers, and the social stigma associated with mental disorders, including depression.

REFERENCE

World Health Organization. http://www.who.int/topics/depression/en/ Accessed on January 10, 2016.

CASE SUMMARY

- Young pregnant woman with history of depression, eating disorder, and substance abuse who presents with ECF volume depletion, hypokalemia, and metabolic alkalosis due to vomiting and diuretic use. Volume and potassium replacement must be initiated, and the underlying causes addressed to prevent recurrence.

- She is actively abusing drugs, placing her and the fetus at risk for multiple complications. Substance abuse treatment referral is warranted.

- The patient needs a referral to an obstetrician for assessment and prenatal care.v

PATIENT DATABASE FORM

Patient Name: Susan Jones Real patient names are not used in this Study Guide.	Weight: 103.4 lb (47 kg)	Location: Urgent Care	Completed by:
Patient MRN:	Height: 64 in (163 cm)	Physician:	
Age (or date of birth): 23 years	Race: Caucasian	Pharmacy:	Pharmacist:
Date of Admission/Initial Visit: 08/01/2015		Patient Occupation: Student, restaurant worker	

Allergies/ Intolerances/ ADRs

☐ No known drug allergies/ADRs

☑ Not known/inadequate information

Drug	Reaction
A common area where information is missing or incomplete. No known drug allergies/ADRs is NOT the same as Not known. No known means the patients has been asked and/or chart reviewed, while Not known means there is missing information.	

HPI, FH, SH, and Additional Information

HPI: Weakness, dizziness, vomiting, diarrhea (?) for ~ 3 days

Appears dry—orthostatic, flat neck veins

Evidence of active IVDU

12 wk pregnant

FH / SH: Smokes ½ ppd, uses marijuana, Hx IVDU (+) dysuria on ROS

> A summary of the key subjective and objective findings from the case.

Additional Information: Hx eating disorder, depression (s/p suicide attempt), PID

Prioritized Medical Problem List		Medication Profile
1	Hypovolemic hyponatremia, d/t vomiting, diuretic use (?)	
2	Hypokalemia with ECG changes	Potassium chloride 40 mEq q am PO
3	Metabolic alkalosis due to #1 and #2	
4	Active substance use with urine (+) cocaine, methamphetamine; no evidence for endocarditis	Methadone 120 mg q day PO
5	12 wk pregnant by exam, (+) urine HCG	Ethinyl estradiol/norethindrone 1 tab PO q day
6	Hx bulimia, appears to be malnourished, diarrhea?, hx depression with s/p suicide attempt × 1	Fluoxetine 20 mg bid PO
		List of medications placed next to problem list to facilitate matching medications with indications. Note that some medications may have multiple indications

Health Maintenance:	Tobacco use
PMH with no therapy needed:	
Inadequate Database:	Indications for trazodone? Indication for omeprazole? Patient has dysuria—r/o UTI? Need allergy/ADE hx; frequency of substance use; adherence with prescribed medications; use of diuretics, laxatives; screen for HIV, viral hepatitis; liver enzymes; previous pregnancies, deliveries

> Get used to including inadequate database or missing information on your problem list so you will remember to follow-up on all missing information.

Vital Signs, Laboratory Data, and Diagnostic Test Results				
	Normal Range or Units			
Date	Having data in tabular form allows following trends over time (date as column heading)	08/01/2015		
Weight	lb (kg)	103.4 (47)		
Temperature	°C	37.1		
Blood Pressure	mm Hg	105/75 lying 70/0 sitting		
Pulse	Not every laboratory test is including on the blank forms, so you will need to add laboratory tests and normal values for tests not already on the form. Normal values may be found in PPP. Make sure you understand the significance of each laboratory test.	110 lying 160 sitting		
Respiratory Rate		12		
Na	135-145 mEq/L (135-145 mmol/L)	126		
K	3.3-4.9 mEq/L (3.3-4.9 mmol/L)	2.1		
Cl	97-110 mEq/L (97-110 mmol/L)	87		
CO_2/HCO_3	22-26 mEq/L (22-26 mmol/L)	32		
BUN	8-25 mg/dL (2.9-8.9 mmol/L)	8 (2.9)		
Serum Creatinine (adult)	male 0.7-1.3 mg/dL; female 0.6-1.1 mg/dL (male 62-115 μmol/L; female 53-97 μmol/L)	0.5 (44)		
Creatinine Clearance (adult)	85-135 mL/min (1.42-2.25 mL/s)	129.9 (2.17)		
Glucose (fasting)	65-109 mg/dL (3.6-6.0 mmol/L)	110 (6.1)		
Total Ca	8.6-10.3 mg/dL (2.15-2.58 mmol/L)	8.7 (2.18)		
Mg	1.3-2.2 mEq/L (0.65-1.10 mmol/L)	1.8 (0.9)		
PO_4	2.5-4.5 mg/dL (0.81-1.45 mmol/L)	3.6 (1.16)		
Hemoglobin	male 13.8-17.2 g/dL; female 12.1-15.1 g/dL (male 138-172 g/L; female 121-151 g/L)	11.6		
Hematocrit	male 40.7-50.3%; female 36.1-44.3% (male 0.407-0.503; female 0.361-0.443)	34.6 (0.346); 7.2 mml/L		
MCV	80.0-97.6 μm³ (80.0-97.6 fl)			
WBC	$4\text{-}10 \times 10^3/\text{mm}^3$ ($4\text{-}10 \times 10^9/\text{L}$)	7.4		
WBC Differential	% polymorphonuclear neutrophils (PMN)/eosinophils/ basophils/lymphocytes/monocytes	////	////	////
Platelet	$140\text{-}440 \times 10^3/\text{mm}^3$ ($140\text{-}440 \times 10^9/\text{L}$)			
Albumin	3.5-5 g/dL (35-50 g/L)	3.2 (32)		
Bilirubin (total)	0.3-1.1 mg/dL (5.13-18.80 μmol/L)			
Bilirubin (direct)	0-0.3 mg/dL (0-5.1 μmol/L)			
AST	11-47 IU/L (0.18-0.78 μkat/L)			
ALT	7-53 IU/L (0.12-0.88 μkat/L)			
Alk phos (adult)	38-126 IU/L (0.13-2.10 μkat/L)			
pH	7.35-7.45	7.56		
PO_2	70-95 mm Hg (9.3-12.6 kPa)	98 (13.0)		

Vital Signs, Laboratory Data, and Diagnostic Test Results				
O$_2$	Saturation (90-110%)	99 (0.99)		
PCO$_2$	35-45 mm Hg (4.7-6.0 kPa)	44 (5.9)		
Urine HCG		Positive		

Additional Notes:
Urine tox screen (+) for cocaine, THC, methamphetamine, HCTZ
ECG: NSR, rate 110, flattened T waves, (+) U wave

This is a free text to add items that do not fit elsewhere or for quick notes to yourself or other clinicians who may be following the patient.

DRUG THERAPY PROBLEM WORKSHEET

> This Worksheet will help you systematically assess the patient for the presence of and potential for all Drug Therapy Problems. After each problem is identified, you will need to assess the significance of each problem, and integrate those problems with your overall Care Plan. Some medications may be associated with multiple problems. Make sure you are as specific as possible in identifying the problem so that appropriate action then can be taken.

Type of Problem	Possible Causes	Problem List	Notes
Correlation between drug therapy and medical problems	Drugs without obvious medical indications	Trazodone, omeprazole	Identified by comparing problem list and medication list
	Medications unidentified		
	Untreated medical conditions		
Need for additional drug therapy	New medical condition requiring new drug therapy		Make sure all new problems are addressed (through all may not require drug therapy).
	Chronic disorder requiring continued drug therapy		
	Condition best treated with combination drug therapy		
	May develop new medical condition without prophylactic or preventive therapy or premedication		
Unnecessary drug therapy	Medication with no valid indication or condition is better treated with nondrug therapy	Pregnancy	Needs prenatal care
	Condition caused by accidental or intentional ingestion of toxic amount of drug or chemical	If dysuria d/t UTI, needs nonteratogenic antimicrobial	
	Medical problem(s) associated with use of or withdrawal from alcohol, drug, or tobacco		
	Taking multiple drugs when single agent as effective		
	Taking drug(s) to treat an avoidable adverse reaction from another medication		
Appropriate drug selection	Current regimen not usually as effective or safe as other choices	Ethinyl estradiol/ norethindrone	Patient is pregnant
	Therapy not individualized to patient	HCTZ contributed to fluid/ electrolyte disorders	Even if a medication is indicated for the problem, it may not be the BEST therapy for that patient.
Wrong drug	Medical problem for which drug is not effective	Need to assess teratogenic effects of all drugs (hormonal contraceptive in pregnancy)	
	Patient has risk factors that contraindicate use of drug		
	Patient has infection with organisms resistant to drug		
	Patient refractory to current drug therapy		
	Taking combination product when single agent appropriate		
	Dosage form inappropriate or medication error		
Drug regimen	PRN use not appropriate for condition		
	Route of administration/dosage form/mode of administration not appropriate for current condition		
	Length or course of therapy not appropriate		
	Drug therapy altered without adequate therapeutic trial		
	Dose or interval flexibility not appropriate		
Dose too low	Dose or frequency too low to produce desired response in this patient		
	Serum drug concentration below desired goal range for indication		
	Timing of antimicrobial prophylaxis not appropriate		
	Medication not stored properly or medication error		

DRUG THERAPY PROBLEM WORKSHEET

Type of Problem	Possible Causes	Problem List	Notes
Dose too high	Dose or frequency too high for this patient	Assess methadone dose with substance abuse provider	Make sure all drug doses have been adjusted for the patient's renal and liver function.
	Serum drug concentration above the desired goal range for indication		
	Dose escalated too quickly	Need for bid fluoxetine	
	Dose or interval flexibility not appropriate for this patient		
	Medication error		
Therapeutic duplication	Receiving multiple agents without added benefit		
Drug allergy/ adverse drug events	History of allergy or ADE to current (or chemically related) agents	Need allergy / ADE history	Allergy / ADE information commonly is missing or incomplete.
	Allergy or ADE history not in medical records	HCTZ and fluid/ electrolyte disorders	
	Patient not using alert for severe allergy or ADE		
	Symptoms or medical problems that may be drug-induced	Fluoxetine and insomnia	
	Drug administered too rapidly		
	Medication error, actual or potential		
Interactions (drug-drug, drug-disease, drug-nutrient, drug-laboratory test)	Effect of drug altered due to enzyme induction/ inhibition, protein binding alterations, or pharmacodynamic change from another drug patient is taking	Fluoxetine and methadone	Slight reduction in methadone clearance; watch QTc
	Bioavailability of drug altered due to interaction with another drug or food	Assessing for interactions is important but make sure you assess for the clinical significance of the interaction in the patient.	Both serotonin modulators
	Effect of drug altered due to substance in food		
	Patient's laboratory test altered due to interference from a drug the patient is taking		
		Fluoxetine and trazodone	
Failure to receive therapy	Patient did not adhere with the drug regimen	Unknown, but likely is nonadherent; likely not taking methadone since not in urine tox	ALWAYS assess adherence. If adherence problems are identified, find out the reasons for poor adherence and possible solutions.
	Drug not given due to medication error		
	Patient did not take due to high drug cost/lack of insurance		
	Patient unable to take oral medication		
	Patient has no IV access for IV medication	Unknown	
	Drug product not available		
Financial impact	The current regimen is not the most cost-effective	Financial or insurance problems are a common reason for poor adherence.	
	Patient unable to purchase medications/no insurance		
Patient knowledge of drug therapy	Patient does not understand the purpose, directions, or potential side effects of the drug regimen	Unknown	Patients often have little understanding about their medications. Make sure you develop an educational plan appropriate for the patient.
	Current regimen not consistent with the patient's health beliefs	Unknown	

PHARMACOTHERAPY CARE PLAN

	Medical Problems	Current Drug Regimen	Therapy Goals, Desired Endpoints	Therapeutic Recommendations	Therapeutic Alternatives	Rationale
1	Hypovolemic hyponatremia	HCTZ use may be contributing factor	Normal hemodynamics (BP, pulse, JVD), improved symptoms (weakness, dizziness); prevent recurrence by treating underlying cause	Normal saline IV 1 L now over 15 min, then 500 mL/h × 2. Repeat until no longer orthostatic; if able to take PO, add oral rehydration solution (ORS) 250 mL q 30 min; promethazine 25 mg PO/IM/PR q 4 h PRN N/V; if pt needs to stop using HCTZ; if pt has diarrhea, order stool culture, R/O laxative abuse; stop using HCTZ	If able to take PO or IV access not available, ORS 500–1000 mL/h as tolerated; metoclopramide 10 mg IV q 6 h PRN nausea	Severe signs and symptoms, presence of vomiting warrant IV fluid; normal saline best for treating ECF depletion, metabolic alkalosis; hyponatremia will correct with volume replacement
	For acute problems, make sure your therapeutic recommendations are carried through to some resolution or stopping point and/or chronic therapy.		Goals and endpoints should be as specific as possible, and should include preventing adverse outcomes as well as seeking positive outcomes.		Therapeutic recommendations and alternatives must be specific (drug, route, dose, frequency, duration).	Your rationale should include why you chose your primary therapy (drug, route, etc.) versus the alternative(s); may include why you did not specifically address certain problems.
2	Hypokalemia	Potassium chloride 40 mEq q AM PO	Normal serum K; normal ECG; no symptoms; prevent recurrence by treating underlying cause	KCl liquid 40 mEq PO now, PO repeat in 2 h; if serum K increasing, change to KCl SR 40 mEq bid × 2 d, then reassess; stop using HCTZ	If unable to take PO, IV KCl 10 mEq/100 mL with 10 mg lidocaine over 1 h × 4 doses	Oral KCl safer than IV if pt able to take; pt has significant K deficit; need K replacement for correction of alkalosis; use liquid KCl for rapid absorption
3	Metabolic alkalosis	Note that some problems are connected to others, and their resolution may be connected to treatment of those related problems.	Normal ABG, electrolytes, ECF volume; prevent recurrence by treating underlying cause	Volume repletion, K replacement, treat vomiting as above; stop using HCTZ; if alkalosis slow to clear or serum Mg drops, provide Mg replacement as MgSO$_4$ 1 g IV in 100 mL NS over 1 h	Alternatives to volume, K replacement as above; no indication for IV HCl administration; could give Mg replacement even though serum Mg in normal range	Alkalosis will resolve with volume and K replacement and with removal of underlying causes; Mg deficiency can prevent resolution of hypokalemia, alkalosis, though serum Mg now normal

PHARMACOTHERAPY CARE PLAN

Medical Problems	Current Drug Regimen	Therapy Goals, Desired Endpoints	Therapeutic Recommendations	Therapeutic Alternatives	Rationale
4 Substance use	Methadone 120 mg q day PO	No use of illicit drugs; avoidance of medical complications of injection use such as skin abscesses or endocarditis Not all problems can be addressed or resolved. Some will require referral to other professionals or institutions.	Hold methadone since pt seems not to be taking and no evidence of narcotic withdrawal; if signs of withdrawal develop, begin methadone 20 mg q day inpatient; if methadone used, watch for potential interactions; blood cultures × 3 to R/O endocarditis; refer back to substance abuse provider after discharge; encourage enrollment in smoking cessation program; test for HIV, hepatitis B and C	Begin methadone 20 mg q day if patient was taking methadone or other opioids chronically	Since urine tox was not positive for methadone, pt likely not taking; narcotic withdrawal not life-threatening, so best to wait to see if withdrawal signs develop and then treat with low dose methadone; while no evidence of endocarditis (fever, murmur), best to R/O with blood cultures especially since she is pregnant
5 Pregnancy, dysuria		Cessation of behavior that is high risk to the fetus; adequate prenatal care	DC ethinyl estradiol/ norethindrone; substance abuse program as per substance abuse provider; refer to OB for full assessment, prenatal care; prenatal vitamin 1 q day; nutrition consult; smoking cessation; need to review all current and future drugs for teratogenic effect		Substance abuse and malnutrition will severely compromise development and health of fetus
		No symptoms; cure UTI if present	Urinalysis; if (+) for UTI, send for culture and start cephalexin 250 mg q 8 h × 7 d, start after all three blood cultures drawn	Amoxicillin-clavulanate 500 mg q 8 h × 7 d	Cephalosporins safe in pregnancy, active against most common organism
6 Eating disorder, depression	Fluoxetine 20 mg bid PO	Normal eating patterns, no use of diuretics or laxatives; normal mood with no s/s depression	If patient has been taking fluoxetine, continue at 20 mg q day; psych consult; if insomnia, withhold hypnotics at this time since may be due to fluoxetine regimen and stimulant use; nutrition consult as above	Change antidepressant to less stimulating agent, i.e., sertraline 50 mg q day	Avoid SSRI withdrawal syndrome if she has been taking fluoxetine; if insomnia, may resolve with change in fluoxetine regimen, stimulant detox

	PATIENT EDUCATION SUMMARY		Summarize your patient education in the type of language you would use with a real patient. Avoid use of medical terms or lingo, and keep in mind the patient's language skills, education background, and culture.
	Medical Problems	**Planned Monitoring and Follow-Up**	**Patient Education Summary Points**
1	Hypovolemic hyponatremia	VS q 15 min × 2 h, then q 1 h while in urgent care. Recheck basic metabolic panel(BMP) in 4 h; pt to self-monitor symptoms, weight daily after discharge; repeat BMP in 2 d Make sure monitoring plan is specific (parameters, frequency) and realistic for the setting.	The problems you are having with your fluid and electrolytes are all related and are causing your weakness and dizziness. There are several reasons why these problems developed, including your vomiting and lack of food and fluid intake and your drug abuse. It appears that you are using an unprescribed diuretic, and that is causing or worsening these problems. Although we can easily treat these problems here, it is important that you take steps so that it does not happen again. You can help prevent this in the future by making sure you eat and drink fluids properly, do not use diuretics, and stop abusing drugs. After we give you some IV fluids, we will be giving you some oral fluids, as well as some oral potassium. It is very important that you take these as directed so that we can get your fluid and electrolyte levels back to normal. We have prescribed a medication, promethazine, for nausea and vomiting. Take it only if you need it and are unable to keep down oral fluids. Sometimes this medication can cause you to be a little drowsy or have a dry mouth. Let us know if that happens.
2	Hypokalemia	BMP in 2 h (recheck in 6 h if IV KCl given); ECG in 4 h	
3	Metabolic alkalosis	BMP, other monitoring as above; recheck serum Mg in 2 h	
4	Substance use	Signs and symptoms of drug withdrawal; temperature q 6 h while in facility, then by pt daily; examine injection sites daily; CBC in 2 d; QTc if on methadone	From your urine screen and looking at your arms we can tell that you are actively abusing drugs. It will be crucial for you and your baby that you stop using immediately. We will refer you back to your substance abuse provider after you are discharged, and we strongly urge that you get involved with a program that will help you stay clean. Since it appears that you have not been using your methadone, we are going to withhold that for the time being. Since injecting drugs can put you (and your baby) at risk for infections like HIV and hepatitis, we are going to test you for those infections. Also, we are going to test you for a bacterial infection of the heart that happens sometimes in people who inject drugs. Smoking tobacco also is very harmful to you and your baby, and we strongly encourage you to stop smoking. Your substance abuse provider can help you with that also.
5	Pregnancy	As per substance abuse provider, OB	We found that you are about 12 wk pregnant. We want to help you have a healthy baby, but the first thing you need to do is stop abusing drugs since they are so harmful to the development of your baby. Also, your nutrition does not appear to be very good, and you need to eat well enough so that your baby can get nutrients. We will refer you to an obstetrician, and we will start you on a prenatal vitamin to be taken every day. Since many medications can harm the baby during pregnancy, make sure all your providers know you are pregnant, and do not take any medication unless you check with your obstetrician or pharmacist. Do not start taking your birth control pills when you get home since you are pregnant.

PATIENT EDUCATION SUMMARY

Medical Problems	Planned Monitoring and Follow-Up	Patient Education Summary Points
	UTI s/s daily; repeat UA after antibiotic completed; stool frequency, consistency	We noticed that you are complaining of some pain or burning when you urinate. This may be caused by a urinary tract infection, and we are going to test you for that. If you do have a urine infection, we will give you an antibiotic for that. Make sure you take every dose since a urine infection can harm your baby as well as you. The antibiotic we will give, cephalexin, will not harm your baby. Sometimes it can cause some diarrhea or skin rashes, so if that happens, please let us know.
6 Eating disorder, depression	As per psych	You had been prescribed fluoxetine (Prozac) for your depression and bulimia. If you have been taking it on a regular basis, we do not want to stop it suddenly. When you take this medication later in the day, sometimes it can cause problems sleeping, so we will give it to you just in the morning. We are going to have a psychiatrist consult with you so that we can determine the best way to manage these problems, with medications and with counseling.

2 Hypertension: Newly Diagnosed

Keri D. Hager   Youssef M. Roman
Robert J. Straka

PATIENT PRESENTATION

Chief Complaint

"My headache won't go away."

History of Present Illness

Alesha Duane is a cheerful 61-year-old African-American woman who presents to clinic for an initial assessment of her ongoing headache over the past week. Alesha states that ibuprofen is not helping to control her headache anymore and acetaminophen never worked well for her. She denies any head trauma or injuries over the past week. Alesha is widowed and lives with her younger sister whom she describes as a great cook. Alesha was diagnosed with hypertension 3 months ago and type 2 diabetes 6 months ago. These diagnoses have caused her distress because she is "no longer able to enjoy her sister's home-cooked meals." Furthermore, she is trying, with limited success, to cut down on her use of salt and sugar as well as dining out at her favorite Chinese restaurant. She also doesn't like having to check her blood sugar during the day per her physician instructions while out with her friends or volunteering at her church. She also admits that she has gone for days without taking her diabetes medication without apparent problems; she comments she wants to avoid using insulin because she doesn't like the thought of injecting herself. She decided to try dietary changes rather than take the antihypertensive (chlorthalidone) she was prescribed 3 months ago.

Past Medical History

Headache
HTN (3 months)
T2DM (6 months)
GERD (4 years)
Gout (6 years)

Family History

Father had hypertension and died of stroke at the age of 53. Mother had T2DM and died in a car accident at the age of 55. She has only one younger sister who has hypertension and was recently diagnosed with breast cancer.

Social History

Alesha is widowed without children. Her husband died of end-stage liver disease. She is a retired bus driver. She likes to stay active, so she goes for short walks with her friends when it is nice outside.

Alcohol/Tobacco/Substance/Caffeine Use

Alesha reports having 4-5 drinks/week; she smokes cigarettes (about half pack per day for the last 30 years), "knows she should quit," and is willing to set a quit date. She drinks about 3-4 cups of coffee a day. She reports no history of illicit drug use.

Allergies/Intolerances/Adverse Drug Events

Metformin

Medications (Current)

Canagliflozin 100 mg po daily (6 months)
Omeprazole 20 mg po daily (3 years)
Allopurinol 100 mg po daily (3 years)
Ibuprofen 200 mg two tablets by mouth prn

Physical Examination

Weight 178 lb. (80 kg)
Height 66 in. (168 cm)
Waist circumference 38 in. (97 cm)

▶ Blood Pressure

Average BP 152/90 mm Hg (three readings in a seated position) (6 months ago)
Average BP 162/98 mm Hg (three readings in a seated position) (3 months ago)
Average BP 156/92 mm Hg (three readings in a seated position) (today)

▶ Vital Signs

P 60 bpm
RR 12/min
Temp: 98.6°F (37°C)
Denies pain

Laboratory History

Fasting Laboratory Results from 6 months Ago

Lipid Panel	mg/dL	mmol/L
Total cholesterol	178	4.60
LDL cholesterol	96	2.48
HDL cholesterol	52	1.34
Triglycerides	150	1.70

Fasting Laboratory Results from Today

Lipid Panel	mg/dL	mmol/L
Total cholesterol	181	4.68
LDL cholesterol	99	2.56
HDL cholesterol	51	1.32
Triglycerides	155	1.75

Fasting Laboratory Results from 6 months Ago

Metabolic Panel	Conventional Units	SI Units
Na	143 mEq/L	143 mmol/L
K	4.5 mEq/L	4.5 mmol/L
Cl	99 mEq/L	99 mmol/L
CO_2	25 mEq/L	25 mmol/L
BUN	15 mg/dL	5.4 mmol/L
SCr	1.3 mg/dL	119.4 μmol/L
Glu	140 mg/dL	7.77 mmol/L
Uric Acid	7.8 mg/dL	463.9 μmol/L
TSH	2.4 IU/mL	2.4 mIU/L
Hb A1c	7.8%	0.078

Fasting Laboratory Results from Today

Na	140 mEq/L	140 mmol/L
K	4.0 mEq/L	4.0 mmol/L
Cl	96 mEq/L	96 mmol/L
CO_2	22 mEq/L	22 mmol/L
BUN	20 mg/dL	7.1 mmol/L
SCr	1.4 mg/dL	123.8 μmol/L
Glu	130 mg/dL	7.22 mmol/L
Uric Acid	7.6 mg/dL	452.1 μmol/L
TSH	2.4 IU/mL	2.4 mIU/L
Hb A1c	8.0%	0.08

Review of Systems

▶ General

Well-appearing, middle-aged, African-American woman in mild distress

▶ Skin

Dry

▶ HEENT

PERRLA, EOMI intact; TMs appear normal

▶ Neck and Lymph Nodes

Thyroid gland smooth; (–) thyroid nodules; (–) lymphadenopathy; (–) carotid bruits

▶ Chest

Clear to auscultation, (–) egophany

▶ Cardiovascular

RRR, normal S_1, S_2; (–) S_3 or S_4

▶ Abdomen

Soft without tenderness, masses, distention; (–) organomegaly

▶ Neurology

Grossly intact; DTRs normal

▶ Genitourinary and Rectal

Examination deferred

Assessment

Sixty-one-year-old African-American female with headache, untreated hypertension, as well as gout and T2DM that are not optimally managed.

Student Work-Up

Missing Information/Inadequate Data

Evaluate:	Patient database
	Drug therapy problems
	Care plan (by problem)

TARGETED QUESTIONS

1. What is the patient's target BP according to the 2014 Evidence-Based Guidelines?

   Hint: See Table 5-3, p. 6 in PPP

2. Which antihypertensive(s) would you consider initiating based on this patient's characteristics and lab values?

   Hint: See p. 5, Table 5-2 in PPP

3. What nonpharmacologic recommendations would you offer this patient to optimize her antihypertensive therapy?

   Hint: See p. 10, and Table 5-5 in PPP

4. How would you educate this patient about the medication(s) selected?

   Hint: See p. 20 in PPP

5. When and what would you monitor after initiating therapy?

   Hint: p. 20 in PPP

FOLLOW-UP

Three weeks later, the patient presents to clinic for a BP checkup. After reviewing the patient's home BP readings and comparing them to the clinic's readings, you notice that the home BP readings are lower than the clinic's readings. What do think can be causing this discrepancy and what course of action should you take to resolve the discrepancy?

🌐 GLOBAL PERSPECTIVE

Hypertension accounts for significant morbidity and mortality and is estimated to affect 1 billion people worldwide. Globally, 51% of all strokes and 45% of ischemic heart disease deaths are attributable to hypertension, and it is the leading risk factor for cause of death worldwide. The prevalence of hypertension in the United States is among the highest in the world. Efforts to increase awareness, risk factor modification, control, and prevention are essential to reduce the global burden of cardiovascular disease. When designing an effective treatment plan for hypertension, individual patient characteristics, including race, comorbidities, the pharmacokinetic and pharmacodynamics properties of antihypertensive agents, and drug costs must be considered.

CASE SUMMARY

- Her current clinical picture is consistent with newly diagnosed HTN, and intervention is indicated.
- Lifestyle modification and pharmacotherapy are warranted to achieve target blood pressure and to reduce other CVD risk factors.
- A variety of therapeutic options are available, and the advantages and disadvantages of each should be considered based on the patient's individual characteristics.

KEY REFERENCES

1. Weber MA, et al. Clinical Practice Guidelines for the Management of Hypertension in the Community: A Statement by the American Society of Hypertension and the International Society of Hypertension. *The Journal of Clinical Hypertension.* 2014;16(1):14-26.

2. James PA, Oparil S, Carter BL, et al. 2014 Evidence-Based Guideline for the Management of High Blood Pressure in Adults: Report From the Panel Members Appointed to the Eighth Joint National Committee (JNC 8). *JAMA.* 2014;311(5):507-520.

For more information on the care plan and facilitator's guide please visit http://www.mhpharmacotherapy.com

3 Uncontrolled Hypertension

Keri Hager   Emily Anastasia
David Parra

PATIENT PRESENTATION

Chief Complaint
"Nothing they did helped my blood pressure."

History of Present Illness
Michael Angelo is a 56-year-old white male who presents to your clinic as a new patient stating "Nothing they did helped my blood pressure. I hope you can do better." He reports that his blood pressure has been "up and down" over the past year despite multiple medication adjustments. He was diagnosed with HTN in his mid-40s, and believes it was fairly well controlled until the past year. Mr. Angelo has no complaints of chest pain, shortness of breath, dizziness, or lightheadedness. He generally feels well with the exception of some lower back pain that was the result of a slip and fall at his place of employment (pizza parlor) last year. He reports that as a result, he was unable to stand for long hours he had to quit his job. Most of his days are spent "lounging around," and he states "if you can get my blood pressure under control, I can start exercising and lose some weight." He brings in all of his pill bottles including an over-the-counter supplement he is considering taking to "jump start some weight loss."

Past Medical History
HTN (diagnosed in his mid 40s)

Type 2 Diabetes Mellitus (diagnosed last year)

Chronic lower back pain (herniated disc at L4-L5, L5-S1)

History of gout (last flare 6 months ago)

Overweight

All immunizations are up to date

Family History
Father aged 78, had a MI at age 56 and coronary artery bypass surgery at 58 years of age. Mother alive and well, aged 76. Twin sister and brother, both aged 48, alive and well.

Social/Work History
Unemployed.

Single, and has lived in Rhode Island since childhood.

Tobacco/Alcohol/Substance Use
Quit smoking (20-year history) after he lost his job, as it was "too expensive." Social drinker, 2-3 beers nightly, (–) illicit drugs.

Allergies/Intolerances/Adverse Drug Events
No known drug allergies

Medications (Current)
Nebivolol 40 mg po q AM

Telmisartan 80 mg po q AM

Amlodipine 10 mg po q AM

Simvastatin 40 mg po q hs

Metformin 1000 mg po bid

Naproxen sodium 220 mg po bid prn pain

Review of Systems
Frequent bilateral body aches and sore muscles that the patient attributes to aging; no chest pain or shortness of breath at rest or with activity; no dizziness, lightheadedness, headaches, or edema.

Physical Examination

▶ *General*

Well-nourished, appears his age, overweight white male in no distress

▶ *Vital Signs*

BP 162/94 mm Hg, P 90 bpm (left-arm, large-sized adult cuff), repeat 164/96 mm Hg, P 88 bpm

RR 14, T 37.4°C

Weight 215 lb. (97.7 kg)

Height 72 in. (183 cm)

BMI 29.2

Pain: rates muscle pain as a 2 on a score of 0-10

▶ *Skin*

(–) rashes or lesions

▶ **HEENT**

PERRLA, EOMI; (–) sinus tenderness; TMs appear normal

▶ **Neck and Lymph Nodes**

(–) thyroid nodules; (–) lymphadenopathy; (–) carotid bruits

▶ **Chest**

Clear to auscultation

Cardiovascular

RRR, normal S_1, S_2; (–) S_3 or S_4

▶ **Abdomen**

Not tender/not distended

▶ **Neurology**

Grossly intact; DTRs normal

▶ **Extremities**

No joint swelling, no edema

▶ **Genitourinary**

Examination deferred

▶ **Rectal**

Examination deferred

Laboratory and Other Diagnostic Tests

	Conventional Units	SI Units
Na	140 mEq/L	140 mmol/L
K	3.9 mEq/L	3.9 mmol/L
Cl	100 mEq/L	100 mmol/L
CO_2	24 mEq/L	24 mmol/L
BUN	10 mg/dL	3.6 mmol/L
SCr	0.8 mg/dL	70.7 µmol/L
Magnesium	1.3 mEq/L	0.65 mmol/L
Uric acid	7 mg/dL	416.4 µmol/L
Glu	104 mg/dL	5.8 mmol/L
Hemoglobin A1c	7.2%	0.072
Total cholesterol	130 mg/dL	3.36 mmol/L
LDL cholesterol	68 mg/dL	1.76 mmol/L
HDL cholesterol	42 mg/dL	1.09 mmol/L
Triglycerides	100 mg/dL	1.13 mmol/L
Urine albumin/ creatinine	1.2 mg/g	0.136 mg/mmol
Hemoglobin	14.6 g/dL	9.05 mmol/L
Hematocrit	43.2%	0.432
MCV	92 µ/m^3	92 fL
WBC	6×10^3 µ/L	6×10^9/L

Platelet	250×10^3 µ/L	250×10^9/L
Albumin	4.5 g/dL	45 g/L
Total bilirubin	0.7 mg/dL	11.97 µmmol/L
Direct bilirubin	0.3 mg/dL	5.1 µmmol/L
AST	25 IU/L	0.417 µkat/L
ALT	30 IU/L	0.5 µkat/L
Alk phos	40 IU/L	0.667 µkat/L

Sleep Study (January 2014): Negative for obstructive sleep apnea

Assessment

Fifty-six-year-old male with T2DM and uncontrolled hypertension despite maximal doses of three antihypertensive agents.

Student Work-Up

Missing Information/Inadequate Data

Evaluate: Patient database

Drug therapy problems

Care plan (by problem)

TARGETED QUESTIONS

1. What stage hypertension does this patient have, and what is his target blood pressure?

    Hint: See Table 5-1 in PPP

2. Does this patient have resistant hypertension, and what are some contributing factors in uncontrolled hypertension?

    Hint: See p. 5 and Table 5-4 in PPP

3. How can this patient participate in his blood pressure management and improve control?

    Hint: See p. 10, Table 5-5 in PPP

4. Based on this patient's individual characteristics, what are the advantages and disadvantages of different therapeutic options for treatment of hypertension?

    Hint: See Table 5-6, 5-7 in PPP

5. What and how will you educate the patient about risks and adverse effects of therapy and follow-up monitoring parameters?

    Hint: See Table 5-6 in PPP

FOLLOW-UP

In-line with, or despite your recommendations at the initial visit, the patient had HCTZ added to his medication regimen.

Four weeks later, the patient returns for follow-up. He brings in his blood pressure log and reports his blood pressure has been much better controlled. His most recent 10-day average reveals an average systolic blood pressure of 134 mm Hg and an average diastolic blood pressure of 82 mm Hg. However, he also reports that he had a gout attack last week and had to go to an urgent care center. He was treated with a steroid injection, and prescribed colchicine and allopurinol. In addition, he was told his potassium and magnesium levels were low, for which he was also prescribed supplements. Because of the gout attack, he had to stop exercising and has yet to resume. He informs you that his muscle aches are much improved, and that his back pain is also improved with physical therapy and acetaminophen. In the office, his seated blood pressure is 132/78 mm Hg with a pulse rate of 68 bpm. However, despite the improvement in blood pressure control, he expresses concern and frustration with the number of total medications he is now taking.

What additional interventions or modifications (if any) would you now make to the patient's anti-hypertensive regimen?

☉ GLOBAL PERSPECTIVE

Although the global burden of hypertension is growing substantially, it does not affect all groups or populations equally. It is estimated that 1 billion adults (333 million in economically developed and 639 million in economically developing countries) have hypertension, with those who reside in economically developing countries being increasingly affected. Furthermore, 80% of worldwide cardiovascular deaths occur in low- to middle-income countries. Efforts to increase awareness, control, and prevention of hypertension are paramount in reducing the global burden of cardiovascular disease. Comprehensive risk-factor modification (diet, lifestyle, tobacco use, cholesterol, obesity, diabetes) are also essential, with special considerations given by region with particular attention to identifying and addressing logistic, socioeconomic, cultural, and resource constraints. In addition the pharmacokinetic and pharmacodynamic properties of antihypertensive agents and adverse event profiles may differ among various populations. For example, blacks are more likely to experience angioedema from ACE inhibitors while Chinese are more likely to experience cough. Finally, differences in drug cost, availability, and national resources may influence the approach to treating hypertension.

CASE SUMMARY

- This patient's clinical picture is consistent with uncontrolled hypertension.
- A thorough investigation into the loss of blood pressure control is warranted with particular attention paid to

medication adherence, ability to afford medications, and social, diet, and lifestyle factors.
- A variety of therapeutic options are available, and should be carefully considered based upon the patient's individual characteristics, preferences, and ability to afford and adhere to the regimen.

REFERENCES

1. James PA, Oparil S, Carter BL, et al. 2014 evidence-based guideline for the management of high blood pressure in adults: report from the panel members appointed to the Eighth Joint National Committee (JNC 8). *JAMA*. Feb 5 2014;311(5):507-520.
2. Weber MA, Schiffrin EL, White WB, et al. Clinical practice guidelines for the management of hypertension in the community: a statement by the American Society of Hypertension and the International Society of Hypertension. *J Clin Hypertens (Greenwich)*. Jan 2014;16(1):14-26.
3. Hermida RC, Ayala DE, Mojon A, Fernandez JR. Influence of circadian time of hypertension treatment on cardiovascular risk: results of the MAPEC study. *Chronobiology international*. Sep 2010;27(8):1629-1651.
4. Antman EM, Bennett JS, Daugherty A, et al. Use of Non-steroidal Anti-inflammatory Drugs An Update for Clinicians: A Scientific Statement From the American Heart Association. *Circulation*. Feb 2007;115:1634-1642.
5. American Diabetes Association. Standards of Medical Care in Diabetes-2015. *Diabetes Care*. 2015;38(Suppl. 1).
6. Stone NJ, Robinson J, Lichtenstein AH, et al. 2013 ACC/AHA Guidelines on the Treatment of Blood Cholesterol to Reduce Atherosclerotic Cardiovascular Risk in Adults: A Report of the American College of Cardiology/American Heart Association Task Force on Practice Guidelines. *Circulation*. Published online Nov 2013.
7. Khanna D, Fitzgerald JD, Khanna PP, et al. 2012 American College of Rheumatology Guidelines for Management of Gout. Part 1: Systematic Nonpharmacologic and Pharmacologic Therapeutic Approaches to Hyperuricemia. *Arthritis Care & Research*. Oct 2012;64(10):1431-1446.

For more information on the care plan and facilitator's guide please visit http://www.mhpharmacotherapy.com

4 Heart Failure

Tien MH Ng   Diana Cao

PATIENT PRESENTATION

Chief Complaint

"I am getting more and more short of breath."

History of Present Illness

JW is a 59-year-old Caucasian male who was brought in to the emergency department by family with a 2-3 day history of shortness of breath, increased lower extremity edema, and decreased urine output. He states that he has been feeling more tired over the last few weeks and he hasn't been able to do as much as he used to. JW used to be able to walk a few blocks without any problems, but he is only able to walk about 20 feet before becoming short of breath in the past few days. He also reports that his legs have become more swollen. JW states that he usually weighs about 160 pounds. JW reports since his divorce 3 weeks ago, he has had a poor diet consisting of mostly take-out or canned food.

The patient is being admitted into the coronary intensive care unit with a preliminary diagnosis of acute decompensated heart failure.

Past Medical History

MI in 2012, s/p drug eluting stent placement

T2DM (6 years)

Heart Failure (2 years)

Family History

Father had hypertension (HTN), type 2 diabetes mellitus (T2DM), coronary artery disease (CAD), and died at age 74. Mother died from breast cancer at age 78.

Social History

Divorced. Lives alone. Works as a high school teacher.

Tobacco/Alcohol/Substance Use

Never smoked; denies alcohol or illicit drug use

Allergies/Intolerances/Adverse Drug Events

No known drug allergies

Medications Prior to Admission

Aspirin 81 mg po daily

Furosemide 20 mg po bid

Metoprolol tartrate 12.5 mg po bid

Enalapril 10 mg po daily

Metformin 850 mg po bid

Review of Systems

Denies pain, fever, chills, nausea, vomiting, or diarrhea. Admits to decreased appetite.

Physical Exam

Weight 181 lb

Height 5'8"

▶ **Vital signs**

Temp 36.8°C, BP 111/58 mm Hg, P 90, RR 22, SO_2 92% on 4L nasal cannula, pain 0/10

▶ **General**

Moderately distressed, unable to lie flat in bed

▶ **HEENT**

(+) JVD

▶ **Chest**

Wet crackles bilaterally at lung bases

▶ **Cardiovascular**

RRR, normal S_1/S_2, (+) S_3, (−) S_4, 3/6 systolic murmur, PMI displaced laterally

▶ **Abdomen**

Soft, NTND, normoactive bowel sounds

▶ **Neurology**

A&O × 4

▶ **Extremities**

Warm, 3+ pitting edema in both lower extremities to the knees, radial and pedal pulses 2+ bilaterally

▶ **Genitourinary**

Deferred

▶ **Rectal**

Deferred

Laboratory Tests (Fasting)

3/30/15

	Conventional Units	SI Units
Na	135 mEq/L	135 mmol/L
K	4.8 mEq/L	4.8 mmol/L
Cl	104 mEq/L	104 mmol/L
CO_2	21 mEq/L	21 mmol/L
BUN	45 mg/dL	16.1 mmol/L
SCr	1.8 mg/dl	159 μmol/L
Glu	148 mg/dL	8.2 mmol/L
Ca	8.9 mg/dL	2.3 mmol/L
Phos	4.0 mg/dL	1.3 mmol/L
Mg	1.8 mEq/L	0.74 mmol/L
WBC	$7.08 \times 10^3/mm^3$	
Hgb	12.0 g/dL	120 g/L
Hct	37.3%	0.373
MCV	93.1 μm³	93.1 fL
MCH	29.7 pg	
MCHC	35.9 g/dL	359 g/L
RDW	13%	0.13
Reticulocyte	0.5%	0.005
Plt	227 $10^3/mm^3$	
Albumin	3.3 g/dL	33 g/L
Bilirubin (total)	1.5 mg/dL	25.7 μmol/L
Bilirubin (direct)	0.5 mg/dL	8.5 μmol/L
AST	61 IU/L	1.01 μkat/L
ALT	76 IU/L	1.3 μkat/L
Alk phos	156 IU/L	2.6 μkat/L
Total cholesterol	183 mg/dL	4.7 mmol/L
Triglycerides	33 mg/dL	0.37 mmol/L
HDL	45 mg/dL	1.2 mmol/L
LDL	131 mg/dL	3.4 mmol/L
TSH	1.56 μIU/mL	1.56 mU/L
INR	1.3	
Hemoglobin A1c	7.8%	0.078
NT-proBNP	22910 ng/mL	2703 pmol/L
Troponin T	0.1 ng/mL	0.1 μg/L

9/14/14

	Conventional Units	SI Units
Na	139 mEq/L	139 mmol/L
K	4.0 mEq/L	4.0 mmol/L

Cl	102 mEq/L	102 mmol/L
CO_2	23 mEq/L	23 mmol/L
BUN	13 mg/dL	8.2 mmol/L
SCr	0.9 mg/dL	79.6 μmol/L
Glu	138 mg/dL	7.7 mmol/L
Ca	8.8 mg/dL	2.2 mmol/L
Phos	3.5 mg/dL	1.1 mmol/L
Mg	1.8 mEq/L	0.74 mmol/L
WBC	$6.88 \times 10^3/mm^3$	
Hgb	12.5 g/dL	125 g/L
Hct	38.5%	0.385
MCV		
MCH		
MCHC		
RDW		
Reticulocyte		
Plt	252 $10^3/mm^3$	
Albumin	3.6 g/dL	36 g/L
Bilirubin (total)	0.7 mg/dL	12 μmol/L
Bilirubin (direct)	0.2 mg/dL	3.4 μmol/L
AST	33 IU/L	0.6 μkat/L
ALT	38 IU/L	0.63 μkat/L
Alk phos	54 IU/L	0.9 μkat/L
Total cholesterol		
Triglycerides		
HDL		
LDL		
TSH		
INR		
Hemoglobin A1c	7.5%	0.075
NT-proBNP		
Troponin T		

Diagnostic Tests

Electrocardiogram: No acute ST-segment changes

Chest Radiograph: Cardiomegaly, pulmonary vascular congestion

Echocardiogram: Hypokinesis of the LV anterolateral wall. LVEF approximately 35%

Assessment

Fifty-nine-year-old male presenting with acute decompensated heart failure.

CO$_2$	24 mEq/L	24 mmol/L
BUN	15 mg/dL	5.4 mmol/L
SCr	1.1 mg/dL	97 μmol/L
Glu	144 mg/dL	7.44 mmol/L

What recommendations would you make at this point?

Student Work-Up

Missing Information/Inadequate Data

Evaluate: Patient database

Drug therapy problems

Care plan (by problem)

TARGETED QUESTIONS

1. What are some other potential signs and symptoms of heart failure congestion not assessed in the case

    Hint: See pp. 69-71 in PPP

2. What is this patient's New York Heart Association functional class (NYHA FC) and ACC/AHA HF stage?

    Hint: See Table 6-5, p. 72 in PPP

3. How do you determine when it is appropriate to start digoxin in a patient with heart failure?

    Hint: See pp. 78-79 in PPP

4. How do ACEIs and β-blockers interfere with the pathophysiology of heart failure to improve patient survival?

    Hint: See pp. 75-78 in PPP

5. What is mineralocorticoid receptor antagonists' (MRAs) place of therapy in heart failure?

    Hint: See pp. 78 in PPP

FOLLOW-UP

One month later, JW returns to clinic for a routine follow up. He states that he has no major complaints at this time. JW reports that he has been eating healthier since hospital discharge. He still gets short of breath after walking a few blocks, which was similar to how he was pre-hospitalization. He denies any significant swelling in his legs. JW is currently on aspirin 81 mg po daily, furosemide 40 mg po bid, enalapril 10 mg po daily, metoprolol succinate 25 mg po daily, atorvastatin 80 mg po daily, and metformin 850 mg po bid.

Vital signs: T 37.4°C, BP 126/84 mm Hg, P 75, RR 16, Wt 162 lbs (74 kg).

Fasting Laboratory Results:

	Conventional Units	SI Units
Na	136 mEq/L	136 mmol/L
K	4.2 mEq/L	4.2 mmol/L
Cl	107 mEq/L	107 mmol/L

REFERENCES

1. Yancy CW, Jessup M, Bozkurt B, et al. 2013 ACCF/AHA guideline for the management of heart failure: A report of the American College of Cardiology Foundation/American Heart Association Task Force on Practice Guidelines. *J Am Coll Cardiol.* 2013 Oct 15;62(16):e147-239.

2. Centers for Disease Control and Prevention. Updated recommendations for the prevention of invasive pneumococcal disease among adults using the 23-valent pneumococcal polysaccharide vaccine (PPSV23). *MMWR.* 2010;59:1102-1106.

3. American Diabetes Association. Standards of medical care in diabetes—2015. *Diabetes Care.* 2015 Jan;38 Suppl 1: S1-93.

4. James PA, Oparil S, Carter BL, et al. 2014 Evidence-based guideline for the management of high blood pressure in adults: report from the panel members appointed to the Eighth Joint National Committee (JNC 8). *JAMA.* 2014 Feb 5;311(5):507-20.

5. Stone NJ, Robinson JG, Lichtenstein AH, et al. 2013 ACC/AHA guideline on the treatment of blood cholesterol to reduce atherosclerotic cardiovascular risk in adults: a report of the American College of Cardiology/American Heart Association Task Force on Practice Guidelines. *J Am Coll Cardiol.* 2014 Jul1;63(25 Pt B):2889-934.

6. Fihn SD, Gardin JM, Abrams J, et al. 2012 ACCF/AHA/ACP/AATS/PCNA/SCAI/STS guideline for the diagnosis and management of patients with stable ischemic heart disease: a report of the American College of Cardiology Foundation/American Heart Association Task Force on Practice Guidelines, and the American College of Physicians, American Association for Thoracic Surgery, Preventive Cardiovascular Nurses Association, Society for Cardiovascular Angiography and Interventions, and Society of Thoracic Surgeons. *J Am Coll Cardiol.* 2012 Dec 18;60(24):e44-e164.

For more information on the care plan and facilitator's guide please visit http://www.mhpharmacotherapy.com

5 Ischemic Heart Disease

Adam Bress   Larisa H. Cavallari
Robert J. DiDomenico

PATIENT PRESENTATION

Chief Complaint

"I used to be able to walk my dog around the neighborhood with no problem, but lately I have been getting pain and heaviness in my chest when I walk uphill. I have to stop about half-way up the hill and rest for the pain to go away."

History of Present Illness

MS is a 54-year-old African-American male who presents to his primary care physician complaining of pain and heaviness in his chest when he walks his dog up the hill near his house. He describes the pain as "heavy" and "pressure-like." He says the symptoms resolve after resting for a few minutes. He denies any associated symptoms including dyspnea, nausea, or vomiting. MS is trying to meet his daily step goal of 10,000 per day, and is worried that the pain will prevent him from reaching his activity goals.

Past Medical History

Hypertension (HTN) (10 years)
Dyslipidemia (5 years)

Family History

Mother died at age 66 from cancer. Father is alive at age 84.
Son, age 15, alive and well.
Daughter, age 17, alive and well

Social History

MS currently lives at home with his wife. He works as an accountant.

Tobacco/Alcohol/Substance Use

(+) Tobacco; quit smoking 15 years ago, Denies illicit drug use; drinks 2 "craft" beers a day.

Allergies/Intolerances/Adverse Drug Events

NKDA

Medications (Current)

Aspirin 81 mg po daily
HCTZ 25 mg po once daily
Simvastatin 20 mg po daily

Review of Systems

Denies current dizziness, chest pain, diaphoresis, or dyspnea; (–) history of syncope, loss of consciousness, seizures, or visual changes.

Physical Examination

▶ *General*

Middle-aged, well-developed, African-American male in no acute distress; conversant and pleasant

▶ *Vital Signs*

BP 130/88 mm Hg, P 65 bpm, RR 19, T 36.9°C
Weight 185 lb. (83.9 kg)
Height 64 in. (162.5 cm)
(–) Pain

▶ *Skin*

Warm and dry; (–) pallor, rashes, or lesions

▶ *HEENT*

PERRLA, EOMI; oral mucosa moist; (–) pharyngeal erythema or exudate

▶ *Neck and Lymph Nodes*

Supple, no tenderness; (–) carotid bruits; (–) jugular vein distension; normal thyroid

▶ *Chest*

Clear to auscultation bilaterally

▶ *Cardiovascular*

RRR; normal S_1, S_2; (–) S_3 or S_4; (–) murmurs, rubs

▶ *Abdomen*

Soft, nontender, nondistended; normal bowel sounds

▶ *Neurology*

Alert and oriented, cranial nerves II–XII intact

▶ *Extremities*

Bilateral lower extremity edema; warm; normal pulses

▶ *Genitourinary*

Examination deferred; per patient: (–) dysuria; (–) hematuria; (–) discharge

▶ *Rectal*

Examination deferred

Laboratory Tests

Fasting, Obtained Prior to Clinic Visit

Laboratory Data, and Diagnostic Test Results

	Conventional Units	*SI Units*
Na	139 mEq/L	139 mmol/L
K	4.0 mEq/L	4.0 mmol/L
Cl	100 mEq/L	100 mmol/L
CO_2	25 mEq/L	25 mmol/L
BUN	12 mg/dL	4.3 mmol/L
SCr	0.8 mg/dL	70.7 µmol/L
Cr clearance	125 mL/min	
Glu (fasting)	69 mg/dL	3.8 mmol/L
Ca	9.0 mg/dL	2.3 mmol/L
Mg	1.0 mEq/L	0.5 mmol/L
Phosphate	2.9 mg/dL	0.94 mmol/L
Hgb	15.6 g/dL	156 mmol/L
Hct	44%	0.44
MCV	95 µm³	95 fL
WBC	$5 \times 10^3/mm^3$	$5 \times 10^9/L$
WBC differential	////	
Platelets	$350 \times 10^3/mm^3$	$350 \times 10^9/L$
Albumin	4 g/dL	40 g/L
Total bilirubin	1.0 mg/dL	17.1 µmol/L
Bilirubin (direct)	0.1 mg/dL	1.7 µmol/L
AST	12 IU/L	0.2 µkat/L
ALT	8 IU/L	0.13 µkat/L
Alkaline phosphatase	38 IU/L	0.63 µkat/L
Total cholesterol	180 mg/dL	4.7 mmol/L
LDL cholesterol (calculated)	105 mg/dL	2.7 mmol/L
HDL cholesterol	45 mg/dL	1.2 mmol/L
Triglycerides	150 mg/dL	1.7 mmol/L

Assessment and Plan

Fifty-four-year-old man with symptoms consistent with chronic stable angina. MS's primary care physician has scheduled a treadmill stress echocardiogram (echo stress test) to evaluate him for ischemic heart disease (IHD) and assess his left ventricular systolic function.

Student Work-Up

Missing Information/Inadequate Data

Evaluate: Patient database

Drug therapy problems

Care plan (by problem)

TARGETED QUESTIONS

1. What symptoms of chronic stable angina does the patient have?

   Hint: See pp. 95-96 in PPP

2. What are the patient's risk factors for IHD?

   Hint: See Table 7-2, p. 93 in PPP

3. What is your assessment of MS's current antihypertensive regimen?

   Hint: See Hypertension chapter 5 in PPP

FOLLOW-UP

One week later, the patient's echo stress test comes back positive for inducible myocardial ischemia (i.e., positive for CAD), and shows mildly decreased left ventricular systolic function (ejection fraction 50%). He is diagnosed with chronic stable angina.

4. What therapy do you recommend to manage the patient's current symptoms of angina?

   Hint: See pp. 97-99 in PPP

5. The patient undergoes a scheduled coronary angiogram with percutaneous coronary intervention (PCI) and placement of a drug-eluting stent in the left anterior descending coronary artery (LAD) one week later. What antiplatelet therapy would you recommend and for what duration?

   Hint: See pp. 100-101 in PPP

6. Now that you have addressed the patient's antianginal medications, what additional medications (other than

those addressed in question 4) would you consider to manage his IHD?

Hint: See pp. 101-106 in PPP

7. What lifestyle modifications are appropriate for this patient?

Hint: See pp. 97-99 in PPP

For more information on the care plan and facilitator's guide please visit http://www.mhpharmacotherapy.com

6 Acute Coronary Syndromes

Sarah A. Spinler

PATIENT PRESENTATION

Chief Complaint

"My chest pressure is gone."

History of Present Illness

LP is a 67-year-old male who presented to the Emergency Department (ED) at 0900 complaining of 1 hour of continuous chest pressure that began while he was driving to work and was not relieved with one antacid tablet. After 30 min he called 911 and was transported to the ED by ambulance.

In the ambulance, he was give 3 SL NTG tablets without relief of chest pressure and one aspirin 325 mg po. An IV line was placed with D5W1/2NS at 80 mL/hr.

In the ED, his VS were BP 150/90 mm Hg, HR 88 bpm regular (0910) and he was afebrile. He was given 2 mg IV morphine sulfate without relief of chest pressure. His 12-lead ECG showed inferior wall ST-segment elevation in leads II, III and AVF (0912). An IV NTG infusion was started at 10 mcg/kg/min. An unfractionated heparin bolus 4000 units IV × 1 was administered and a continuous infusion started at 1050 units/hr and the patient was transported to the cardiac catheterization lab (0920).

In the cath lab, coronary angiography revealed a 99% right coronary artery (RCA) lesion and the patient underwent percutaneous coronary intervention (PCI) and a bare metal stent (BMS) placed. (0955) A post-PCI echocardiogram revealed inferior wall motion dyskinesis, normal valvular function and a left ventricular ejection fraction of 55%. Unfractionated heparin was discontinued post-PCI and ticagrelor 180 mg po × 1 administered in the post-procedure room. (1030).

The patient was transferred to the cardiac intensive care unit (CCU) post-procedure (1045).

Past Medical History

HTN (5 years)

Family History

Father with stroke at age 65 years; sister with type 2 diabetes mellitus; mother alive at age 85 years without atherosclerotic vascular disease (ASCVD).

Social History

Retired former newspaper reporter

Tobacco/Alcohol/Substance Use

Nonsmoker. Denies use of alcohol or illicit drugs

Allergies/Intolerances/Adverse Drug Events

None

Medications (Current)

NTG 10 mcg/min IV

Medications Taken Prior to Admission

HCTZ 25 mg po once daily

ASA 325 mg po once daily

Received influenza vaccine 10/14; pneumococcal vaccine 2 years ago

Review of Systems

Previous 10/10 chest pressure now 0/10; (–) nausea, abdominal pain, or headache; + pain at groin cath site

Physical Examination

▶ **General**

Sixty-seven-year-old male in less distress

▶ **Vital Signs**

BP 140/90 mm Hg, P 88 bpm, RR 17, T 37°C

Weight 87 kg

Height 71 in. (180 cm)

Denies chest pain or pressure

▶ **HEENT**

Normal; (–) AV nicking, (–) papilledema

▶ **Chest**

Clear to A&P, JVD 4 cm, PMI left midclavicular line 4th intercostal space

▶ **Cardiovascular**

RRR, normal S_1, S_2, (–) S_3 or S_4, (–) M/R/G

▶ **Abdomen**

Not tender/not distended, normal bowel sounds

▶ **Neurologic**

A&O × 3, cranial nerves II-XII intact

▶ **Genitourinary**

Deferred

▶ **Rectal**

(–) Occult blood

▶ **Extremities**

No bruits, pulses 2+, (–) edema

Laboratory Tests

Laboratory Data, and Diagnostic Test Results

Date : 08/15/15 (0915)

	Conventional Units	SI Units
Na	140 mEq/L	140 mmol/L
K	3.9 mEq/L	3.9 mmol/L
Cl	105 mEq/L	105 mmol/L
CO_2/HCO_3	24 mEq/L	24 mmol/L
BUN	16 mg/dL	5.7 mmol/L
SCr	1.0 mg/dL	88.4 μmol/L
Cr Clearance	88 mL/min	
Glu	90 mg/dL	5 mmol/L
Ca		
Mg		
Phosphate		
Hgb	14.8 g/dL	9.2 mmol/L
Hct	44%	0.44
MCV		
WBC		
WBC differential	////	////
Platelets	$220 \times 10^3/mm^3$	$220 \times 10^9/L$
Albumin		
Total bilirubin		
Bilirubin (direct)		
AST		
ALT		
Alkaline phosphatase		

Troponin-T	0.05 ng/mL	0.05 μg/L
LDL cholesterol	95 mg/dL	2.5 mmol/L
HDL cholesterol	35 mg/dL	0.91 mmol/L
Triglycerides	100 mg/dL	1.13 mmol/L

Date: 08/15/15 (1130)

	Conventional Units	SI Units
Na	141 mEq/L	141 mmol/L
K	4.1 mEq/L	4.1 mmol/L
Cl	104 mEq/L	104 mmol/L
CO_2/HCO_3	24 mEq/L	24 mmol/L
BUN	16 mg/dL	5.7 mmol/L
SCr	1.1 mg/dL	97.2 μmol/L
Cr Clearance	80 mL/min	
Glu	88 mg/dL	4.9 mmol/L
Ca	9.0 mg/dL	2.3 mmol/L
Mg	2.0 mEq/L	0.5 mmol/L
Phosphate	2.9 mg/dL	0.82 mmol/L
Hgb	14.0 g/dL	8.7 mmol/L
Hct	42%	0.42
MCV		
WBC	$6.2 \times 10^3/mm^3$	$6.2 \times 10^9/L$
WBC differential	////	////
Platelets	$261 \times 10^3/mm^3$	$261 \times 10^9/L$
Albumin		
Total bilirubin	0.8 mg/dL	13.7 μmol/L
Bilirubin (direct)	0.2 mg/dL	3.4 μmol/L
AST	20 IU/L	0.33 μkat/L
ALT	22 IU/L	0.37 μkat/L
Alkaline phosphatase	60 IU/L	1 μkat/L
Troponin-T	1.9 ng/mL	1.9 μg/L
LDL cholesterol		
HDL cholesterol		
Triglycerides		

Nonfasting, Obtained in the ED

ECG: In ED showed sinus tachycardia with 2 mm ST elevation in leads II, II and AVF; normal PR, QRS, and QTc intervals; post-PCI ECG shows NSR with resolution of ST elevation, no Q waves.

Assessment

Sixty-seven-year-old male with signs, symptoms, and laboratory tests consistent with ACS.

Student Work-Up

Missing Information/Inadequate Data

Evaluate: Patient database

Drug therapy problems

Care plan (by problem)

🌐 GLOBAL PERSPECTIVE

According to the World Health Organization, cardiovascular diseases (CVDs) are the leading cause of death globally. MI is the most common type of fatal CVD, and almost 30% of deaths worldwide are caused by CVD. Almost 80% of CVD deaths occur in low- and middle-income countries. More than 20 million people survive MIs each year, requiring secondary preventive care.

TARGETED QUESTIONS

1. What type of ACS is this?

   Hint: See p. 112 in PPP

2. What signs and symptoms of ACS does this patient have?

   Hint: See p. 114 in PPP

3. What are this patient's risk factors for developing CHD?

   Hint: See Table 8-1 in PPP

4. What is the minimal duration of time that dual antiplatelet therapy should be continued?

   Hint: See pp. 125-128 and Table 8-3 in PPP

5. How is the dose of the β-blocker titrated?

   Hint: See pp. 129-130 and Table 8-3 in PPP

FOLLOW-UP

The patient presents to his cardiologist 2 weeks following discharge. His BP is 142/90 mm Hg, pulse 55 bpm, and he is afebrile. His chemistry panel includes potassium of 4.2 mEq/L (4.2 mmol/L) and SCr 1.07 mg/dL (95 μmol/L). What recommendations would you make to the physician regarding his pharmacotherapy regimen?

   Hint: See Table 8-3 in PPP

For more information on the care plan and facilitator's guide please visit http://www.mhpharmacotherapy.com

7 Atrial Fibrillation

Toby C. Trujillo

PATIENT PRESENTATION

Chief Complaint
"I have chest pain and I feel short of breath."

History of Present Illness
Darryl Williams is a 64-year-old male who presents to the emergency department (ED) with complaints of chest pain and shortness of breath (SOB). The patient states that with the chest pain he was nauseated and sweaty, and the pain was not associated with exertion. He took a dose of nitroglycerine (NTG) which did not help but once paramedics arrived another NTG dose relieved his chest pain and he presented to the ED within 1 hour after his initial episode of chest pain. He denies any exertional chest pain and states that his SOB has been increasing in conjunction with an increase in leg swelling. The patient states he is adherent to his medications. He occasionally feels fatigued and notices a rapid heart rate when he is active in his yard. Last check-up with his primary care physician (PCP) noted he was in normal sinus rhythm. He has had several hospitalizations within the last 2-3 years secondary to atrial fibrillation with rapid ventricular response.

Past Medical History
AF

Hypertension (HTN)

Heart failure (HF) (EF 45% 1 month ago)

Dyslipidemia

Coronary Artery Disease (CAD) (s/p PCI and stent placement 3 years ago)

GERD (gastroesophageal reflux disease)

Family History
Father had CAD and died of an myocardial infarction (MI) at age 63. Mother died of a stroke at age 74. He has one younger brother and sister who are healthy.

Social History/Work History
Married and lives with his wife of 27 years.

Tobacco/Alcohol/Substance Use
Occasional glass of wine with dinner; (–) tobacco or illicit drug use

Allergies/Intolerances/Adverse Drug Events
No known drug allergies

Medications (Current)
Warfarin 2.5 mg po once daily

Metoprolol tartrate 25 mg po twice daily

Atorvastatin 40 mg po once daily

HCTZ 25mg po once daily

Aspirin 81 mg po daily

Ranitidine 150 mg po once daily

Centrum Silver vitamin po once daily

Nitroglycerin 0.4 mg sublingually as needed for chest pain

Review of Systems
Constitutional: Positive for activity change and unexpected weight gain. Negative for chills, diaphoresis and fatigue

Respiratory: Positive for SOB and wheezing

Cardiovascular: Positive for chest pain and bilateral leg swelling. Negative for palpitations

Neurological: Positive for light-headedness and headaches. Negative for dizziness and numbness

Physical Examination

▶ **General**

Well-appearing, elderly Caucasian male in mild distress. He is oriented to person, place and time.

▶ **Vital Signs**

BP 111/78 mm Hg P 105 bpm RR 20 T 36.5°C

Weight 185 lb. [83.9.0 kg (dry weight 80 kg)]

Height 68 in. (173 cm)

▶ **Skin**

Warm and dry

▶ **HEENT**

PERRLA, mucosal membranes dry

▶ **Neck and Lymph Nodes**

(+) JVD; (–) carotid bruits

► **Chest**

Wheezes present (RLL and LLL)

► **Cardiovascular**

Irregularly irregular rhythm; slightly tachycardic; no murmurs, rubs, or gallops

► **Abdomen**

Not tender, not distended; (−) he-patomegaly

► **Neurology**

Alert and oriented × 3

► **Extremities**

Bilateral 1+ pitting edema

► **Genitourinary**

Examination deferred

► **Rectal**

Examination deferred

Laboratory Tests
Fasting, Drawn Today

	Conventional Units	SI Units
BNP	270 ng/L	31.86 pmol/L
Troponin T	0 ng/ml	0 ug/L
Na	140 mEq/L	140 mmol/L
K	4.1 mEq/L	4.1 mmol/L
Cl	104 mEq/L	104 mmol/L
CO_2	22 mEq/L	22 mmol/L
BUN	22 mg/dL	7.9 mmol/L
SCr	1.6 mg/dL	141 μmol/L
Glu	84 mg/dL	4.7 mmol/L
Ca	8.9 mg/dL	2.23 mmol/L
Mg	1.8 mEq/L	0.90 mmol/L
Phosphate	3.8 mg/dL	1.23 mmol/L
Hgb	15.9 g/dL	159 g/L; 9.86 mmol/L
Hct	42.8%	0.428
WBC	$7.9 \times 10^3/mm^3$	$7.9 \times 10^9/L$
Albumin	3.8 g/dL	38 g/L
AST	26 U/L	0.43 μkat/L
ALT	24 U/L	0.40 μkat/L
Prothrombin	20 s	
INR	1.5	
Total cholesterol	170 mg/dL	4.40 mmol/L

LDL cholesterol	104 mg/dL	2.69 mmol/L
HDL cholesterol	38 mg/dL	0.98 mmol/L
Triglycerides	145 mg/dL	1.64 mmol/L

Assessment

Sixty-four-year-old male with a past medical history of atrial fibrillation on warfarin, CAD status post PCI and stent placement, HTN, hyperlipidemia (HLD) who presents with atrial fibrillation with rapid ventricular rate and mild HF exacerbation.

Student Work-Up

Missing Information/Inadequate Data

Evaluate:
Patient database
Drug therapy problems
Care plan (by problem)

TARGETED QUESTIONS

1. What underlying etiologies are present in this patient for the development of AF?

   Hint: See p. 144 in PPP

2. How should this patient's AF be classified?

   Hint: See Table 9-5, p. 146. in PPP

3. Should this patient undergo emergent electrical cardioversion at this time?

   Hint: See p. 145 in PPP

4. Should the patient receive a direct oral anticoagulant (dabigatran, rivaroxaban, apixaban, edoxaban) instead of warfarin for prevention of stroke?

   Hint: See pp. 150-151 in PPP

5. Should the patient receive antiarrhythmic drug therapy at this time?

   Hint: See pp. 146-148 in PPP

FOLLOW-UP

Five weeks later, the patient returns for follow-up. He continues to experience SOB, dyspnea on exertion (DOE), and occasional palpitations. His current vitals reveal a BP of 125/80 mm Hg and a HR of 78 bpm. Today his INR is 2.7 (3 weeks ago, it was 2.2). What antiarrhythmic agent would be recommended for LL at this time to restore and maintain normal sinus rhythm?

Hint: See pp. 146-148 in PPP

⊙ GLOBAL PERSPECTIVE

As of 2015, four different direct oral anticoagulants (DOACs) had received regulatory approval in various jurisdictions around the world for stroke prevention in nonvalvular atrial fibrillation. While vitamin K antagonist such as warfarin remain the most prevalent modality used in atrial fibrillation patient worldwide, the DOACs have made significant strides with respect to overall usage. Given the convenience the DOACs offer compared to warfarin, utilization is likely to increase in the future. Although each of the agents (dabigatran, rivaroxaban, apixaban, edoxaban) are approved for use in both the United States (Food and Drug Administration) and the European Union (European Medicines Agency), clinicians need to be cognizant of differences in the labeling for each agent depending on the jurisdiction. For example, in the RELY trial[1], both a 150 mg and 110 mg twice daily dose were investigated against warfarin for stroke prevention in atrial fibrillation. However, only the 150 mg dose is available in the U.S., while the 110 mg dose is also available in Europe and other jurisdictions. This distinction is pertinent as it changes available treatment options available to clinicians as the 110 mg may be a preferred option for patients who are at higher risk of bleeding. Additional differences such as dose adjustment for renal dysfunction or drug-drug interactions may also be present. Clinicians should ensure they are familiar with prescribing guidelines not only in their own jurisdiction, but also other jurisdictions worldwide in the event they manage patients who are traveling or spend significant time abroad.

REFERENCE

1. Connolly SJ, Ezekowitz MD, Yusuf S, et al. Dabigatran versus warfarin in patients with atrial fibrillation. N Engl J Med 2009;361:1139-1151.

CASE SUMMARY

- DW's current clinical picture is consistent with a recurrence of atrial fibrillation with rapid ventricular rate.
- Current rate control therapy may be considered inadequate given the presentation of symptoms with the recurrence of atrial fibrillation.
- Patient is currently receiving therapy for stroke prevention, but there is a need to question whether current therapy is appropriate. In addition, consideration of alternative options may be appropriate as well.
- Aspirin therapy is indicated for secondary CAD prevention, but also increases the risk of bleeding when co-administered with therapeutic anticoagulation. Consideration for stopping aspirin should be evaluated as patient is 3 years removed from PCI.

For more information on the care plan and facilitator's guide please visit http://www.mhpharmacotherapy.com

Deep Venous Thrombosis

Aimee B. Chevalier

PATIENT PRESENTATION

Chief Complaint

"I have pain in my right leg. It is swollen and I took extra water pills but that didn't help."

History of Present Illness

Donald James is a 52-year-old African-American male presenting to the emergency department (ED) with c/o right lower extremity (RLE) pain and swelling for the past week. He admits to taking extra "water pills" since he had swelling but also reports he ran out of losartan 2 weeks ago. DJ denies any current lower left extremity (LLE) swelling. He reports his RLE pain began at work and has gotten progressively worse over the past few days. He cannot complete his bus route due to pain. DJ denies any injury or trauma to the RLE and denies recent travel. He also denies chest pain (CP), shortness of breath (SOB), fatigue, headache (HA), visual changes. No bleeding history reported.

Past Medical History

Hypertension (HTN)

Osteoarthritis

Obesity

Depression

Family History

Father: Myocardial infarction (MI) aged 60 years, deceased

Mother: a-fib with embolic cerebrovascular accident (CVA), on warfarin

Social History

DJ has worked in construction (20 years), now a City Transit bus driver (9 years). Married (25 years). Lives with wife and has three adult children.

Tobacco/Alcohol/Substance Use

(+) half-1 ppd (25 years), quit for 5 years but restarted 1 ppd 3 years ago

(+) Social drinker, 3-4 drinks/week (weekends only)

(−) Denies illicit drug use

Allergies/Intolerances/Adverse Drug Events

Lisinopril (rash)

"antibiotic" (hives)

Medications (Current)

HCTZ 25 mg po daily

Losartan 100 mg po daily

Naproxen 500 mg po bid prn

Acetaminophen/Codeine #3 1 tab po q 6 h prn

Sertraline 50 mg po daily

St. John's Wort po daily

Capsaicin cream to knees prn

Men's Health Vitamin po daily

Review of Systems

B/L knee pain/stiffness not relieved by current therapy.

Physical Examination

▶ **General**

Obese, African-American male in pain

▶ **Vital Signs**

BP 152/86 mm Hg, P 72 bpm, RR 16, T 36.9°C

Weight 265 lb. (120 kg)

Height 72 in. (183 cm)

Pain 8/10 in RLE

▶ **Skin**

(−) Rashes or lesions; (−) trauma to RLE;

(+) warmth and erythema of RLE

▶ **HEENT**

PERRLA, EOMI

▶ **Neck and Lymph Nodes**

(−) Thyroid nodules; (−) lymphadenopathy;

(−) carotid bruits

▶ **Chest**

Clear to auscultation

▶ **Cardiovascular**

RRR, normal S_1, S_2; (–) S_3 or S_4

▶ **Abdomen**

Obese, nontender/nondistended; (–) organomegaly; (+) bowel sounds

▶ **Extremities**

1+ pitting edema; tenderness to palpation in RLE; (+) Homan's RLE; (+) pedal pulses

▶ **Neurology**

Grossly intact; DTRs normal

▶ **Genitourinary**

Examination deferred

▶ **Rectal**

Examination deferred

Laboratory Tests/Imaging

	Conventional Units	SI Units
Na	135 mEq/L	135 mmol/L
K	4.7 mEq/L	4.7 mmol/L
Cl	101 mEq/L	101 mmol/L
CO_2	23 mEq/L	23 mmol/L
BUN	15 mg/dL	5.4 mmol/L
SCr	1.2 mg/dL	106 µmol/L
Glu	98 mg/dL	5.4 mmol/L
Hgb	14 g/dL	140 d/L; 8.68 mmol/L
Hct	41.5%	0.415
WBC	$10 \times 10^3/mm^3$	$10 \times 10^9/L$
MCV	92.6 µm³	92.6 fL
PLT	$191 \times 10^3/mm^3$	$191 \times 10^9/L$
AST	24 IU/L	0.40 µkat/L
ALT	25 IU/L	0.41 µkat/L
Alk phos	98 IU/L	1.63 µkat/L
D-dimer	714 ng/mL	714 µg/L

Venous Duplex Exam Results:

LLE: no evidence of DVT

RLE: acute occluding thrombus in the posterior tibial vein with extension to popliteal vein

Assessment

DJ is a 52-year-old obese African-American male, with multiple risk factors for DVT, who has symptoms and diagnostic imaging consistent with DVT of the RLE.

Student Work-Up

Missing Information/Inadequate Data

Evaluate: Patient database

Drug therapy problems

Care plan (by problem)

TARGETED QUESTIONS

1. What signs and symptoms of acute DVT does DJ have? What objective information helps lead to the diagnosis? Which model can be used to determine a patient's probability of having an acute DVT?

   Hint: See pp. 165-167, Table 10-2 in PPP

2. What risk factors does this patient have for the development of DVT? Are any of DJ's risk factors modifiable? List other risk factors that may place a person at risk for DVT.

   Hint: Table 10-1 in PPP

3. The emergency room attending wants to discharge DJ to home. What therapeutic options exist for the treatment of his acute DVT? List some advantages/disadvantages of each option.

   Hint: See pp. 169-186 in PPP

4. Which therapy will you recommend and for how long? What parameters will you monitor to evaluate the efficacy and safety of the therapy you have chosen?

   Hint: See pp. 187-189 in PPP

5. For the therapy you have chosen, what general educational information will you provide DJ?

   Hint: See pp. 189-190 in PPP

FOLLOW-UP

DJ completed his treatment for RLE DVT and has been doing well for the past 3 years. Unfortunately, his osteoarthritis has progressed and he has elected to have a left total knee arthroplasty next month. Does he require DVT prophylaxis? If so, what will you recommend and for how long? What models can be used to assess the risk of DVT in hospitalized patients?

Hint: See pp. 168-172 in PPP

✪ GLOBAL PERSPECTIVE

The incidence of DVT is difficult to measure given the large number of asymptomatic cases (estimated at 50% or more). Differences have been noted in VTE incidence among various ethnic groups. In epidemiologic studies, Asian Pacific Islanders and Hispanics were found to have a lower VTE risk than Caucasians or those of African descent. Although not fully understood, one explanation may be due to variations in the prevalence of genetic factors that predispose an individual (or population) to VTE. One example is factor V Leiden mutation, which is the main cause of activated protein C resistance. This mutation is the most common genetic risk factor for VTE and occurs at a much higher rate in Caucasians (5%) vs. Asians (0.5%). Another common defect is prothrombin G20210A mutation that is also primarily found in Caucasians (2-4%) vs. African Americans (0.4%). It is rarely found in other groups. These genetic factors, and potentially others, are one reason differences in risk and incidence of VTE are found between ethnic groups.

CASE SUMARY

- DJ's clinical picture is consistent with DVT.
- Several options are available for the treatment of DVT. Careful evaluation of patient specific factors (i.e., renal and liver function, bleeding risks, current medications) and the advantages/disadvantages of the potential therapies will guide the treatment choice.
- Rationale for treatment, anticipated length of therapy, and medication education Is important at the start of therapy. Ongoing assessment of adherence, efficacy and safety should be performed.
- DJ may require anticoagulation prophylaxis in situations of increased VTE risk (i.e., surgery, prolonged periods of immobility).

For more information on the care plan and facilitator's guide please visit http://www.mhpharmacotherapy.com

9 Ischemic Stroke

Susan R. Winkler

PATIENT PRESENTATION

Chief Complaint

"I was discharged from the hospital last week after having a stroke."

History of Present Illness

John Peters is a 61-year-old African-American male who presents to the neurology clinic today accompanied by his wife. He was discharged from the local hospital 5 days ago and is here for follow-up with a neurologist. He suffered an acute ischemic stroke 10 days ago and was taken by ambulance to the emergency department (ED). On arrival in the ED, he was experiencing speech difficulties and weakness in his right arm that began approximately 2 hours prior. A CT scan confirmed an ischemic stroke without hemorrhagic conversion. He received IV recombinant tissue plasminogen activator (rt-PA) in the ED 3 hours after the acute onset of symptoms and was admitted to the intensive care unit for monitoring. He had an assessment by a physical therapist and speech therapist prior to hospital discharge after a 5-day hospital stay. He continues to have residual weakness in his right arm and was discharged on warfarin 2.5 mg orally daily.

Past Medical History

Hypertension (HTN) (10 years)
Dyslipidemia (15 years)

Family History

Father is 86 years old and has a history of myocardial infarction (MI) at age 67. Mother is 82 years old and has osteoarthritis and hypertension. He has one brother who is in good health. He has an adult son and daughter who are healthy.

Social/Work History

He works full-time as an auto mechanic. He has two children aged 31 and 33.

Tobacco/Alcohol/Substance Use

He drinks 1-2 glasses of wine or 2-3 cans of beer on the weekends. He has smoked 1 pack per day for 37 years. Has made many quit attempts without success. He smokes his first cigarette within 30 minutes of waking up.

Allergies/Intolerances/Adverse Event History

Varenicline caused episodes of nausea

Medications (Current)

Atorvastatin 80 mg, 1 tablet po every morning
Lisinopril 40 mg, 1 tablet po every morning
HCTZ 25 mg, 1/2 tablet every morning

Prior Medication Use

Nicotine patch 21 mg, apply once daily for 4-6 weeks, patient discontinued use due to continued smoking
Aspirin 81 mg, 1 tablet po daily
Varenicline 1 mg, 1 tablet twice daily, discontinued due to nausea

Review of Systems

Denies headache; (−) confusion; (−) trouble swallowing or speaking; (+) right arm weakness

Physical Exam

▸ **General**

African-American male appearing calm in no apparent distress; no speech deficits noted; + right arm weakness

▸ **Vital Signs**

BP 156/88 mm Hg, P 76, RR 14, T 37°C
Weight 207.2 lb. (94.0 kg)
Height 72 in. (182.9 cm)
Complaining of mild pain, pain score 2 out of 10

▸ **Skin**

Warm and dry to touch

▸ **HEENT**

PERRLA, EOMI; no nystagmus; slight right-sided facial droop

▸ **Neck and Lymph Nodes**

(−) Carotid bruits; (−) lymphadenopathy

▸ **Chest**

Clear to auscultation

▶ *Cardiovascular*

RRR, normal S_1, S_2; (–) S_3; (+) S_4

▶ *Abdomen*

Soft, nontender, nondistended; (+) BS; (–) organomegaly

▶ *Neurology*

A&O × 3; slight right-sided facial droop; strength RUE 3/5; RLE 4/5; LUE 5/5; LLE 5/5; DTRs 2+ throughout; normal Babinski reflex

▶ *Extremities*

No cyanosis, clubbing, or edema; pulses 1+ bilaterally

▶ *Genitourinary*

Examination deferred

▶ *Rectal*

Examination deferred

Laboratory Tests

	Conventional Units	SI Units
Na	141 mEq/L	141 mmol/L
K	4.4 mEq/L	4.4 mmol/L
Cl	104 mEq/L	104 mmol/L
CO_2	23 mEq/L	23 mmol/L
BUN	12 mg/dL	4.28 mmol/L
SCr	0.9 mg/dL	79.56 µmol/L
Glu	98 mg/dL	5.44 mmol/L
Ca	8.7 mg/dL	2.18 mmol/L
Mg	1.7 mEq/L	0.85 mmol/L
Phosphate	3.2 mg/dL	1.03 mmol/L
Hgb	14.5 g/dL	145 g/L; 8.99 mmol/L
Hct	46.0%	0.46
WBC	$6.2 \times 10^3/mm^3$	$6.2 \times 10^9/L$
Platelets	$260 \times 10^3/mm^3$	$260 \times 10^9/L$
aPTT	27.2 s	
Total cholesterol	202 mg/dL	5.22 mmol/L
LDL cholesterol	113 mg/dL	2.92 mmol/L
HDL cholesterol	41 mg/dL	1.06 mmol/L
Triglycerides	240 mg/dL	2.71 mmol/L

Diagnostic Tests

(completed in ED two weeks prior)
ECG: NSR

Head CT Scan: (–) hemorrhage noted; no areas of hyperintensity

Carotid Doppler: Mild plaque in the left internal carotid artery, <50% obstruction noted

Assessment

Sixty-one-year-old African-American male presenting to the clinic after a recent hospitalization for an acute left-sided ischemic stroke. The patient received rt-PA (alteplase) in the emergency department. The patient has a history of hypertension and dyslipidemia and is a current smoker.

Student Work-up

Missing Information?

Evaluate:	Smoking History and Quit Attempts
	Medication History
	Medication Adherence

TARGETED QUESTIONS

1. What nonmodifiable risk factors for ischemic stroke are evident in this patient?

   Hint: See Table 11-1 in PPP

2. What modifiable risk factors for ischemic stroke are evident in this patient?

   Hint: See Table 11-1 in PPP

3. What are the available options for antiplatelet therapy for secondary stroke prevention?

   Hint: See pp. 200-201 in PPP

4. What long-term nonpharmacologic therapy would be appropriate in this patient for secondary stroke prevention?

   Hint: See p. 201 in PPP

5. What long-term therapy would be appropriate in this patient for the management of stroke risk factors?

   Hint: See pp. 199-200 in PPP

FOLLOW-UP

The patient returns for a follow-up visit in two weeks. His blood pressure (BP) is 138/84 mm Hg and he states he is smoking about half pack of cigarettes per day. How would you manage Mr. Peters's BP and other risk factors at this point?

   Hint: See pp. 199-201 in PPP

☉ GLOBAL PERSPECTIVE

Stroke has decreased to the fifth leading cause of death in the United States; however, it remains a major cause of long-term disability. Strokes occur more commonly in people 65 years and older, with the stroke risk doubling every decade after 55 years. Worldwide, stroke is the second most common cause of death after ischemic heart disease. Globally, a symptomatic stroke occurs every two seconds resulting in approximately 20 million strokes and 5.7 million deaths annually. Large disparities exist between countries in access to care and in models of health care delivery. Lower income countries have the greatest risks due to cerebrovascular disease. The World Stroke Organization has developed the Stroke Quality Action Plan as a pathway from the initial symptoms through rehabilitation after stroke. The incidence of stroke is expected to increase over the next decade due to the aging of the population.

CASE SUMMARY

- Sixty-one-year-old African-American male patient with recent acute left-sided ischemic stroke, s/p alteplase treatment 10 days ago. Patient is presenting for his follow-up clinic visit.

- Management of risk factors and choice of antiplatelet agent important for secondary stroke prevention.

For more information on the care plan and facilitator's guide please visit http://www.mhpharmacotherapy.com

10 Dyslipidemia

Jeannie Kim Lee   Kristina De Los Santos

PATIENT PRESENTATION

Chief Complaint

"My doctor sent me here for you to check my cholesterol."

History of Present Illness

Liliana Martinez is a 74-year-old Hispanic female referred to the pharmacy clinic for lipid evaluation and management. She is feeling well, but she has had a few episodes of dizziness and headache in the past week that she attributes to low blood sugar. Last appointment with her primary care provider was 1 month ago when the dose of her metformin was increased. Based upon laboratory tests taken at her primary care appointment, the provider felt she would benefit from a pharmacist evaluation of her atherosclerotic cardiovascular disease risk and need for statin therapy. LM has longstanding HTN and was started on prescription medications several years ago. She questions the safety of prescription medications as "they are not natural," and is resistant to taking any additional medications.

Past Medical History:

Hypertension (HTN) (20 years)

Type 2 diabetes (5 years)

Obesity (22 years)

Depression (5 years)

Hypothyroidism (15 years)

Family History

Father died from cancer at age 60. Mother died from complications of cardiovascular disease and diabetes at age 75. Sister is 65 and has hypertension, diabetes, and a history of breast cancer. Brother is 68 and has hypertension, benign prostatic hyperplasia (BPH), and dyslipidemia.

Social History

LM is Catholic and has lived in Tucson, Arizona her entire life. She is bilingual (Spanish and English). She is widowed, and has two children aged 40 and 38. She is a retired lawyer. She spends her time volunteering as an interpreter and with her grandchildren.

Tobacco/Alcohol/Substance Use:

Lifetime nonsmoker; drinks wine with dinner; has never used illicit drugs.

Allergies/Intolerances/Adverse Drug Events:

NKDA; Intolerance to atorvastatin (muscle aches)

Medications History (Current)

Metformin 850 mg po bid

Glyburide 5 mg po bid

Lisinopril/HCTZ 20 mg/12.5 mg po q 24 h

Sertraline 25 mg po q 24 h

Levothyroxine 0.112 mg po q 24 h

Prior Medication Use

Atorvastatin 80 mg po q 24 h × 4 years

Review of Systems

(–) Headache, dizziness, light-headedness (currently); (–) chest pain, palpitations; (–) constipation, diarrhea, nausea; (–) edema; (–) hyperglycemic symptoms; (–) hypothyroid symptoms; (–) hyperthyroid symptoms; (+) depressed mood; (+) hypoglycemic symptoms.

Physical Exam (from PCP Visit 1 month Ago):

▶ **General**

Well-appearing, elderly, Hispanic female in no acute distress

▶ **Vital Signs**

BP 135/80 mm Hg, P 72, RR 14, T 36.2°C, pain 0/10

Weight 210 lb. (95.5 kg)

Height 63 in. (160 cm)

▶ **Skin**

Intact; (–) rashes or lesions

▶ **HEENT**

PERRLA, EOMI; trace periorbital edema; (–) sinus tenderness; TMs appear normal

▶ **Neck and Lymph Nodes**

Thyroid gland normal; (–) thyroid nodules; (–) lymphadenopathy; (–) carotid bruits

▶ **Chest**

Clear to auscultation

▸ *Cardiovascular*

RRR, normal S_1, S_2; (–) S_3 or S_4

▸ *Abdomen*

Not tender/not distended; (–) organomegaly

▸ *Neurology*

Grossly intact; DTRs normal

▸ *Genitourinary*

Examination deferred

▸ *Rectal*

Examination deferred

Laboratory Tests

Fasting Obtained 2 Weeks Ago

	Conventional Units	SI Units
Na	140 mEq/L	140 mmol/L
K	4.2 mEq/L	4.2 mmol/L
Cl	102 mEq/L	102 mmol/L
CO_2	25 mEq/L	25 mmol/L
BUN	18 mg/dL	6.4 mmol/L
SCr	1.2 mg/dL	106 µmol/L
Hgb A1c	9.5%	0.095 (fraction)
Glucose	130 mg/dL	7.2 mmol/L
TSH	3.5 µU/ml	3.5 mU/L
Total cholesterol	237 mg/dL	6.13 mmol/L
LDL cholesterol	134 mg/dL	3.46 mmol/L
HDL cholesterol	46 mg/dL	1.19 mmol/L
Triglycerides	285 mg/dL	3.2 mmol/L
AST	16 IU/L	0.27 µkat/L
ALT	14 IU/L	0.23 µkat/L

Assessment

Seventy-four-year old female with dyslipidemia as well as DM, HTN, hypothyroidism, obesity and depression.

Student Work-Up

Missing Information/Inadequate Data

Evaluate:	Patient database
	Drug therapy problems
	Care plan (by problem)

TARGETED QUESTIONS

1. What risk factors for arteriosclerotic cardiovascular disease (ASCVD) does LM have?

   Hint: See Tables 12-7 and 12-8 in PPP

2. Would LM benefit from any therapeutic lifestyle changes? If yes, specify.

   Hint: See Table 12-6 in PPP

3. What is LM's ASCVD risk and treatment goal? Does she need statin therapy?

   Hint: See Tables 12-4 and 12-5, and Figure 12-6 in PPP

4. Which medication would you choose for LM, and how would you plan her monitoring and follow-up?

   Hint: See Tables 12-4, 12-10, 12-11, and Figure 12-6 in PPP

5. What education does LM require to be successful with her treatment plan?

   Hint: See Table 12-6 and 12-11 in PPP

FOLLOW-UP

Six years later, LM returns for follow-up. She had a stroke 1 year ago, and her cognition has declined. She has lost 20 lbs. and her diabetes and hypertension are under control. Her fasting laboratory tests include:

Total cholesterol 131 mg/dL (3.39 mmol/L)

LDL cholesterol 60 mg/dL (1.55 mmol/L)

HDL cholesterol 41 mg/dL (1.06 mmol/L)

Triglycerides 150 mg/dL (1.7 mmol/L)

How would the treatment plan change? How should her cholesterol be managed as her age and cognitive decline progress?

Hint: See pages 218 in PPP

⟳ GLOBAL PERSPECTIVE

Clinicians must be aware that various ethnic groups may vary in their risk and presentation for chronic heart disease (CHD). For instance, South Asians, who make up 25% of the global population, have a three- to five-fold increased risk of cardiovascular morbidity and mortality as compared with other ethnic groups. Despite their significantly higher risk of CHD due to a high prevalence of risk factors, they are less likely to receive preventative statin treatment due to their low baseline serum cholesterol levels compared with Caucasian patients. In addition, there is a paucity of data for statin treatment in South Asian patients. For South Asians living in the United States, the U.S. Food and Drug Administration (U.S. FDA) recommends that the starting dose of rosuvastatin be 5 mg (instead of 10 mg) due to a pharmacokinetic study that showed South Asians had a 1.6- to 2.3-fold increased exposure to rosuvastatin compared with Caucasian patients.

CASE SUMMARY

- LM's current clinical picture is consistent with chronic dyslipidemia.
- All patients may benefit from lifestyle modifications. Initial goals and treatment vary widely on the basis of risk factors. Medication therapy is indicated as determined by the 2013 AHA/ACC Blood Cholesterol Guideline and the National Lipid Association recommendations.
- The intensity of statin therapy stratified by degree of risk as indicated by ACC/AHA Blood Cholesterol Guideline should be applied to patients with ASCVD risks for primary prevention.

For more information on the care plan and facilitator's guide please visit http://www.mhpharmacotherapy.com

11 Hypovolemic Shock and Metabolic Acidosis

Wood G. Christopher   Joseph M. Swanson

PATIENT PRESENTATION

Chief Complaint

Severe nausea, vomiting, and diarrhea

History of Present Illness

A 65-year-old male patient just arrived in the emergency department (ED). He had worsening nausea and diarrhea over the past 2 days. However, over the past 8 hours those symptoms have worsened, and now the patient has been vomiting approximately every 60-90 minutes.

Past Medical History

Hypertension (20 years)
Heart failure (10 years)
Osteoarthritis (25 years)

Family History

Father had "heart disease"

Social/Work History

Noncontributory

Tobacco/Alcohol/Substance Use

Approximately 6 beers per day; denies tobacco use

Allergy/Intolerance/Adverse Event History

None

Medication History

▶ Current

None yet. The patient just arrived.

▶ Prior

Carvedilol 12.5 mg orally twice daily.
Losartan 50 mg orally once daily.
Furosemide 20-40 mg orally daily as needed for weight gain/edema/shortness of breath.

Review of Systems/Physical Exam

▶ General

Height 5'9" (175 cm)
Weight 90 kg (198 lb.)
He feels "lightheaded" and "weak" and can't stand up on his own.

▶ Vital Signs

BP 80/40 mm Hg, HR 130, RR 22, T 35.0°C (95.0°F)
Urine output: 0 mL since Foley placed 5 minutes ago

▶ Skin

Pale and cool

▶ HEENT

Normal

▶ Neck and Lymph Nodes

Flat neck veins

▶ Chest

Shallow, rapid breathing. Breath sounds normal.

▶ Cardiovascular

ECG and heart sounds normal except for tachycardia. Also is hypotensive.

▶ Abdomen

Severe nausea. The patient's last episode of diarrhea and emesis were both approximately 30 minutes ago. A nasogastric tube is being placed.

▶ Neurology

Awake and oriented × 3 upon arrival but now confused and lethargic after 5-10 minutes in the ED.

▶ Extremities

No edema, redness or other swelling

► *Genitourinary*

A urinary catheter has just been placed. The patient reports that he has not urinated in the past several hours.

► *Rectal*

Positive for occult blood

Laboratory and Other Diagnostic Tests:

	Conventional Units	SI Units
Na	142 mEq/L	152 mmol/L
K	2.9 mEq/L	2.9 mmol/L
Cl	100 mEq/L	100 mmol/L
HCO_3	16 mEq/L	16 mmol/L
BUN	35 mg/dL	12.5 mmol/L
Creatinine	1.8 mg/dL	160 μmol/L
Glucose	110 mg/dL	6.1 mmol/L
Lactate	5 mEq/L	5 mmol/L
Hemoglobin	9.5 g/dL	5.9 mmol/L
Hematocrit	29%	
Platelets	$289 \times 10^3/\mu L$	$289 \times 10^9/\mu L$
PTT	52 seconds	
INR	1.8	
Arterial blood gas	pH 7.19	
$PaCO_2$	33 mm Hg	4.4 kPa
PaO_2	90 mm Hg	12 kPa
SaO_2	92%	
Base excess	−5.2	

Assessment

The patient is in hypovolemic shock with electrolyte and acid-base abnormalities, requiring immediate therapy.

Student Work-up

Missing Information/Inadequate Data

Evaluate: Patient database

Drug therapy problems

Care plan (by problem)

TARGETED QUESTIONS

1. What appears to be the cause of hypovolemic shock in this patient? In addition, what important information is missing from the patient's past medical history and history of present illness that could help determine the etiology and underlying cause of this shock episode?

   Hint: See Table 13-1 and p. 229, 232 in PPP

2. Discuss the current clinical and laboratory derangements in this patient and the immediate treatment goals in the first hour.

   Hint: pp. 231-232 in PPP

3. What should be administered for initial therapy of this patient's hypovolemic shock? Discuss the various crystalloid, colloid, blood product, and vasopressor options.

   Hint: See Figure 13-3, Table 13-3 and pp. 232-237 in PPP

4. What acid-base disorder(s) does the patient have, what are the likely causes, and what is the most appropriate management?

   Hint: See Table 28-1, Figure 28-1, Table 28-4 and p. 446 in PPP

5. What are the specific treatment goals for this patient's hypovolemic shock and associated abnormalities within the first 24 hours?

   Hint: See p. 238 in PPP

FOLLOW-UP

It is 2 hours later and the initial therapies have been administered. It was discovered that the patient had a bleeding gastric ulcer that was repaired endoscopically. The patient is still sedated from that procedure. A pulmonary artery catheter has been placed and the current values are: PAOP 12 mm Hg, CI 2.2 L/min/m², SvO_2 65%. The patient's current vital signs are: BP 95/55, HR 115, RR 16, urine output 20 mL over the last hour. The most relevant repeat laboratory values are: SCr 2.0 (177 μmol/L), hematocrit 32%, INR 1.9., lactate 4.8 mEq/L (4.8 mmol/L), arterial pH 7.22.

What should be administered at this time? Also discuss the remaining treatment options for hypovolemic shock (inotropes, sodium bicarbonate, activated Factor VII, tranexamic acid, glucocorticoids).

Hint: See Figure 13-3 and p. 237 in PPP

⚘ GLOBAL PERSPECTIVE

Hypovolemic shock, especially related to trauma and hemorrhage, is a leading cause of morbidity and mortality for younger populations regardless of country or ethnic group. The incidence of violence-related trauma (e.g., gunshot wounds) as well as other trauma (e.g., motor vehicle accidents, work-related injuries) varies widely based on multiple sociopolitical factors. Treatment of hypovolemic shock will vary around the world primarily related to the availability of health care infrastructure (ambulance services, capable emergency departments and trauma centers, diagnostic imaging and surgery), as well as transportation issues in areas with decentralized populations and poor infrastructure. Tranexamic acid use in trauma patients may also vary. This agent was studied in Europe and developing countries as a low cost, simple intervention that could be used in most any country. However, the United States has been relatively slow to adopt its use, partially because of poor experiences from U.S. centers and applicability of the foreign data to U.S. patients. An important cultural factor in some patients will be a social and/or religious prohibition against receiving blood products, complicating therapy in patients with hemorrhagic shock.

CASE SUMMARY

- Rapid assessment of the type and severity of hypovolemic shock, and rapid restoration of systolic blood pressure are key components of initial therapy.

- Ongoing therapy in the first 24 hours focuses on continued volume resuscitation and reversal of organ dysfunction.

For more information on the care plan and facilitator's guide please visit http://www.mhpharmacotherapy.com

12 Chronic Asthma

Alexis E. Horace   Susan M. Sirmans

PATIENT PRESENTATION

AB is a 43-year-old male who reports to your ambulatory care clinic this morning with shortness of breath (SOB) and coughing. He also says that he has a sore throat. He states that he did not have asthma as a child, however he has taken allergy medicine and had the occasional "allergy shot" throughout the years. Since relocating to Louisiana for his career, his allergies have gotten much worse. Last spring he was started on albuterol and fluticasone inhalers. He says that he did not have to use the fluticasone inhaler during the winter, but has recently started using both inhalers for the past 2 months. He reports that his SOB started a few weeks ago when he was jogging with his running group, and ran by a lawn mower that was emitting dust and pollen into the air. AB says that he had to stop shortly after running through the dust and was unable to continue the exercise. Taking his rescue inhaler once he reached his car provided only partial relief. He complains that he has been unable to keep up with his running partner since then and has not been able to run at his normal speed for the entire week, despite taking both inhalers. AB reports using his fluticasone inhaler 2 times a day, two puffs in one breath, and his albuterol inhaler more than 4 times a week. The patient experiences symptoms >3 days a week, and feels that his physical activity is limited. He says that when he is walking normally or participating in daily activities his breathing is "OK" but he feels slight chest tightness. He worries that with the pollen count being the worst it's been in years, he may have an asthma attack. He also complains of itchy eyes and sneezing. AB denies night-time symptoms. He's mostly concerned about his ability to train for a half-marathon that is 2 months away.

Chief Complaint

"I'm having trouble breathing and I can't run like I normally do."

History of Present Illness

As above

Past Medical History

Allergic rhinitis (allergies increase during pollen season) × 30 years

Hypothyroidism (4 years)

Hypertension (3 years)

Asthma (diagnosed at the age of 42, currently using medications prescribed from last spring)

Family History

Mother has hypothyroidism and hypertension, father has hypertension and diabetes.

Social/Work History

He doesn't have any children. Lives at home with his fiancé and one dog. He works as a paralegal for a law firm and trains for half-marathons in his free time.

Tobacco/Alcohol/Substance Abuse

He denies current tobacco and alcohol use. However, his fiancee smokes occasionally and sometimes in the house.

Allergy/Intolerance/Adverse Event History

Milk protein allergy

Aspirin sensitivity

Medication History

Albuterol HFA 90 mcg 1-2 puffs every 4-6 hours as needed for shortness of breath

Fluticasone 44 mcg two puffs every 12 hours

Levothyroxine 75 mcg po daily

Multivitamin po daily

Review of Systems

Unremarkable except for what's noted above.

Physical Examination

▶ **General**

Well-developed, well-nourished white male in no acute distress

▶ **Vital Signs**

BP 139/75, P 75, RR 20, T 38°C

Weight 180 lb. (81.8 kg)

Height 72 in. (196 cm)

Denies pain

▶ **HEENT**

Red, watery eyes. Rhinorrhea w/mucosal swelling. Positive for nasal polyps. Throat has slightly raised white lesions with red tender borders.

▶ **Chest**

Sibilant rhonchi (wheezing). Prolonged phase of forced exhalation.

▶ **Cardiovascular**

RRR, S_1 and S_2 normal, no rubs, gallops, or murmurs.

Laboratory and Other Diagnostic Tests.

(%) Predicted	Prealbuterol	Postalbuterol
FEV$_1$	75% [0.75]	88% [0.88]
FVC	94% [0.94]	100% [1]
FEV1/FVC	0.80	0.88

Asthma Control Test Score: 17

Assessment

43-year-old male with signs, symptoms, and diagnostic tests consistent with uncontrolled asthma.

Student Work-Up

Missing Information/Inadequate Data

Evaluate:	Patient database
	Drug therapy problems
	Care plan (by problem)

Additional Information:

Self discontinued carvedilol when he started training for half-marathons; fiancee occasionally smokes inside the house.

TARGETED QUESTIONS

1. How would you assess the patient's asthma severity and control?

   Hint: Table 14-1, Figure 14-6 in PPP

2. How would you counsel a patient regarding trigger avoidance for asthma?

   Hint: p. 244 in PPP

3. How should the patient's current asthma treatment be modified?

   Hint: Table 14-5 and Table 14-6, Figure 14-6 in PPP

4. What are important counseling points for optimizing metered dose inhaler technique?

   Hint: Figure 14-1, p. 244 in PPP

FOLLOW-UP

4 weeks later the patient returns to clinic for follow-up. The patient states that his chest no longer feels tight and the coughing has stopped. AB is using his inhaler 2 times a week 15 minutes before his longer runs. What changes, if any, would you make to his current asthma treatment?

🌐 GLOBAL PERSPECTIVE

An estimated 334 million individuals worldwide are affected by asthma. The prevalence of asthma in children and adults has increased over the past several decades and continues to increase fastest in low- and middle-income countries. One in every 250 deaths worldwide can be attributed to asthma. Asthma prevalence rates increase as regions become more westernized and more urbanized. Asthma in developing regions of the world, including Africa, Central and South America, Asia and the Pacific Basin has increased significantly. The wide variation in regional prevalence of asthma in China has been attributed to the rate of economic development and associated lifestyle changes. Risk factors associated with the increasing global prevalence of asthma include sedentary life habits, high-fat diets, reduced dietary intake of antioxidant vitamins, passive tobacco smoke exposure, indoor/outdoor allergen exposure and pollution. Before the global burden of asthma can be significantly reduced, asthma must be recognized as a significant cause of morbidity, mortality and economic costs. Economic and political factors that limit the access to health care and the availability of essential medications to low and middle income countries must be addressed. Although the World Health Organization has added two inhaled corticosteroids and one bronchodilator to the Essential Medicine List, surveys indicate that many countries do not have these critical medications on their national Essential Medicine lists. The same countries do not provide these medications gratis or at reduced rates. In addition, national medicine regulatory agencies in low-income countries have limited capacity to assure that inhalers available are of high quality. Increased availability of quality asthma medications, especially inhaled corticosteroids, can reduce asthma severity, symptoms, dramatically reduce hospitalizations, and reduce overall costs of care in resource-poor areas. However, studies have shown that patients in resource-poor regions may discontinue inhaled corticosteroids because they perceive them as ineffective when compared to inhaled bronchodilators. Therefore, patients with asthma require ongoing asthma education that emphasizes the importance of continuing inhaled corticosteroids. Indoor pollution, outdoor pollution and tobacco smoking must be reduced. Proven and cost-effective approaches to reducing the morbidity and mortality associated with asthma must be more widely implemented. The focus of management in some areas of the world has been on acute management of life threatening asthma exacerbations. A greater focus on the routine management of asthma is essential. Treatment strategies that have been adapted to address local societal, economic and healthcare environments have markedly reduced asthma burden in certain countries. To that end, the World Health Organization published guidelines for the management of asthma in low-income settings. Education of healthcare providers is also important since studies have shown that providers do not consistently adhere to guidelines when assessing asthma severity or prescribing inhaled corticosteroids.

CASE SUMMARY

- His presentation is consistent with asthma that is not well controlled.

- His current inhaler regimen should be "stepped up" or increased to a medium-dose inhaled corticosteroid.

- Patient is suffering from oral candidiasis caused by his steroid inhaler, and he should be counseled on all required steps for administration.

For more information on the care plan and facilitator's guide please visit http://www.mhpharmacotherapy.com

13 Acute Asthma Exacerbation

Hanna Phan   Allison Mruk

PATIENT PRESENTATION

It is November 5, currently in the emergency department (ED).

Chief Complaint

"I couldn't catch my breath during basketball practice."

History of Present Illness

Peter Davis is a 14-year-old Caucasian male who presents to the ED with an 8-hour history of increased work of breathing and wheezing unrelieved by albuterol treatments (metered dose inhaler, MDI) at home. Patient was out playing basketball and began having difficulty keeping up with his teammates. Peter was pulled out of the game to catch his breath; however, with little improvement, he was taken home to retrieve his forgotten albuterol inhaler. He received two puffs of albuterol every 4 hours with minimal relief, so he was taken to the ED.

Past Medical History

Mild persistent asthma (diagnosed age 7 years)

GERD (gastroesophageal reflux disease, diagnosed age 12 years)

Allergic rhinitis and atopy (diagnosed age 8 years)

Last ED visit for asthma exacerbation was 1 month ago

Family History

Mother has mild persistent asthma. Father has allergic rhinitis and type 2 diabetes mellitus. No siblings.

Social/Work History

Lives at home with parents. There is a cat at home which sleeps with patient in bed. States he forgets to take his beclomethasone about 3 days a week (review of refill history notes he refills his beclomethasone about every other month).

Tobacco/Alcohol/Substance Abuse

Denies tobacco, alcohol, and drug use. Patient exposed to secondhand smoke. Both parents smoke cigarettes, but claim to try to smoke outside as much as possible.

Allergies/Intolerance/Adverse Drug Events

Peanut allergy (anaphylaxis)

Medication History

▶ **Current Medications**

- Albuterol 2.5 mg nebulized every 20 minutes, received 2 doses at this time

▶ **Prior to Admission**

- Albuterol HFA MDI 90 mcg 1-2 puffs every 4-6 hours prn shortness of breath/wheezing
- Beclomethasone HFA MDI 80 mcg 2 puffs inhaled twice daily
- Omeprazole 20 mg po once daily
- Cetirizine 10 mg po once daily
- Montelukast 10 mg po once daily
- Epinephrine pen 0.3 mg IM prn allergic reaction

Immunizations

Routine childhood vaccines reported to be up to date, with last influenza vaccination last fall season.

Review of Systems

Acute respiratory distress, (+) inspiratory and expiratory wheeze, SOB. Able to speak in short phrases, but not complete sentences. Denies fever/chills.

Physical Examination

▶ **General**

Patient appears anxious and presents in respiratory distress. Patient is unable to speak in full sentences without gasping for air. Increased work of breathing, bilateral wheezing, and some intercostal retractions noted.

▶ **Vital Signs**

BP 125/73, HR 112, RR 32, Temp 36.9°C, O_2 saturation 86% on RA

Weight 132 lb. (60 kg)

Height 63 in. (160 cm)

BMI 23.4 (88th percentile for age)

▶ **Chest**

Diffuse wheezes bilaterally during inspiration and expiration; no crackles or rhonchi noted

▶ **Cardiovascular**

Tachycardic, RRR. No murmurs present

▶ **Abdomen**

Normal, active bowel sounds. Soft, nontender, and nondistended

▶ **Neurology**

Alert and oriented × 3

Laboratory Tests

September (3 months ago, Fasting)

	Conventional Units	SI Units
IgE level	325 ku/L (812.5 ng/mL)	<400 ku/L or <167 ng/mL
Na	136 meq/L	136 mmol/L
K	3.5 meq/L	3.5 mmol/L
Cl	107 meq/L	107 mmol/L
CO_2	22 meq/L	22 mmol/L
Ca	9.2 mg/dL	2.3 mmol/L
BUN	8 mg/dL	2.9 mmol/L
Albumin	4.2 g/dL	420 g/L
SCr	0.5 mg/dL	44.2 µmol/L
Glucose	97 mg/dL	5.4 mmol/L

Diagnostic Studies

Current: Chest x-ray (CXR) normal lung fields, shows no infiltrates or signs of heart failure. ECG shows sinus tachycardia.

Other Tests

Spirometery (3 months ago)

FVC 3.68 L (pre-bronchodilator)

FVC % predicted 96% (pre-bronchodilator)

FEV_1 3.18 L (pre-bronchodilator)

FEV_1 % predicted 89% (pre-bronchodilator)

FEV_1/FVC % predicted 93% (pre-bronchodilator)

FVC 3.98 L (post-bronchodilator)

FVC % predicted 98% (post-bronchodilator)

FEV_1 3.31 L (post-bronchodilator)

FEV_1 % predicted 94% (post-bronchodilator)

FEV_1/FVC % predicted 96% (post-bronchodilator)

Peak Expiratory Flow (PEF)

Personal best: 340

September, 3 months ago: 310

November, current: 120

Assessment

This is a 14-year-old Caucasian male who presents with an acute asthma exacerbation.

Student Work-Up

Missing Information/Inadequate Data

Evaluate: Patient database

Drug therapy problems

Care plan (by problem)

TARGETED QUESTIONS

1. What is this patient's acute asthma exacerbation severity?

   Hint: See Table 14-1 in PPP

2. What initial therapy should Peter receive in the emergency department?

   Hint: See Figure 14-4, pp. 252-254 in PPP

3. What adjunctive medication(s) should be utilized if patient has minimal improvement with initial therapy? What is/are the mechanism(s) of action?

   Hint: See p. 252 in PPP

4. What parameter(s) should be monitored to ensure successful treatment of patient's acute asthma exacerbation?

   Hint: See Figure 14-4, pp. 257-258 in PPP

5. What medications and patient education should be included in this patient's treatment plan upon discharge?

   Hint: See pp. 257-258, Tables 14-3 and 14-4 in PPP

FOLLOW-UP

Peter comes to his pediatrician for follow up 4 weeks later. In the past 2 weeks, his Mom notes that he has had daytime asthma symptoms 2-3 days/week, night-time awakenings due to cough weekly, and used albuterol for rescue about 2 times per week. Upon further questioning about the patient's history, Mom instructed her son to stop taking his daily inhaled corticosteroid because she thought his asthma was improving due to concern of chronic use and stunted growth.

How would you classify Peter's asthma control today, based on this information? Would you make any changes to his asthma medications? What counseling information would you provide mom and her son regarding Peter's asthma medications?

Hint: See Table 14-6 in PPP

🌀 GLOBAL PERSPECTIVE

Asthma is a common disease among children and adults. According to the World Health Organization (WHO), about 235 million people suffer from asthma, making it the most common noncommunicable disease among children. Asthma is a public health problem in both high- and low-income countries. Most asthma-related deaths occur in low- and low-middle income countries. The WHO monitors the magnitude of asthma and geographic trends worldwide with an emphasis on poor and disadvantaged populations. Primary prevention and improving access to cost-effective medicines remain main objectives to decrease the asthma burden worldwide.[1]

CASE SUMMARY

- This patient's clinical picture is consistent with a severe asthma exacerbation requiring additional therapies to manage his exacerbation.

- Selection of common and adjunctive therapy for an asthma exacerbation is based on available care guidelines and updated literature.

- Patient factors including insurance (i.e., access to medications and medical care), patient/caregiver concerns, and adherence should be taken into account when selecting asthma controller therapy.

- Patient/caregiver education regarding medications, the asthma action plan, inhaler technique, and medication adherence is important in controlling asthma and preventing asthma exacerbations.

KEY REFERENCES/READINGS

The World Health Organization. Facts about asthma. Available at: http://www.who.int/mediacentre/factsheets/fs307/en/. Accessed May 30, 2015.

For more information on the care plan and facilitator's guide please visit http://www.mhpharmacotherapy.com

14 Chronic Obstructive Pulmonary Disease

Nicole D. Verkleeren, Pharm.D., BCPS

PATIENT PRESENTATION

Chief Complaint

"He won't stop coughing. He kept me up all night – AGAIN!" – per the patient's wife

History of Present Illness

Dieter McDouglan is a 61-year-old male who was reluctantly brought to the hospital-based walk-in clinic early this morning by his wife. She is concerned because he has been coughing for most of the night for several nights, and she states that the last time he was coughing like this, he was admitted to the hospital for 4 days. The patient does not admit to being bothered by the cough, but does eventually admit that he had been abnormally short of breath yesterday while fielding balls at his grandson's baseball practice. Additionally, he did use his albuterol inhaler 2 times last evening, and kept it at bedside and used it "several" times overnight. In the last 6 months, he has been treated for 2 other COPD exacerbations, the most recent being the inpatient admission 3 weeks ago. At the time of discharge, he was started on fluticasone/salmeterol. Previously, he had used olodaterol daily and albuterol as needed.

Past Medical History

COPD (diagnosed 2 years ago)

Benign prostatic hyperplasia (BPH) (diagnosed 2 years ago)

Post-traumatic stress disorder after combat in Vietnam

Right below knee amputation due to combat injury

Cutaneous candidiasis of right stump (recurrent)

Left lower extremity deep vein thrombosis in 2009 after knee replacement surgery

Family History

Father died at age 85 of lung cancer. Mother is alive and well at age 89. Twin brother killed in combat in Vietnam. Sister is alive and healthy at age 55.

Social History

Married and lives with his wife of 31 years. Son and 12-year-old grandson are local and visit often. He is on disability, but maintains an active volunteer schedule leading a support group for veterans 5 days a week at the VA hospital. He also supervises recess at his grandson's school, and acts as an assistant coach for his baseball and soccer teams.

Tobacco/Alcohol/Substance Use

Former heavy smoker with a 36-year history, quit in the early 1980s

Drinks 1-2 beers per week

No illicit drug use

Allergies/Intolerances/Adverse Drug Events

Heparin (heparin-induced thrombocytopenia)

Amoxicillin (anaphylaxis)

Medications (Prior to Admission)

Fluticasone/salmeterol 250 mcg/50 mcg 1 in. hour q 12 h

Albuterol MDI 1-2 puffs q 4-6 h prn SOB (used more frequently over the last night)

Tamsulosin 0.4 mg once daily

Paroxetine 40 mg once daily

OTC antifungal cream applied to stump twice daily as needed

OTC ibuprofen 400 mg q 4-6 h prn pain

Prior Medication Use

Olodaterol 2 in. hours once daily (stopped 3 weeks ago)

Warfarin, dosed per INR results (stopped in 2009)

Influenza vaccine (most recently received last fall)

Review of Systems

(+) fatigue; (−) nasal congestion or drainage; (+) SOB, cough with increased thick, tan, sputum production; (−) fever; (+) chest tightness; (−) chest pain; (−) muscle pain/weakness; (+) mild shoulder pain after baseball practice; (−) constipation; (+) sick contacts; (−) recent travel; (−) anxiety or mood changes; (−) nocturia, frequency, or urgency

Physical Exam

▶ **General**

Physically fit, somewhat ill-appearing white male

▶ **Vital Signs**

BP 125/76 mm Hg, P 85, RR 18, T 37.0°C

Weight 190 lb. (86.4 kg)

Height 72 in. (182.9 cm)

2/10 musculoskeletal pain in right shoulder

▶ **Skin**

Warm, dry, and intact

▶ **HEENT**

PERRLA, EOMI; TMs appear normal.

▶ **Neck and Lymph Nodes**

(–) lymphadenopathy, (–) thyromegaly, (–) JVD

▶ **Chest**

(+) rhonchi, (–) crackles. Lung sounds distant. Bilateral wheezes on inspiration and expiration.

▶ **Cardiovascular**

RRR, normal S_1, S_2; (–) S_3 or S_4; no murmurs, rubs, or gallops

▶ **Abdomen**

Nontender, nondistended; (–) organomegaly.

▶ **Neurology**

A&O × 3, CN II-XII intact

▶ **Extremities**

Reveals right below knee amputation with prosthesis. Stump is slightly erythematous with some scaling. Left lower extremity is cool, no cyanosis, no clubbing, no edema, radial and pedal pulses 2+; (–) joint swelling or tenderness bilaterally.

Laboratory Tests

	Conventional Units	SI Units
Na	141 mEq/L	141 mmol/L
K	3.9 mEq/L	3.9 mmol/L
Cl	108 mEq/L	108 mmol/L
CO_2	26 mEq/L	26 mmol/L
Glu	107 mg/dL	5.9 mmol/L
WBC	$11.2 \times 10^3/mm^3$	$11.2 \times 10^9/L$
Neutrophils	$9.1 \times 10^3/mm^3$	$9.1 \times 10^9/L$
Lymphocytes	$0.9 \times 10^3/mm^3$	$0.9 \times 10^9/L$
Bands	$1.2 \times 10^3/mm^3$	$1.2 \times 10^9/L$
Hgb	14.1 mg/dL	8.7 mmol/L
Hct	41.1%	0.411
Plts	$279 \times 10^3/mm^3$	$279 \times 10^9/L$
D-dimer	157 ng/mL	157 µg/L
BUN	19 mg/dL	6.7 mmol/L
SCr	0.8 mg/dL	70.7 µmol/L

Diagnostic Tests

Chest x-ray shows mild hyperinflation of the lungs; (–) infiltrates, effusion

ECG reveals normal sinus rhythm, no ST-segment changes or T-wave inversion

Pulse oximetry shows oxygen saturation 94% (0.94)

Assessment

Sixty-one-year-old man with signs, symptoms, and laboratory tests consistent with a COPD exacerbation that can be treated as an outpatient.

Student Work-Up

Missing Information/Inadequate Data

Evaluate: Patient database

Drug therapy problems

Care plan (by problem)

TARGETED QUESTIONS

1. What signs and symptoms of a COPD exacerbation does the patient have?

   Hint: See pp. 262-263 in PPP

2. What factor(s) may have precipitated this patient's exacerbation?

   Hint: See pp. 269-270 in PPP

3. What are the pharmacologic therapies that should be instituted for this patient's COPD exacerbation?

   Hint: See p. 270 in PPP

4. Why might anticholinergics be avoided in this patient?

   Hint: What side effect of anticholinergics might worsen an underlying condition in this patient? See p. 265 in PPP

5. What characteristics of this patient's presentation make him a good candidate for outpatient management?

   Hint: What characteristics of an exacerbation warranting admission to the hospital does this patient lack? See p. 269 in PPP

FOLLOW-UP

A week later, the patient is seen by his primary care physician (PCP) for follow-up. His symptoms have improved back to his baseline, and he is back to his normal activities. What changes, if any, would you recommend to the PCP for his COPD maintenance therapy? What pieces of patient education on the disease and his medications may have the most impact on this patient's outcomes?

> *Hint: Into which GOLD patient category does this patient fit? See Figure 15-2 in PPP*

🌐 GLOBAL PERSPECTIVE

Causes of COPD vary among geographic areas. In high- and middle-income countries, tobacco smoke is the leading risk factor for COPD. Lower-income countries can attribute the majority of COPD cases to indoor air pollution, commonly from the use of biomass fuels for heating and cooking. Biomass fuels used for cooking are to blame for the high prevalence of COPD among nonsmoking women in the Middle East, Africa, and Asia.

CASE SUMMARY

- His clinical presentation is appropriate to provide outpatient treatment of his COPD exacerbation.
- His underlying medical conditions (BPH, e.g.), must be taken into consideration when designing a drug therapy regimen and establishing therapeutic goals and monitoring.
- Recent changes to the patient's pharmacotherapy are relevant in assessing the potential cause(s) of his exacerbation and in formulating a maintenance therapy plan.

For more information on the care plan and facilitator's guide please visit http://www.mhpharmacotherapy.com

15 Cystic Fibrosis

Hanna Phan   Nicole M. Varner

PATIENT PRESENTATION

Admitted November 18 at 12:00 from CF clinic (currently day 2 of hospitalization, November 19).

Chief Complaint

"I don't feel good; I am coughing more and have no appetite. I am coughing up thicker stuff than usual."

History of Present Illness

Andy Koff is a 14-year-old Caucasian-Hispanic male with cystic fibrosis (CF). His father brought him to the clinic for worsening respiratory symptoms for the past 10 days resulting in subsequent direct admission for acute CF exacerbation. For the past week, has had increased cough with dark-green colored sputum, shortness of breath (SOB), and lethargy. He has lost 10 pounds since his last CF clinic visit (3 months ago) and is having stools (4-5 stools per day) that are foul smelling and greasy.

Past Medical History

Diagnosed with CF at age 10 months via newborn screen, confirmed by sweat chloride testing and genotyping.

Previous hospitalizations: he is hospitalized approximately every 2 to 3 months for acute pulmonary CF exacerbations.

He was diagnosed with asthma and allergic rhinitis at age 5 years.

He has pancreatic insufficiency requiring enzyme supplementation and cystic fibrosis-related diabetes (CFRD, diagnosed at age 12 years).

CF genotype: ΔF508 homozygous.

Family History

He has 1 younger 12-year-old brother who also has CF (ΔF508 heterozygous) who is hospitalized about once a year for acute CF exacerbations.

Social/Work History

Andy is a freshman at a local high school. He lives with his father and brother. He is nonadherent to his medications and airway clearance. He admits that he forgets taking his pancreatic enzymes about 1-2 times per week and does not do his chest physiotherapy as often as he is supposed to. Also admits that he does not check his blood sugar or take his insulin like he knows he is supposed to. When asked about other medications, he states "I'm good about taking other pills, it's just my enzymes and insulin shots that I forget." His father works full time and Andy does not participate in any sports or extracurricular activities outside of school.

Tobacco/Alcohol/Substance Use

Admits to smoking 1-2 cigarettes a few times per week. Denies alcohol and illicit drug use.

Allergies/Intolerances/Adverse Drug Event History

Vancomycin—flushing not prevented by premedicating with diphenhydramine and 2 hour extended infusion duration

Sulfamethoxazole/trimethoprim—rash

Medication History

► *Current Medications*

- Airway clearance via percussion and postural drainage bid
- Albuterol 2.5 mg nebulized every 4-6 hours PRN
- Dornase alfa 2.5 mg nebulized daily
- Fluticasone 110 mcg MDI HFA 2 puff inhaled without spacer bid
- Mometasone 50 mcg nasal spray 1 spray each nostril daily
- Cetirizine 10 mg po daily
- Insulin lispro 1 unit for every 10 g of carbohydrates, before meals and 1 unit for every BG 50 mg/dL if FSBG > 150 for correction dose, subcutaneously
- Insulin glargine 8 units subcutaneously every evening
- Pancreatic enzyme (Creon) 12,000 units (8 capsules po with meals and 4 caps po with snacks)
- Vitamin A-D-E-K supplement (Aquadek) 1 gelcap po bid
- Regular multivitamin 1 tablet po daily
- Cefepime 1000 mg IV every 8 hours
- Tobramycin 100 mg IV every 8 hours
- Tobramycin inhalation solution (Tobi) 300mg nebulized bid
- Vancomycin 1000 mg IV every 8 hours infused over 3 hours

▶ **Prior to Admission**

Airway clearance via high frequency chest wall oscillation vest daily (prescribed bid)

Albuterol 2.5 mg nebulized bid

Dornase alfa 2.5 mg nebulized daily

Fluticasone 110 mcg MDI HFA 2 puff inhaled without spacer bid

Mometasone 50 mcg nasal spray 1 spray each nostril daily

Cetirizine 10 mg po daily

Azithromycin 500 mg po every Monday, Wednesday, and Friday

Insulin lispro 1 unit SC for every 10 g of carbohydrate before meals and 1 unit for every BG 50 mg/dL if FSBG > 150 for correction dose

Insulin glargine 8 units SC every evening

Pancreatic enzyme (Creon) 12,000 units (8 capsules po with meals and 4 capsules po with snacks)

Vitamin A-D-E-K supplement (Aquadek) 1 gelcap po bid

Gummy multivitamin 1 po daily

Tobramycin inhalation solution (Tobi) 300 mg nebulized bid, 28 days on/off alternating with aztreonam, currently "on" month

Immunizations

Routine childhood vaccines reported to be up to date, with last influenza vaccination last fall season.

Review of Systems

Positive for lethargy, increased cough frequency, and thick sputum production (reported as dark green in color); increased stool frequency (noted that it floats versus well-formed, sinking). Denies fever/chills.

Physical Examination

▶ **General**

Lean adolescent male, in acute respiratory distress and noted steatorrhea.

▶ **Vital Signs**

HR 95, BP 110/70 mm, RR 18, Temp: 36.7°C

Height 65 in. (165.1 cm)

Weight: 88 lb. (40 kg)

BMI 14.7

O2 sats: 86% on RA, 97% with 1.5 L nasal cannula

▶ **Skin/Extremities**

Clubbing noted with no cyanosis; capillary refill <2 seconds

▶ **HEENT**

EOMI, PERRLA

▶ **Neck and Lymph Nodes**

(–) lymphadenopathy

▶ **Chest**

Crackles in both upper lobes, greater than lower lobes, poor airway movement throughout

▶ **Cardiovascular**

RRR, no murmurs, rubs, or gallops

▶ **Abdomen**

Nondistended, nontender, normal bowel sounds. Normal diet but he is not very hungry most days and often doesn't feel like eating anything. Does drink 1-2 cups of coffee every morning.

▶ **Neurology**

Grossly intact; DTRs normal; A&O × 4

▶ **Genitourinary**

Examination deferred. UOP: good, approximately 2.2 mL/kg/hr

▶ **Rectal**

Examination deferred

Laboratory Tests

November 19 (Current Admission, Fasting)

	Conventional Units	SI Units
Na	137 meq/L	137 mmol/L
K	3.7 meq/L	3.7 mmol/L
Cl	109 meq/L	109 mmol/L
CO_2	24 meq/L	24 mmol/L
Ca	9.2 mg/dL	2.3 mmol/L
BUN	12 mg/dL	4.3 mmol/L
Albumin	3.2 g/dL	32 g/L
SCr	0.7 mg/dL	61.88 µmol/L
Glucose	140 mg/dL	12.21 mmol/L
Hgb A1c	8%;	0.08 (fraction)
WBC	$7.8 \times 10^3/\mu L$	$7.8 \times 10^9/L$
Neutrophils	60%	
Lymphs	$1.9 \times 10^3/\mu L$	$1.9 \times 10^9/L$
Monos	5%	3-6
Eosinophil	4%	(0-5)
Basophil	1%	0-3
Hgb	11 g/dL	6.82 mmol/L
Hct	41%	0.41
Plt	$264 \times 10^3/\mu L$	$264 \times 10^9/L$
PT	14.6 secs	
INR	1.2	

AST	25 IU/L	0.42 µkat/L
ALT	29 IU/L	0.43 µkat/L
Alk Phos	155 IU/L	2.58 µkat/L
Gamma glutamyl transferase (ggt)	15 units/LL	0.25 µkat/L
	9-26 units/L	0.15-0.43 µkat/L
Total bilirubin	0.3 mg/dL	5.13 µmol/L
Vitamin A (retinol)	0.06 µg/dL	0.002 µmol/L
	0-0.1 µg/L	0-0.003 µmol/L
Vitamin E (alpha tocopherol)	8.1 mg/L	188 µmol/L
	5.5-18 mg/L	127.7-418 µmol/L
Vitamin E (gamma-tocopherol)	0.4 mg/L	9.3 µmol/L
	0-6 mg/L	0-139 µmol/L
Vitamin D (25-OH total)	21 ng/ML	52.4 nmol/L
	30-60 ng/ML	75-150 nmol/L
Serum IgE	45 ku/L or IU/ML (112.5 ng/mL)	(<400 ku/L or <1000 ng/mL)

Cultures and Susceptibilities:

June 30 (4 months ago), Respiratory Sputum:

2+ *pseudomonas aeruginosa*, mucoid

Susceptible: tobramycin (MIC 4), amikacin (MIC ≤ 4) meropenem (MIC 4), cefepime (MIC 4)

Intermediate: pipercillin/tazobactam (MIC 32), ciprofloxacin (MIC 2)

Resistant: gentamicin (MIC 8), aztreonam (MIC 16)

2+ *pseudomonas aeruginosa*, non-mucoid

Susceptible: tobramycin (MIC ≤ 2), amikacin (MIC ≤ 4), cefepime (MIC 4)

Intermediate: meropenem (MIC 8), aztreonam (MIC 8)

Resistant: gentamicin (MIC 8), pipercillin/tazobactam (MIC > 64), ciprofloxacin (MIC > 2)

1+ *staphylococcus aureus*

Susceptible: oxacillin, doxycycline, vancomycin

resistant: erythromycin, clindamycin, trimethoprim/sulfa

11/18 (current admission) respiratory sputum:

Final results pending

Gram stain—negative

3+ Gram-negative rods, non-lactose fermenting

Other Tests

Spirometry

11/18 (at clinic)

FVC 3.36 L (pre-bronchodilator)

FVC % predicted 83% (pre-bronchodilator)

FEV₁ 2.38 L (pre-bronchodilator)

FEV₁ % predicted 67% (pre-bronchodilator)

FVC 3.45 L (post-bronchodilator)

FVC % predicted 85% (post-bronchodilator)

FEV₁ 2.45 L (post-bronchodilator)

FEV₁ % predicted 69% (post-bronchodilator)

8/15 (3 months ago)

FVC 3.6 L

FVC % predicted 89%

FEV₁ 2.7 L

FEV₁ % predicted 76% (baseline)

Assessment

Based on the physician's assessment, Andy is diagnosed with an acute CF pulmonary exacerbation.

Student Work-Up

Missing Information/Inadequate Data

Evaluate: Patient database)

Drug therapy problems

Care plan (by problem)

TARGETED QUESTIONS

1. Describe pharmacokinetic differences specific to patients with CF that would affect Andy's antibiotic dosing.

   Hint: See pp. 280-281 in PPP

2. What should be monitored, including therapeutic drug monitoring goals, during Andy's antibiotic course (i.e., laboratory tests, clinical signs/symptoms)?

   Hint: See Table 16-3 and pp. 282-283 in PPP

3. How does the effect of hypertonic saline differ from dornase alfa? Would it provide additional benefit for Andy with regard to his pulmonary manifestation of CF?

   Hint: See Table 16-1 and p. 278 in PPP

4. Would high-dose ibuprofen be appropriate to start as chronic therapy for Andy? Why or why not?

   Hint: See p. 279 in PPP

5. What is the most appropriate order of administration for Andy's inhaled therapies? Why?

   Hint: See p. 278 and Table 16-1 in PPP

FOLLOW-UP

Andy returns to clinic 2 months after being discharged for his CF exacerbation. You interview him and find out that he is getting better at taking his enzymes, airway clearance, and inhaled therapies. His mother asks you about the "new pills for CF" and if they are useful for Andy as they "would be easier for him to take every day compared to everything he has to do right now." What is the most appropriate response to his mother's question?

Hint: See p. 282 in PPP

🌐 GLOBAL PERSPECTIVE

Cystic fibrosis is an autosomal recessive genetic disorder that has variable incidence worldwide. Because it more commonly diagnosed in Caucasian populations, approximately 1:3500 in the United States and 1:2000-3000 in the European Union are new diagnoses with CF. Prevalence in other racial and ethnic groups in the United States is considerably less, with 1:15,000 and 1:30,000, in African-American and Asian-American populations, respectively. With advances in newborn screening and awareness of CF worldwide, the previously reported prevalence of CF in geographic regions such as the Middle East (1:5800 to 15,876), Asia (1:40,000 to 350,000), and Africa (1:7056) are likely to increase.[1] The approach to and availability of specific care for patients with CF is variable internationally, with a standardized approach to care (e.g., drug therapy, multidisciplinary care) most notable in the United States, Canada, and the European Union.[2,3]

CASE SUMMARY

- The patient's current clinical picture is consistent with an acute pulmonary exacerbation secondary to cystic fibrosis and he should be started on increased frequency of airway clearance and systemic antimicrobials. He also presents with classic symptoms of pancreatic insufficiency with his increase in stool output and steatorrhea.

- Selection of appropriate empiric antimicrobial therapy should be based on previous culture and susceptibility history and patient-specific factors including medication allergies or intolerances, organ function and recent antimicrobial use.

- Difference in pharmacokinetics of antimicrobials should be considered when determining drug therapy dose in patients with cystic fibrosis.

- Cystic fibrosis is a multi-organ systemic disease; thus, other possible comorbidities should be considered and managed including pancreatic insufficiency and CF-related diabetes.

KEY REFERENCES/READINGS

1. World Health Organization. The molecular genetic epidemiology of cystic fibrosis. Available at: http://www.who.int/genomics/publications/en/hgn_wb_04.02_report.pdf. Accessed May 22, 2015.
2. Cystic Fibrosis Foundation. Available at: http://www.CFF.org. Accessed May 22, 2015.
3. European Cystic Fibrosis Society. Available at: https://www.ECFS.eu. Accessed May 22, 2015.

For more information on the care plan and facilitator's guide please visit http://www.mhpharmacotherapy.com

16 Gastroesophageal Reflux Disease

Jeannie Kim Lee   Stephanie Davis

PATIENT PRESENTATION

Chief Complaint

"I keep waking up in the middle of the night with burning in my chest and cannot go back to sleep."

History of Present Illness

Tommy Burning is a 66-year-old man who presents to his primary care clinic complaining of waking up at night with a burning sensation in his chest. He also notices more severe symptoms when he eats out with his friends at Monster Burger on Friday after 09:00 PM. He also eats nachos and hot wings and drinks beer while watching sports with friends on Sunday nights. He reports daily occurrence of acidic taste in his mouth and stomach discomfort. He has recently had knee pain and has not been active after he comes home from work at call center for an insurance company. He states he drinks a pot of coffee throughout the day to keep him awake during the calls and to ease his cough that has been chronic for the past few months. States he is frustrated that he has been gaining weight and has become a "couch potato." He mentioned that he has switched to light beer and has not made any other lifestyle changes. He has been taking Tagamet for a week, but it has not helped him sleep through the night.

Past Medical History

Hypertension (HTN) (10 years)

Osteoarthritis (5 years)

Benign prostatic hyperplasia (BPH) (6 years)

Tobacco use (50 years)

Dyslipidemia (10 years)

Family History

Father had myocardial infarction (MI) at age 70 and died at age 73.

Mother had diabetes mellitus (DM), HTN, and congestive heart failure (CHF) and died at age 72.

Patient has two living brothers. One had a MI at age 69 and the other has had DM and HTN since age 46.

Social/Work History

TB is an African-American male raised in Georgia. He is married and lives with his wife of 45 years. He and his wife have two daughters and one son, aged 42, 39 and 36. He works as a sales representative for an automobile insurance company.

Tobacco/Alcohol/Substance Use

Tobacco half ppd × 20 years; 5-6 beers each weekend; (–) illicit drug use

Allergy/Intolerance/Adverse Event History

NKDA; no history of intolerance or adverse event

Medication History

▸ Current Medications

Tamsulosin 0.4 mg po q 24 h

Cimetidine 300 mg po q 12 h

HCTZ 25 mg po q 24 h

Amlodipine 10 mg po q 24 h

KCl 10 mEq po q 24 h

Simvastatin 80 mg po q 24 h

Ibuprofen 400 mg po q 8 h prn pain

Nettle root extract 4 gm po q 24 h

▸ Prior Medication Use

Unknown

Review of Systems

(–) headache, dizziness, cough, vision changes, C/D/N/V, LE edema, muscle pain and weakness, hematuria, melena, urinary frequency or urgency; (+) burning in the chest, not radiating and no pressure, right knee pain, abdominal cramps after eating large meals, fatigue

Physical Exam

▸ General

Well-appearing, older, and overweight African-American man in no acute distress

▶ **Vital Signs**

BP 129/72 mm Hg, P 71, RR 14, T 36.2°C, Pain 0/10

Weight 201 lb. (91.4 kg)

BMI 28.8 kg/m²

Height 70 in. (177 cm)

▶ **Skin**

Dry-appearing skin and scalp; (–) rashes or lesions

▶ **HEENT**

PERRLA, EOMI; (–) periorbital edema; (–) sinus tenderness, TMs appear normal

▶ **Neck and Lymph Nodes Thyroid Gland**

Normal; (–) thyroid nodules; (–) lymphadenopathy; (–) carotid bruits

▶ **Chest**

Clear to auscultation

▶ **Cardiovascular**

RRR, normal S_1, S_2; (–) S_3 or S_4

▶ **Abdomen**

Not tender/not distended; (–) organomegaly

▶ **Neurology**

Grossly intact; DTRs normal

▶ **Extremities**

Appears normal

▶ **Genitourinary**

Examination deferred

▶ **Rectal**

Examination deferred

Laboratory and Other Diagnostic Tests

Fasting Obtained 6 days ago

	Conventional Units	SI Units
Na	140 mEq/L	140 mmol/L
K	4.2 mEq/L	4.2 mmol/L
Cl	101 mEq/L	101 mmol/L
CO_2	22 mEq/L	22 mmol/L
BUN	8.2 mg/dL	2.9 mmol/L
SCr	1.2 mg/dL	91.56 μmol/L
Glucose	109 mg/dL	6.0 mmol/L
Ca	8.2 mg/dL	2.05 mmol/L
Mg	1.6 mEq/L	0.80 mmol/L
Phosphate	4.0 mg/dL	1.29 mmol/L
Hemoglobin	13.9 g/dL	139 g/L; 8.63 mmol/L
Hematocrit	40.1%	0.401
PLT	$221 \times 10^3/mm^3$	$221 \times 10^9/L$
WBC	$7.9 \times 10^3/mm^3$	$7.9 \times 10^9/L$
neutrophils (PMN)	49.9%	49.9%
eosinophils	0.7%	0.7%
basophils	0.2%	0.2%
lymphocytes	36.8%	36.8%
monocytes	8.8%	8.8%
MCV	81 μm³	81 fL
Albumin	4.2 g/dL	42 g/L
Bilirubin (total)	0.5 mg/dL	8.55 μkat/L
Bilirubin (direct)	0.1 mg/dL	0.70 μkat/L
AST	18 IU/L	0.30 μkat/L
ALT	18 U/L	0.30 μkat/L
TC	162 mg/dL	4.19 mmol/L
TG	148 mg/dL	1.67 mmol/L
HDL	37 mg/dL	0.96 mmol/L
LDL	96 mg/dL	2.48 mmol/L

Assessment

Sixty-six-year-old male with symptoms consistent with GERD.

Student Work-Up

Missing Information/Inadequate Data

Evaluate: Patient database

Drug therapy problems

Care plan (by problem)

TARGETED QUESTIONS

1. What typical and atypical symptoms of GERD does the patient have?

   Hint: See p. 286 in PPP

2. Which of the patient's lifestyle and medications make the GERD symptoms worse?

   Hint: See pp. 288-289 and Table 17-1 in PPP

3. What medications decrease lower esophageal sphincter pressure?

   Hint: See Table 17-1 in PPP

4. What would be the drug of choice for the patient's acid suppression therapy, and how long should the patient be treated?

   Hint: See Table 17-2 and pp. 289-290 in PPP

5. What risks and adverse effects of therapy would you discuss with the patient?

   Hint: See pp. 289-290 in PPP

FOLLOW-UP

Six weeks later, Tommy returns for his second follow-up. He decreased his tobacco use to three cigarettes per day after meals. He has started pool exercise 3 times a week and has lost 4 lbs (1.8 kg). He now eats a grilled chicken sandwich instead of a burger on Friday nights and now munches on peanuts and popcorn instead of the hot wings and nachos. He is taking his proton pump inhibitor (PPI) every morning on an empty stomach and has not had GERD symptoms for the past 2 weeks. Would you consider a change in his current acid suppression therapy? If yes, what change would you recommend? What are possible complications of long term use of PPIs?

Hint: See Table 17-2, pp. 289-290 in PPP

☯ GLOBAL PERSPECTIVE

Genetic variations among patients may change PPI effectiveness because of an alteration in their ability to metabolize drugs through the cytochrome p-450 (CYP450) enzyme system. It is unclear which patients have a polymorphic gene variation that makes them slow or fast metabolizers. Drug interactions with omeprazole are associated more often with those who are considered "slow metabolizers." Asian populations have a greater number of PPI rapid metabolizers compared to Caucasian populations. Rapid metabolizers may not receive optimal therapeutic effect from PPI therapy. PPIs may differ in the extent of drug–drug interaction related to the CYP450 enzyme system. For example, esomeprazole is metabolized more readily by CYP3A4 enzymes and may be affected less by the patient's genotype. Therefore, patients on PPI therapy should be monitored routinely for drug interactions and associated drug-related problems.

CASE SUMMARY

- Patient's current clinical picture is consistent with GERD, presenting with typical and atypical symptoms warranting acid suppression therapy.

- An initial PPI trial (e.g., omeprazole 20 mg daily is reasonable) of 8 weeks, along with lifestyle modification, can determine the diagnosis of GERD.

- Overuse of PPI agents should be avoided, especially in the elderly, with serious complications related to prolonged and high-dose PPI use.

For more information on the care plan and facilitator's guide please visit http://www.mhpharmacotherapy.com

17 Peptic Ulcer Disease

Michael D. Katz

PATIENT PRESENTATION

Chief Complaint

"My stomach has been so upset. I'm queasy and it burns, but if I eat something it feels worse."

History of Present Illness

HP is a 28-year-old Chinese-American woman who presents to her local hospital's ED complaining of feeling a little weak and dizzy, with nausea (no vomiting), lethargy, and epigastric pain—described as "burning" off and on during the day, but especially after eating. She has recently moved to this area from another state to complete her post graduate year 2 (PGY2) pharmacy residency training and has yet to establish a primary care provider. She has experienced symptoms like this off and on before, but not this severe. She denies any melena, frank blood in stool, throwing up blood, chest pain, or any other symptoms. Because of the nausea she has not eaten or drunk much in the last 3 days. She calls herself a "Type A" personality and a workaholic. Sometimes when she "gets stressed out" she gets a headache that is relieved with ibuprofen. Her only other complaint is that she feels cold all the time.

Past Medical History

Hypothyroidism (4 years)

Family History

Her father is 66 has a history of hypertension (HTN) and hyperlipidemia, Mother is alive and well at age 62. She has two siblings.

Social History

The patient is engaged and planning her wedding. She works as a PGY2 pharmacy resident.

Tobacco/Alcohol/Substance Use

Does not drink alcohol; (–) tobacco or illicit drug use

Allergies/Intolerances/Adverse Drug Events

Penicillin (unknown reaction as a child)

Alcohol (flushing, nausea)

Medications (Current)

Ibuprofen 200-400 mg prn HA

Levothyroxine 25 mcg po qday

Calcium carbonate 500 mg po qday

Review of Systems

Nausea and epigastric pain as listed above; (–) changes in bowel habit or change in color/consistency of stool; dizzy and tired × 2 days, as listed above; anorexia, as listed above; (–) tinnitus, vertigo, or infections; (+) occasional HA

Physical Examination

▶ *General*

Well-appearing thin Asian woman, with minimal distress

▶ *Vital Signs*

BP 110/68 mm Hg, P 64 (sitting), BP 104/62 mm Hg, P 78 (standing), RR 12, T 37.2°C

Weight 106 lb. (48.1 kg)

Height 65 in. (165 cm)

Epigastric pain 3/10

▶ *HEENT*

PERRLA, EOMI; (–) sinus tenderness; TMs appear normal

▶ *Skin*

Decreased skin turgor

▶ *Neck and Lymph Nodes*

Thyroid gland smooth; (–) thyroid nodules; (–) lymphadenopathy; (–) carotid bruits; flat neck veins

▶ *Chest*

Clear to auscultation

▶ *Cardiovascular*

RRR, normal S_1, S_2; (–) S_3 or S_4

▶ *Breasts*

Examination deferred

► *Abdomen*

Not tender/not distended; (+) epigastric pain, sl worse on deep palpation

► *Neurology*

Grossly intact; DTRs normal

► *Genitourinary*

Examination deferred

► *Rectal*

Normal rectal tone; minimal stool in rectal vault that is occult blood (−)

Laboratory Tests

Obtained While in ED

	Conventional Units	SI Units
Na	136 mEq/L	136 mmol/L
K	3.9 mEq/L	3.9 mmol/L
Cl	100 mEq/L	100 mmol/L
CO_2	24 mEq/L	24 mmol/L
BUN	18 mg/dL	6.43 mmol/L
SCr	0.5 mg/dL	44.2 μmol/L
Glucose	89 mg/dL	4.9 mmol/L
Ca	9.4 mg/dL	2.35 mmol/L
Mg	1.8 mEq/L	0.90 mmol/L
Phosphate	3.8 mg/dL	1.23 mmol/L
Hemoglobin	11.8 g/dL	7.32 mmol/L (118 g/L)
Hematocrit	35.4%	0.354
WBC	$8.2 \times 10^3/mm^3$	$8.2 \times 10^9/L$
MCV	$79 \ \mu m^3$	79 fL
Platelets	$247 \times 10^3/mm^3$	$247 \times 10^9/L$
H. pylori serology	(+)	
TSH	4.2 μIU/mL	4.2 mIU/L
Stool for occult blood	(−)	

The patient undergoes endoscopic esophagoduodenoscopy (EGD) which reveals a nonbleeding shallow ulcer with no visible vessel in the proximal duodenum. Rapid urease test of the ulcer biopsy is *H. pylori* +

Assessment

Twenty eight-year-old woman with history, signs, symptoms, and laboratory tests consistent with PUD and *H. pylori* infection. She appears to have ECF volume depletion due to poor intake. She also has a history of hypothyroidism that may not be optimally treated.

Student Work-Up

Missing Information/Inadequate Data

Evaluate:
Patient database
Drug therapy problems
Care plan (by problem)

TARGETED QUESTIONS

1. What signs and symptoms of PUD does this patient have?
   Hint: See p. 297 in PPP

2. What treatment regimen for *H. pylori* infection would you select in this patient? What specific parts of the patient database would guide your decision?
   Hint: See pp. 299-301 in PPP

3. What medications should be *avoided* in this patient to treat her HA?
   Hint: See p. 298 in PPP

4. What risks and adverse effects of therapy would you discuss with this patient?
   Hint: See pp. 299-301 in PPP

5. Would you make any changes in her hypothyroid therapy?
   Hint: See pp. 685-686 in PPP

FOLLOW-UP

The patient is referred to a new primary care physician to establish care and for follow-up. The patient is seen 5 days after completing *H. pylori* eradication therapy, though she is still taking the PPI. Although she feels somewhat better, she still complains of epigastric pain after meals. However, this pain is diminished and the nausea she felt before has abated. She is eating and drinking normally at this time. Urea breath test is + for *H. pylori*. The patient confirms that she was adherent to the original *H. pylori* eradication regimen. What actions would you take?

Hint: See p. 300 in PPP

For more information on the care plan and facilitator's guide please visit http://www.mhpharmacotherapy.com

18 Ulcerative Colitis

Brian A. Hemstreet

PATIENT PRESENTATION

Chief Complaint

"I'm having a lot of bowel movements and stomach pain, and it's interfering with my work."

History of Present Illness

Devin Stark is a 32-year-old man who presents to his gastroenterologist complaining of 2 to 3 watery bowel movements per day with intermittent blood. He also reports intermittent abdominal pain, which is often associated with the bowel movements and the urge to use the restroom immediately. He has also noticed the presence of a low-grade fever on some days. These symptoms started about 7 weeks ago and since then he has experienced a 7-pound (3.2 kg) unintentional weight loss. He reports no sick contacts and has not traveled internationally over the last year. He works as a sales manager for a medical device manufacturer and travels 2-3 days per week via car and airplane as he has a large sales territory. These symptoms have caused him significant distress, particularly on longer flights and car rides. He has been using Pepto-Bismol intermittently for his symptoms, and after seeing his primary care provider 2 weeks ago, he underwent a colonoscopy and was told that his results are consistent with ulcerative colitis (UC).

Past Medical History

UC (affecting the rectum, sigmoid colon, and descending colon diagnosed via colonoscopy 2 weeks ago)

Asthma (13 years ago)

Hypothyroidism (2 years ago)

Family History

Mother had colon cancer at the age of 58, and is still alive following total colectomy. Father is alive at the age of 64 with dyslipidemia. He has one younger sister with no significant medical history.

Social History

Single with no children. Works as sales manager for a medical device company. Sexually active.

Tobacco/Alcohol/Substance Use

Occasional alcohol use; (–) tobacco use, (–) illicit drug use.

Allergies/Intolerances/Adverse Drug Events

Penicillin (rash after receiving amoxicillin)

Medications (Current)

Pepto-Bismol 2 caplets 2-3 times/day as needed

Synthroid 0.125 mg daily

ProAir HFA MDI 2 inhalations prn

Advair 250 mcg/50 mcg 1 inhalation twice daily

Acetaminophen 325 mg as needed for pain or headache

Review of Systems

Occasional headache (HA) and muscle aches relieved with acetaminophen, (–) fatigue, (–) shortness of breath (SOB), (+) watery bowel movements with crampy abdominal pain and intermittent blood, (+) weight loss, (–) rash or yellowing of skin, (+) subjective intermittent low-grade fever

Physical Examination

▸ *General*

Well-appearing, young Caucasian man in no acute distress

▸ *Vital Signs*

BP 128/71 mm Hg, P 88, RR 15, T 37.2°C

Weight 155.6 lb. (70.5 kg)

Height 72 in. (182 cm)

Denies pain

▸ *Skin*

Dry and intact, no rashes or lesions noted.

▸ *HEENT*

PERRLA, EOMI; (–) sinus tenderness; TMs appear normal.

▸ *Neck and Lymph Nodes*

Thyroid gland smooth, no thyromegaly (–) thyroid nodules; (–) lymphadenopathy; (–) carotid bruits.

▸ *Chest*

Clear to auscultation

▸ *Cardiovascular*

RRR, normal S_1, S_2; (–) S_3 or S_4

Laboratory Tests

Fasting, Obtained 14 days ago

	Conventional Units	SI Units
Na	135 mEq/L	135 mmol/L
K	3.5 mEq/L	3.5 mmol/L
Cl	99 mEq/L	99 mmol/L
CO_2/HCO_3	27 mEq/L	27 mmol/L
BUN	20 mg/dL	7.14 mmol/L
SCr	1.1 mg/dL	97.2 µmol/L
Cr Clearance	92 mL/min	0.88 mL/s
Glu	100 mg/dL	5.5 mmol/L
Ca	9.3 mg/dL	2.33 mmol/L
Mg	1.0 mEq/L	0.5 mmol/L
Phosphate	2.0 mg/dL	0.646 mmol/L
Hgb	14.0 g/dL	8.68 mmol/L
Hct	41%	0.41
MCV	90 µm³	
WBC	7.2 × 10³/mm³	
Platelets	330 × 10³/mm³	330 × 10⁹/L
Albumin	3.8 g/dL	38 g/L
Total bilirubin	0.7 mg/dL	11.97 µmol/L
Bilirubin (direct)	0.2 mg/dL	3.42 µmol/L
AST	23 IU/L	0.38 µkat/L
ALT	27 IU/L	0.45 µkat/L
CRP	1.8 mg/dL	18 mg/L

Assessment

Thirty-two-year-old man with signs, symptoms, and laboratory tests consistent with active UC.

Student Work-Up

Missing Information/Inadequate Data

Evaluate: Patient database

Drug therapy problems

Care plan (by problem)

TARGETED QUESTIONS

1. What signs and symptoms of UC does the patient have?

   Hint: See p. 309 in PPP

2. How would you assess the appropriateness of this patient's Pepto-Bismol use?

   Hint: See p. 310 in PPP

3. How would you assess and classify the extent and severity of the patient's UC at this point in time?

   Hint: See p. 309 in PPP

4. How does the disease extent and location affect your selection of drug therapy for this patient?

   Hint: See pp. 313-314 in PPP

5. What are potential pharmacotherapeutic intervention(s) that could be made at this time to manage this patient's UC?

   Hint: See Table 19-4 in PPP

FOLLOW-UP

The patient is seen again in clinic 6 months later. His symptoms have not significantly improved and he continues to experience difficulty with symptom control and interference with his work and daily activities. He has been adherent to his prescribed therapies thus far and has required two 10-day courses of oral prednisone during this time for disease flares. What recommendations would you make regarding alterations in this patients drug therapy?

   Hint: See p. 314 in PPP

⟳ GLOBAL PERSPECTIVE

The available treatment options for moderate to severe in inflammatory bowel disease have continued to expand with the approval of additional biologic agents for use in ulcerative colitis (UC). The tumor-necrosis factor alpha (TNF-α) inhibitors infliximab, adalimumab, and golimumab and the anti-integrin agent vedolizumab are available options in the United States. These agents, while effective, are associated with the potential significant adverse effects and high overall costs. Given that one of the main barriers to widespread use of these agents is high drug costs, patients in developing countries may have limited access to these agents. Patient assistance programs offered through the drug manufacturers continue to be important mechanisms by which patients with limited financial resources may gain access, and should be explored for drugs that are approved for use in the respective country. In addition, infliximab and vedolizumab are both intravenously administered and thus require that patients receive the therapies in an infusion center. As we continue to gain more and more effective therapies for UC, the ability of patients to access these therapies should always be a consideration when choosing which agents are appropriate for the patient.

CASE SUMMARY

- His current signs, symptoms, and supporting diagnostic tests support a diagnosis of UC.

- The main treatment goals are induction and maintenance of remission and avoidance of long-term complications.
- Appropriate patient education reading his UC and associated treatments should be implemented to ensure maximal effectiveness.

For more information on the care plan and facilitator's guide please visit http://www.mhpharmacotherapy.com

19 Nausea and Vomiting

Vanessa E. Millisor   Sheila M. Wilhelm

PATIENT PRESENTATION

Chief Complaint

"I have been throwing up all night and I feel horrible."

History of Present Illness

JR is a 68-year-old Caucasian female with extensive stage small-cell lung cancer with complaints of nausea and vomiting after receiving her first cycle of chemotherapy with carboplatin (AUC: 5 mg/mL*min) IV on day 1 and etoposide 100 mg/m^2 on days 1, 2, and 3 of a 21-day cycle.

Prior to day 1 chemotherapy, she was given antiemetic prophylaxis with ondansetron 32 mg IV and dexamethasone 20 mg IV. In addition, she received dexamethasone 8 mg IV on days 2 and 3, prior to chemotherapy. For breakthrough nausea and vomiting, ondansetron 4 mg IV every 6 hours and diphenhydramine 25 mg IV every 6 hours were available as needed.

The first day of chemotherapy went well, however the patient had three episodes of vomiting on day 2 of therapy and two additional episodes on day 3 of chemotherapy, prior to discharge. Upon discharge on day 3, she was given a prescription for dexamethasone 8 mg po daily for 2 days and ondansetron 4 mg po as needed for nausea and vomiting. She is currently day 5 into her first cycle and presenting to the emergency department (ED) with nausea and vomiting (reports 5-6 episodes per day). She reports taking her dexamethasone as instructed at home on day 4 in the morning without issues, but she vomited immediately after the dose this morning and believes the dose was not absorbed.

Past Medical History (PMH)

Type 2 diabetes mellitus (T2DM) (10 years)

GERD (1 year)

Neuropathy (5 years)

Gastroparesis (3 years)

Family History

Father died from myocardial infarction (MI) at age 67. Mother died from lung cancer at age 70. One younger brother with heart failure and T2DM.

Social/Work History

Lives at home with husband of 45 years, both retired. She has three children.

Tobacco/Alcohol/Substance Use

Thirty pack-year smoking history, rare alcohol intake, no illicit drug use

Allergy/Intolerance/Adverse Event History

NKDA

Medication History

▶ Current Medications

Prior to Admission:

Insulin glargine 30 units SQ at bedtime

Insulin regular 5 units SQ with meals

Gabapentin 300 mg po at bedtime

Calcium carbonate 500 mg po prn acid reflux

Ondansetron 4 mg po q 6 h prn N/V

Dexamethasone 8 mg po daily × 2 days

▶ Prior Medication Use

Carboplatin (AUC: 5 mg/mL*min) IV on day 1 of chemotherapy

Etoposide 100 mg/m^2 on days 1, 2, and 3 of chemotherapy

Ondansetron 32 mg IV on day 1 of chemotherapy

Dexamethasone 20 mg IV on day 1 of chemotherapy, 8 mg on days 2 and 3

Ondansetron 4 mg IV every 6 hours as needed (total of 6 doses used while inpatient)

Diphenhydramine 25 mg IV every 6 hours (total of 3 doses used while inpatient)

Review of Systems

Exam (+) for stomach pain, decreased urination, joint pain, muscle pain, dizziness, fatigue

Exam (–) for diarrhea, signs of infections

Physical Exam

▶ *General*

Ill-appearing elderly female, anxious, marked pallor

▶ *Vital Signs (Include Pain as 5Th Vital Sign)*

BP 109/55; P 98; RR 14; T 35.9°C

Weight 110 lb. (50 kg)

Height 60 in. (152.4 cm)

Pain 5/10 (abdominal)

▶ *Skin*

Decreased turgor, dry mucous membranes, dry skin, no rash

▶ *HEENT*

PERRLA, EOMI; TMs appear normal, erythematous throat

▶ *Neck and Lymph Nodes*

Unremarkable

▶ *Chest*

Clear to auscultation

▶ *Breasts*

Examination deferred

▶ *Cardiovascular*

Reduced JVP, RRR, normal S_1, S_2, (–) S_3 or S_4

▶ *Abdomen*

Tender, nondistended; (–) organomegaly

▶ *Neurology*

Lassitude, dizziness, normal DTRs

▶ *Extremities*

Unremarkable

▶ *Genitourinary*

Examination deferred

▶ *Rectal*

Examination deferred

Laboratory and Other Diagnostic Tests (Obtained on Presentation)

	Conventional Units	SI Units
WBC	$5.6 \times 10^3/\mu L$	$5.6 \times 10^9/L$
Hgb	12.1 g/dL	7.5 mmol/L
Hct	36%	0.36
Plt	$225 \times 10^3/\mu L$	$225 \times 10^3/mm^3$

Na	138 mEq/L	138 mmol/L
K	3.3 mEq/L	3.3 mmol/L
Cl	95 mEq/L	95 mmol/L
CO_2	35 mEq/L	35 mmol/L
BUN	45 mg/dL	45 mmol/L
SCr	1.58 mg/dL	140 µmol/L
Glu	235 mg/dL	13 mmol/L
Ca	8.6 mg/dL	2.15 mmol/L
Mg	1.8 mEq/L	0.9 mmol/L
Phos	2.3 mEq/L	2.3 mmol/L
Alb	2.3 g/dL	23 g/L

CT abdomen (–)

Assessment

Chemotherapy-induced refractory nausea and vomiting (N/V) and resulting volume depletion.

Student Work-Up

Missing Information/Inadequate Data

Evaluate: Patient database

Drug therapy problems

Care plan (by problem)

TARGETED QUESTIONS

1. Does this patient have simple or complex nausea and vomiting?

   Hint: See p. 324 in PPP

2. Did the patient receive the appropriate antiemetic prophylaxis for this chemotherapy regimen?

   Hint: See Table 20-4 in PPP

3. Does this patient have any comorbidities that could contribute to her current clinical presentation?

   Hint: See Table 20-1 in PPP

4. How should this patient's breakthrough nausea and vomiting be treated?

   Hint: See p. 329 in PPP

5. How would you counsel the patient regarding N/V therapy?

   Hint: See Table 20-2 in PPP

FOLLOW-UP

The patient's chemotherapy-induced nausea and vomiting (CINV) resolves with your recommended interventions. How would you change antiemetic prophylaxis used for her next cycle of chemotherapy?

Hint: See p. 329 in PPP

☉ GLOBAL PERSPECTIVE

Tropisetron and ramisetron are 5-HT3 antagonists that are not available in the United States. Tropisetron is approved in other countries for prevention of chemotherapy-induced nausea and vomiting and has been shown to have similar efficacy and toxicity as ondansetron. Ramosetron is approved for management of CINV, and like palonosetron, it has a higher binding affinity to 5-HT3 receptors and longer half-life than other 5-HT3 antagonists, therefore potentially having improved efficacy in delayed nausea and vomiting than other 5-HT3 antagonists. Outside of the United States, it is used most commonly for postoperative nausea and vomiting (PONV).

Domperidone is an antiemetic and prokinetic agent, similar to metoclopramide, which is available outside of the United States. Due to minimal passage across the blood brain barrier, it exhibits less central nervous system (CNS) side effects such as extrapyramidal symptoms (EPS) than metoclopramide. This medication should be avoided in patients with QT prolongation.

CASE SUMMARY

- A patient presents with refractory nausea/vomiting despite adequate prophylaxis for a moderately emetogenic chemotherapy regimen.

- Carboplatin may act as a highly emetogenic chemotherapy agent in some patients and antiemetic prophylaxis should be adjusted in high-risk patients, such as those who experience nausea and vomiting following carboplatin dosing despite adequate prophylactic therapy.

- Medications chosen to treat breakthrough nausea and vomiting should have different mechanisms of action than those used for the prevention of nausea and vomiting and be tailored to address patient specific factors (e.g., gastroparesis, anxiety).

For more information on the care plan and facilitator's guide please visit http://www.mhpharmacotherapy.com

20 Diarrhea

Yolanda McKoy-Beach   Clarence E. Curry, Jr.

PATIENT PRESENTATION

Chief Complaint

"I have had diarrhea for about a week."

History of Present Illness

Adriana Ortiz is a 72-year-old Latino female who is a native of El Salvador. She has lived in the United States for 18 years and has not made a return visit since leaving due to financial difficulties. However, recently her daughter was able to purchase a ticket for her to travel to El Salvador for 1 month. Mrs. Ortiz reports she really enjoyed herself. She had access to many fruits and vegetables she is unable to get in the United States and she purchased foods from street vendors like she did 20 years ago. Additionally, Adrianna reports that while visiting she acquired the Chikungunya virus, and became ill. She saw a physician in El Salvador when she initially became ill and believes the illness resolved during her stay there. Today, she comes to clinic and reports bouts of loose stools, abdominal cramping, and nausea since she arrived back in the U.S. 4 days ago. She started self-treatment with Pepto-Bismol 2 days ago following the dosing instructions on the bottle and continues to have symptoms, but they appear to be milder. Adriana does not believe the problems she is now experiencing is related to the Chikungunya virus or from anything that she ate while visiting El Salvador. She states today she feels weak and tired, but she is not sure if it is from the 6-hour trip back to the U.S. or the diarrhea. As a result of Mrs. Ortiz symptoms, the clinician prescribes ciprofloxacin 500 mg twice daily for 5 days and obtains stool cultures. Mrs. Ortiz is also instructed to drink frequent small amounts of water to replenish her fluid losses.

Past Medical History

Type 2 diabetes mellitus (T2DM) (diagnosed 2 years ago)

Hypertension (HTN) (diagnosed 3 years ago)

Dyslipidemia (diagnosed last year)

Family History

Father and mother are both deceased

Has a 40-year-old daughter (+) hypertension (+) dyslipidemia but otherwise in good health

She has two grandchildren: one male age 14 years and one female age 20 years

Social History

Originally a native of El Salvador; has been in the United States for 18 years.

The patient has a seventh-grade education; she is a non-smoker; she has no health insurance and receives prescription medications through a national chain pharmacy's $4.00 generic drugs program or through drug manufacture's patient assistance program.

Tobacco/Alcohol/Substance Use

Denies tobacco, alcohol, and illicit substance use

Medication History (Current)

Metformin 1000 mg po daily

Losartan 25 mg po daily

Aspirin 81 mg po daily

Simvastatin 40 mg po every night

Bismuth Subsalicylate (Pepto-Bismol) 30 ml or 2 tabs po every 30-60 minutes as needed up to 8 doses (patient self-treated with this medication)

Ciprofloxacin 500 mg po twice daily (medication initiated the day of clinic visit)

Allergies/ Intolerances/Adverse Drug Reactions

Lisinopril (cough)

Physical Examination

▶ *General*

Well-nourished female in no acute distress

▶ *Vital Signs*

BP 141/90 mm Hg, HR 77 bpm, RR 18, T 38°C (101.4°F)

Weight 152 lb. (69 kg)

Height 62 in. (157.5 cm)

BMI 27.8 kg/m^2

Denies pain

▶ *HEENT*

PERRLA, EOMI

▶ *Cardiovascular*

RRR; S_1 and S_2 normal; no S_3 or S_4

▶ *Chest*

Clear to auscultation and percussion

▶ *Abdomen*

No hepatomegaly or splenomegaly; nontender, distended; normoactive bowel sounds

▶ *Genitourinary*

Within normal limits

▶ *Rectal*

No fissures or hemorrhoids; palpable stool; heme (–)

▶ *Neurology*

Alert and oriented × 3

Laboratory and Diagnostic Tests

Urinalysis: Clear and colorless

Stool culture: Pending

Assessment

Seventy-two year-old female with signs and symptoms of diarrhea.

Student Work-Up

Missing Information/Inadequate Data

Evaluate: Patient database

Drug therapy problems

Care plan (by problem)

TARGETED QUESTIONS

1. What signs and symptoms of diarrhea does the patient have?

   Hint: See p. 339 in PPP

2. What questions are important to ask when faced with a patient presenting like Mrs. Ortiz?

   Hint: See p. 338 in PPP

3. Are the present signs and symptoms indicative of traveler's diarrhea? Is antibiotic therapy needed?

   Hint: See pp. 338-339 in PPP

4. Should this patient be treated for dehydration?

   Hint: See p. 339 in PPP

5. How might common treatments used to alleviate the diarrhea be counterproductive?

   Hint: See p. 340 in PPP

FOLLOW-UP

One week later, a follow-up phone call to the patient informed her that the stool culture was positive. During the call, the patient indicated that the diarrhea had ended. She was reminded that the antibiotic given her was sufficient to resolve the problem if she had taken it as directed. She assured the clinician that she had. She was advised to contact the office if any new symptoms occurred. What advice should be given to Mrs. Ortiz about future travel to El Salvador?

   Hint: See pp. 340-341 in PPP

CASE SUMMARY

- Seventy-two-year-old woman who traveled to El Salvador and developed diarrhea.

- Diarrhea is not severe, and no evidence of severe dehydration or volume depletion.

- Patient was treated empirically with ciprofloxacin, with stool culture result reportedly positive for unstated micro-organism.

For more information on the care plan and facilitator's guide please visit http://www.mhpharmacotherapy.com

21 Constipation

Beverly C. Mims   Clarence E. Curry, Jr.

PATIENT PRESENTATION

Chief Complaint

"When I have a bowel movement, only small hard pieces of stool are produced. This has been going on for about two weeks now."

History of Present Illness

Robert Brooks is a 71-year-old male who presented to his primary care physician's (PCP) office complaining of constipation. RB lives alone in his own home and was an active golfer and gardener until 2 weeks ago when he suffered bruised ribs and right arm after a fall over a rug in his home. He stated that since his fall, he has been watching a lot of television and that he no longer cooks for himself. His daughter prepares all of his meals.

Past Medical History

Superficial generalized muscle soreness more on the right side with some bruising S/P fall

Hypertension

Benign prostatic hyperplasia (BPH)

Family History

Father is deceased. Mother is alive at age 95, lives with daughter and has hypertension and osteoarthritis. One sister age 62 has hypertension and hypercholesterolemia.

Social History

Widower, has 1 son aged 48 and 2 daughters aged 45 and 40.

Tobacco/Alcohol/Substance Use

Drinks beer once or twice a week, (–) tobacco, and (–) illicit drug use

Allergies/Intolerances/Adverse Drug Events (ADEs)

NKDA

Medications (Current)

Docusate/Senna 3 tablets po daily for several months until recently

Amlodipine 10 mg po once daily

Triamterene/HCTZ 37.5 mg/25 mg po every morning

Ibuprofen 600 mg po every 8 hours, as needed for pain

Tamsulosin 0.4 mg po once daily

Review of Systems

Generalized muscular aches and pains S/P fall are relieved with ibuprofen; noticed change in bowel habits after he ran out of his docusate plus senna tablets last week; feels like he has to have a bowel movement and cannot.

Physical Examination

Well-developed, thin older man, who appears to be in discomfort

▶ **Vital Signs**

BP 160/90 mm Hg, P 90, RR 20, T 37.0°C

Weight 220 lb. (100 kg)

Height 74 in. (188 cm)

▶ **Skin**

Dry-appearing skin; intact; some superficial bruises on right arm and side

▶ **HEENT**

PERRLA, EOMI

▶ **Neck and Lymph Nodes**

Supple w/o JVD, bruits or thyromegaly

▶ **Chest**

Clear to auscultation; some guarding on the right side

▶ **Cardiovascular**

Elevated BP; no gallops, murmur, rub, click, or irregularity

▶ **Abdomen**

No scars, lesions or rashes, round hardened, tender, some guarding, hypoactive bowel sounds, no visible pulsations, no bruits.

▶ **Neurology**

Grossly intact; DTRs normal

▶ *Genitourinary*

Deferred

▶ *Rectal*

Anal sphincter pressure normal; small hard pieces of stool present in rectum; (–) external hemorrhoids

Laboratory Tests

	Conventional Units	SI Units
Na	138 mEq/L	130 mmol/L
K	4.2 mEq/L	4.2 mmol/L
Cl	100 mEq/L	100 mmol/L
CO_2	24 mEq/L	24 mmol/L
BUN	10 mg/dL	3.57 mmol/L
Scr	1.0 mg/dL	88.4 μmol/L
Glu	100 mg/dL	5.6 mmol/L
Ca	9.7 mg/dL	2.4 mmol/L
Mg	1.6 mEq/L	0.8 mmol/L
Phosphate	3.2 mg/dL	1.03 mmol/L
Hgb	14.7 g/dL	147 g/L
Hct	38.6%	0.386
WBC	$8 \times 10^3/mm^3$	8
Albumin	4.0 g/dL	40 g/L
Stool Occult Blood	(–)	

Assessment

Seventy-one year old man in moderate distress and discomfort, consistent with constipation/fecal impaction.

Student Work-up

Missing Information/Inadequate Data

Evaluate: Patient database

                 Drug therapy problems

                 Care plan (by problem)

TARGETED QUESTIONS

1. How does this patient fit the demographic and risk profile of a patient with constipation?

   Hint: See pp. 333-334 in PPP

2. What symptoms of constipation does this patient have?

   Hint: See p. 334 in PPP

3. What medications and comorbid conditions present can cause or worsen constipation?

   Hint: See Table 21-1 in PPP

4. What nonpharmacologic therapy should be employed in a treatment approach for this patient?

   Hint: See p. 334 in PPP

5. What adverse effects and risk factors associated with laxative products should be considered as you prepare to recommend a treatment option?

   Hint: See pp. 335-336 in PPP

FOLLOW-UP

Two weeks later, the patient returns to the provider's office for follow-up. RB reported that he feels much better and reports the absence of hard stools. He states that he regularly sets time aside to have a bowel movement every other day.

How can constipation be avoided in the future? (Keep in mind that an older patient may not have a bowel movement every day.)

   Hint: See p. 334 in PPP

⊕ GLOBAL PERSPECTIVE

Constipation occurs all over the world. At one time or another as much as 12% or more of the world's population has experienced constipation. Inhabitants of developed countries report higher rates of constipation than those living in developing countries. Around the world, many people choose to treat constipation without the aid of commercially available laxatives. In many parts of the world, some people attempt to self-treat constipation by altering their diets. For constipation relief in various cultures, the ingestion of fruit such as pear, mango, guava, prune, and papaya is favored. Herbal remedies are also popular, including the use of buckthorn, flaxseed, aloe, fenugreek, and beetroot. Some locales favor homeopathic remedies such as bryonia, calcarea carbonica, lycopodium, or nux vomica.

CASE SUMMARY

- Seventy-one-year-old male patient presented to his primary care provider complaining of altered stool frequency and consistency.

- RB's constipation does not appear to be due to organic causes.

- In recent past, RB took docusate plus senna laxatives daily and stopped when he ran out of the product after experiencing a fall.

- RB's presenting medication regimen includes several medications associated with constipation as an adverse effect.

For more information on the care plan and facilitator's guide please visit http://www.mhpharmacotherapy.com

22 Cirrhosis and Portal Hypertension

Laurajo Ryan

PATIENT PRESENTATION

Chief Complaint

"I think he ate the trash."

History of Present Illness

LT is a 59-year-old white male who was brought to the emergency department (ED) by ambulance after being found semiconscious by his wife. She states he smelled strongly of alcohol when she found him slumped at the kitchen table, but what really worried her was the vomit on his shirt that contained what looked like coffee grounds. LT is currently nonresponsive to verbal commands, but does respond sluggishly to painful stimuli. His wife states that he was in his regular state of health until about 10 days ago when he began complaining of severe pain in his right ankle and first toe. He self-treated with ibuprofen for several days, but the pain became intolerable so he sought care at a local acute care clinic where he was diagnosed with gout. The clinic prescribed indomethacin and prednisone, which according to his wife provided moderate pain relief. She said he has been drinking more than normal this past week for "pain relief." She is not sure if he has been taking his routine medications.

Past Medical History

Hepatitis C cirrhosis after blood transfusion (17 years)

Long-standing ascites with numerous therapeutic paracentesis procedures

Single episode of variceal bleeding (2 years ago)

Gout

Family History

Noncontributory

Social History

Lives with wife

Works for the city on road maintenance crew

Tobacco/Alcohol/Substance Use

Remote tobacco use (quit 30 years ago), no illicit drugs, drinks 12-18 beers daily with "occasional" shots on the weekends.

Allergies/Intolerances/Adverse Drug Events (ADEs)

NKDA

Medications (Home Regimen)

Propranolol 10 mg po q 12

Spironolactone 200 mg q am

Furosemide 20 mg q am

Indomethacin 50 mg TID × 1 week

Review of Systems

(+) Nausea, vomiting, hematemesis; patient currently obtunded

Physical Examination

▶ **General**

Patient only arousable to painful stimuli

▶ **Vital Signs**

BP 76/52 mm Hg, HR 118 bpm, RR 18, T 39.3°C

Weight 236 lb. (107.3 kg)

Height 69 in. (175 cm)

▶ **Skin**

Dry and jaundiced, with spider angiomata on the upper trunk

▶ **HEENT**

PERRLA, EOMI, (+) scleral icterus

▶ **Chest**

Clear to auscultation bilaterally

▶ **Cardiovascular**

Regular rhythm, tachycardic; no murmurs, rubs, or gallops

▶ **Abdomen**

Obese, distended abdomen with (+) fluid wave, unable to assess for hepatomegaly/splenomegaly due to obesity; (+) caput medusae, umbilical hernia

▶ **Neurology**

Obtunded; GSC 9

▶ **Extremities**

Bilateral lower extremity edema to knees

▶ **Genitourinary**

Examination deferred

▶ **Rectal**

Examination deferred

Laboratory Tests

	Conventional Units	SI Units
Na	128 mEq/L	128 mmol/L
K		
Cl		
CO$_2$/HCO$_3$	27 mEq/L	27 mmol/L
BUN	12 mg/dL	4.3 mmol/L
SCr	1.2 mg/dL	106 μmol/L
Cr Clearance		
Glu		
Ca		
Mg		
Phosphate		
Hgb	8.4 g/dL	84 g/L
Hct	26%	0.26
MCV	103 μm^3	103 fL
WBC	11 × 10^3/mm^3	11 × 10^9/L
WBC Differential	64/26/8/1/1	
Platelets	79 × 10^3/mm^3	79 × 10^9/L
Albumin	2.8 g/dL	28 g/L
Total bilirubin	2.4 mg/dL	41 μmol/L
Bilirubin (direct)		
AST	52 IU/L	0.87 μkat/L
ALT	23 IU/L	0.38 μkat/L
Alk phos (adult)	89 IU/L	1.48 μkat/L
Ammonia	132 mcg/dL	
PT/INR	2.1	

Assessment

Fifty-nine-year-old man with a history of cirrhosis and ascites presents with acute hematemesis.

⊙ GLOBAL PERSPECTIVE

In the United States, the majority of cirrhosis cases are caused by overconsumption of alcohol and/or infection with the hepatitis C virus. Worldwide, the primary cause of cirrhosis is hepatitis B; according to the World Health Organization, approximately 2 billion people worldwide are infected. Hepatitis B is preventable by vaccination, and in those countries (such as the United States) that have implemented vaccination programs beginning in infancy, rates of hepatitis B have dropped dramatically. Cirrhosis related to alcohol consumption has increased in industrialized countries, and hepatitis C-related cirrhosis is increasing in many countries since a vaccine is not yet available. In the United States, the prevalence of hepatitis C actually began to decrease in 1992 and has since plateaued despite the lack of a vaccine.

TARGETED QUESTIONS

1. What are the signs/symptoms cirrhosis and portal hypertension in this patient? What is/are the cause(s) in this patient?

   Hint: See pp. 353-354 in PPP

2. How should LT's gastrointestinal bleeding be treated?

   Hint: See pp. 356-357 in PPP

3. What can reduce LT's risk of repeat variceal bleeding?

   Hint: See pp. 356-357 in PPP

4. What are the potential sources of acute mental status change in this patient, and how should they be treated?

   Hint: See pp. 354, 358-359 in PPP

5. When should the beta blocker be restarted?

   Hint: See pp. 356-357 in PPP

6. What specific counseling would you provide LT to decrease his future risk of complications, including management of his gout?

   Hint: See pp. 351, 358-360 in PPP. Also see Gout chapter

CASE SUMMARY

- Fifty-nine-year-old man with a history of cirrhosis and varices due to hepatitis C and possibly alcohol who now presents with upper GI bleeding and altered mental status.

- Recently diagonosed with gout and treated with NSAID.

23 Hepatitis B

Juliana Chan

PATIENT PRESENTATION

Chief Complaint

"I was referred for liver treatment."

History of Present Illness

Mr. Bradley Takada is a 39-year-old Asian male referred for further evaluation of his hepatitis B virus (HBV). He is naïve to HBV treatment. He feels well with no complaints and denies dark urine, pale stools, or yellow eyes or skin. He was born in the United States and parents are from Japan.

Past Medical History

Hepatitis B (diagnosed 2 years ago)
Hypertension (HTN)

Surgical History

None

Family History

Mother has hepatitis B. Father has HTN.

Social History

He is married and has 1 son. Married for 15 years and had 4 sexual partner in his lifetime.

He currently works as a cook. Has insurance but a very high deductible and co-pay.

Tobacco/Alcohol/Substance Use

No use of illicit drugs. He drinks on social occasions. No history of tobacco use.

Allergies/Intolerances/Adverse Drug Events

NKDA

Medications (Current)

HCTZ 50 mg daily

Review of Systems

(–) Chest pain, shortness of breath (SOB), weight loss, weight gain, dysuria, melena, or hematochezia.

Physical Examination

▶ *General*

The patient is a well-developed, alert and oriented, well looking Asian man.

▶ *Vital Signs*

BP 128/88 mm Hg, P 82, RR 19, T 37°C

Weight 150 lb. (68.2 kg)

Height 65 in. (165.1 cm)

Pain scale: 0 out of 10

▶ *Skin*

There are no spider angiomata or palmar erythema.

▶ *HEENT*

Eyes anicteric, normal.

▶ *Neck and Lymph Nodes*

Thyroid not palpable.

▶ *Chest*

Clear to auscultation and percussion.

▶ *Cardiovascular*

RRR, no murmurs or gallops.

▶ *Abdomen*

(+) Bowel sounds. (–) Ascites. Liver and spleen not palpable.

▶ *Neurology*

(–) Asterixis

▶ *Extremities*

(–) Peripheral edema

Laboratory Tests

Date : 02/14/2012

	Conventional Units	SI Units
Na	138 mEq/L	138 mmol/L
K	4.4 mEq/L	4.4 mmol/L
Cl	104 mEq/L	104 mmol/L
CO_2/HCO_3	26 mEq/L	26 mmol/L
BUN	23 mg/dL	8.211 mmol/L
SCr	1.3 mg/dL	114.92 µmol/L
Cr Clearance	71.67 mL/min	0.69 mL/s
Glu	110 mg/dL	6.105 mmol/L
Ca		
Mg		
PO_4		
Hgb	14.5 g/dL	145 g/L; 8.99 mmol/L
Hct	43.1%	0.43
MCV		
WBC	$6.1 \times 10^3/mm^3$	
WBC differential	////	////
Platelets	$117 \times 10^3/mm^3$	
Albumin	3.8 g/dL	38 g/L
Total bilirubin	1.2 mg/dL	20.5 µmol/L
Bilirubin (direct)		
AST	67 IU/L	1.11 µkat/L
ALT	68 IU/L	1.13 µkat/L
Alkaline phosphatase	64 IU/L	1.07 µkat/L
HBsAg	positive	
HBeAg		
Anti-HBc total		
HBV DNA quant		

Date : 02/21/2013

	Conventional Units	SI Units
Na	137 mEq/L	137 mmol/L
K	4.3 mEq/L	4.3 mmol/L
Cl	104 mEq/L	104 mmol/L
CO_2/HCO_3	26 mEq/L	26 mmol/L
BUN	25 mg/dL	8.925 mmol/L
SCr	1.5 mg/dL	132.6 µmol/L
Cr Clearance	63.6 mL/min	0.612 mL/s
Glu	140 mg/dL	7.77 mmol/L
Ca	8.6 mg/dL	2.15 mmol/L
Mg		
PO_4		
Hgb	14.3 g/dL	143 g/L; 8.86 mmol/L
Hct	42%	0.42
MCV		
WBC	$5.2 \times 10^3/mm^3$	
WBC differential	////	////
Platelets	$100 \times 10^3/mm^3$	
Albumin	3.8 g/dL	38 g/L
Total bilirubin	1.2 mg/dL	20.5 µmol/L
Bilirubin (direct)		
AST	68 IU/L	1.13 µkat/L
ALT	71 IU/L	1.18 µkat/L
Alkaline phosphatase	64 IU/L	1.07 µkat/L
HBsAg	positive	
HBeAg	positive	
Anti-HBc total	positive	
HBV DNA quant	8, 845, 116	

Imaging

Abdominal ultrasound 03/03/2013

Findings: The liver demonstrated uniform echotexture. No focal intrahepatic mass lesions or evidence of biliary dilation. The common duct measures 2 mm. Doppler reveals appropriate directional flow in the portal hepatic venous system. There is no evidence of cholelithiasis, gallbladder wall thickening, or pericholecystic fluid. The pancreatic head and body are within normal limits. Pancreatic tail is not visualized secondary to shadowing from bowel gas. No evidence of hydronephrosis in the right kidney. Mild splenomegaly present.

Impression: Negative liver ultrasound for hepatocellular carcinoma. Mild splenomegaly.

Assessment

Thirty-nine-year-old asymptomatic Asian man with chronic HBeAg (+) hepatitis B with detectable HBV DNA level.

Student Work-Up

Missing Information/Inadequate Data

Evaluate:
- Patient database
- Drug therapy problems
- Care plan (by problem)

TARGETED QUESTIONS

1. What signs and symptoms of hepatitis B does the patient have?

   Hint: See p. 374 in PPP

2. What are the goals of therapy for the treatment of Hepatitis B?

   Hint: See pp. 374, 378 in PPP

3. What preventative measure can be taken to prevent the spread of hepatitis B and minimize the progression of the liver disease?

   Hint: See pp. 376-377 in PPP

4. What are the adverse effects of hepatitis B therapy you would need to discuss with the patient prior to starting treatment?

   Hint: See pp. 378-379 in PPP

5. On the basis of the patient's laboratory results, what pharmacological recommendation would you make at this time?

   Hint: See pp. 378-379 in PPP

FOLLOW-UP

Approximately 2 years later, Mr. Takada continues to be asymptomatic from his hepatitis B infection. He had been doing well for the past year and returns for follow-up and results of his laboratory tests.

How long should you treat this patient based on these laboratory results?

   Hint: See p. 382 in PPP

🌐 GLOBAL PERSPECTIVE

Despite having an effective vaccine to prevent the spread of hepatitis B infection, this disease continues to affect more than 2 billion people worldwide. Chronic hepatitis B affects close to 400 million people and 500,000-700,000 may die due to complications associated with the liver disease. Approximately 75% of chronic HBV cases occur in Asia. The hepatitis B–related mortality rate in Asian immigrants to the United States is seven times greater than individuals who are Caucasian. Although the treatment armamentarium for hepatitis B has grown significantly over the past decade, at present, the agents available are only effective in suppressing HBV levels and delaying the progression of liver disease to cirrhosis. These agents may not be readily available to patients in developing countries. Since most of these HBV infections are acquired at birth from mothers infected with HBV, providing immunization to include the hepatitis B vaccine with or without immune globulin at birth is the most effective measure to prevent chronic hepatitis B disease.

CASE SUMMARY

- The patient has HBV and naïve to HBV therapy. He has elevated HBV DNA levels and LFTs. Reviewing his platelet counts and ultrasound report, the patient has advance liver disease. He is an ideal candidate for HBV therapy.

- Entecavir is the drug of choice because it has a lesser chance of causing further renal abnormalities compared to tenofovir. Patient's renal condition must be evaluated as his Cr levels are elevated. Pegylated interferon may be also be considered if the patient is willing to self-administer an injection every week for at least 52 weeks and all other medical conditions are stable at baseline.

- Patient with hepatitis B is at risk of developing hepatocellular carcinoma and esophageal varices thus should be followed by a hepatologist.

- Treatment for HBV should be continued until HBeAg seroconversion has been attained along with undetectable HBV DNA levels. Once anti-HBe appears, complete an additional 6 months of hepatitis B therapy.

For more information on the care plan and facilitator's guide please visit http://www.mhpharmacotherapy.com

UPDATED PATIENT LABORATORY DATA

	HBV DNA Quant. (Normal Range: <20 IU/mL)	HBsAg	HBcAg	HBeAg	Anti-HBs	Anti-HBe	Cr mg/dL (µmol/L)	ALT IU/L (µkat/L)
7/5/2013	136,644	+		+	−	−	1.5 (132.6)	50 (0.83)
10/8/2013	2,135						1.6 (141.4)	39 (0.65)
1/30/2014	910						1.5 (132.6)	28 (0.47)
7/13/2014	51	+	+	+	−	−	1.4 (123.8)	20 (0.33)
11/4/2014	29						1.4 (123.8)	19 (0.32)
2/8/2015	41							
5/29/2015	<20	+	+	+	−	−	1.5 (132.6)	21 (0.35)
8/21/2015	<20		+	−	−	+	1.4 (123.8)	20 (0.33)

24 Hepatitis C

Juliana Chan

PATIENT PRESENTATION

Chief Complaint
"I would like to be treated for my hepatitis C."

History of Present Illness
Mr. Nick Bally is a 53-year-old Caucasian male, with complaints of fatigue. He is feeling well otherwise and is at the clinic because the primary care physician referred him to the liver doctor for further medical evaluation of his hepatitis C.

Past Medical History
Hepatitis C (2010)
Hypertension (HTN) (2011)
Hyperlipidemia (2010)
Depression

Surgical History
Coronary angioplasty with stents placed (12/2014)
Nephrolithotripsy (2009)

Family History
Mother died at age 90
Father died at age 91
Two brothers and 1 sister with negative past medical history

Social History
Happily married for 21 years. Has 1 daughter and 1 son. He works as real estate agent.

Tobacco/Alcohol/Substance Use
He used intravenous drugs including heroin and cocaine at the age of 18 and quit at age 19. He denies drinking "a lot" of alcohol. He admits to drinking at least 1 glass of wine with meals over the past 6 years. He smokes tobacco, half ppd

Allergies/Intolerances/Adverse Drug Events
Penicillin: hives

Medications (Current)
Losartan 50 mg daily
Pravastatin 40 mg daily
Trazodone 150 mg daily
St. John's Wort
Multivitamin daily

Review of Systems
Complains of fatigue frequently

Physical Examination

▶ **General**

The patient is not in acute distress.

▶ **Vital Signs**

BP 134/90 mm Hg, P 84, RR 20, T 37.1°C
Weight 260 lb. (118.2 kg)
Height 71 in. (180.34 cm)
Pain scale: 0 out of 10

▶ **Skin**

(+) Palmar erythema and no spider angiomas on anterior chest.

▶ **HEENT**

Normocephalic, atraumatic; sclerae anicteric, no gross lesions.

▶ **Neck and Lymph Nodes**

Thyroid not enlarged

▶ **Chest**

Clear to auscultation

▶ **Cardiovascular**

RRR, normal S_1, S_2

▶ **Abdomen**

(+) Bowel sounds, obese

▶ **Neurology**

(−) Asterixis; alert and oriented × 3; DTRs WNL

Extremities: Trace edema bilaterally present. Dry skin, no open sores.

Laboratory Tests

Fasting, Obtained on 2/21/2015

	Conventional Units	SI Units
Na	144 mEq/L	144 mmol/L
K	4.3 mEq/L	4.3 mmol/L
Cl	108 mEq/L	108 mmol/L
CO_2/HCO_3	29 mEq/L	29 mmol/L
BUN	7 mg/dL	2.5 mmol/L
SCr	0.9 mg/dL	80 μmol/L
Cr Clearance		
Glu	132 mg/dL	7.3 mmol/L
Ca	8.6 mg/dL	2.15 mmol/L
Mg		
Phosphate		
Hgb	15.2 g/dL	152 g/L; 9.43 mmol/L
Hct	45.1%	0.451
MCV		
WBC	$2.1 \times 10^3/mm^3$	
WBC Differential	////	
Platelets	$100 \times 10^3/mm^3$	$100 \times 10^9/L$
Albumin	3.3 g/dL	33 g/L
Total bilirubin	1.2 mg/dL	20.5 μmol/L
Bilirubin (direct)		
AST	42 IU/L	0.7 μkat/L
ALT	45 IU/L	0.7 μkat/L
Alkaline phosphatase	126 IU/L	2.1 μkat/L
Total cholestrol	134 mg/dL	3.47 mmol/L
LDL cholesterol	78 mg/dL	2.02 mmol/L
HDL cholesterol	33 mg/dL	0.85 mmol/L
Triglycerides	116 mg/dL	1.31 mmol/L
HCV RNA quant	9,525,641 IU/mL	
HCV genotype	3a	

Imaging and Other Studies

Liver biopsy: 03/2010   Mild chronic hepatitis consistent with hepatitis C virus (HCV) infection, grade 2 fibrosis, stage 2 disease

Histologic activity index   Portal inflammation: 2, piecemeal necrosis: 2, lobular inflammation: 2, fibrosis: 2

CT of the abdomen with and without contrast: 03/2015

The liver appears to be heterogeneous. The spleen is enlarged. There is no evidence of ascites. A patent portal vein is present.

Assessment

Mr. Bally is a 53-year-old asymptomatic Caucasian man with hepatitis C, genotype 3a disease with normal ALT levels and a baseline HCV RNA level of 9,525,641 IU/mL (or kIU/L).

Student Work-Up

Missing Information/Inadequate Data

Evaluate: Patient database

Drug therapy problems

Care plan (by problem)

TARGETED QUESTIONS

1. What signs and symptoms of HCV does the patient have?

   Hint: See p. 374 in PPP

2. What are the goals of therapy for the treatment of HCV?

   Hint: See pp. 374, 379-380, in PPP

3. What preventative measure can be taken to prevent the spread of HCV and minimize the progression of the liver disease?

   Hint: See p. 379 in PPP

4. What are the adverse effects of HCV therapy you would need to discuss with the patient prior to starting treatment?

   Hint: See pp. 379-382 in PPP

5. Should the patient receive HCV treatment?

   Hint: This patient has several comorbidities, which include depression, HTN, and hyperlipidemia. More importantly, he had recently had a coronary angioplasty with stents placed. At this time, post procedure, how does the patient feel? Is he experiencing any cardiac symptoms? Has he been cleared for HCV therapy to include ribavirin? Additionally, the patient is on medications that can interact with the hepatitis C medications. These drug interactions must be addressed prior to starting HCV therapy. The HCV medications have many adverse effects that may develop during the course of treatment and could possibly worsen these comorbidities. It would be prudent to treat and stabilize all medical conditions prior to initiating any HCV medications.

FOLLOW-UP

The patient started HCV treatment and returns today for week 5 follow-up. He complains of significant fatigue, headaches and occasional chest pains. He also states that he is itching more now and never had this type of complaint prior to starting treatment.

Laboratory Tests
Fasting, Obtained at week 4 of HCV Therapy

	Conventional Units	SI Units
Na	142 mEq/L	142 mmol/L
K	3.9 mEq/L	3.9 mmol/L
Cl	105 mEq/L	105 mmol/L
CO_2	29 mEq/L	29 mmol/L
BUN	9 mg/dL	3.2 mmol/L
SCr	1 mg/dL	88 µmol/L
Glu	170 mg/dL	9.4 mmol/L
Ca	8.3 mg/dL	2.08 mmol/L
HCV RNA quant	undetectable	undetectable
Hgb	11.2 g/dL	112 g/L; 7.08 mmol/L
Hct	36.7%	0.367
WBC	$3.1 \times 10^3/mm^3$	$3.1 \times 10^9/L$
ANC	$2.2 \times 10^3/mm^3$	$2.2 \times 10^9/L$
Platelets	$102 \times 10^3/mm^3$	$102 \times 10^9/L$
Albumin	3.4 g/dL	34 g/L
Total bilirubin	1.3 mg/dL	22.2 µmol/L
AST	35 IU/L	0.58 ukat/L
ALT	32 IU/L	0.53 ukat/L

6. Why is the patient complaining of these symptoms? Is the patient responding to the HCV regimen? What action should be taken at this time? What other laboratory test(s) should be obtained at this time?

   Hint: See pp. 379-38 in PPP and www.hcvguidelines.org

🜨 GLOBAL PERSPECTIVE

Hepatitis C may affect anyone in the world. There is a higher prevalence of HCV infections in non-Hispanic blacks compared with non-Hispanic whites. Genotype plays an important role in determining the likelihood of the patient's response to hepatitis C treatment. Approximately 75% of those infected with HCV in the United States have genotype 1, and about 14% and 5% have genotypes 2 and 3, respectively. Genotype 4 is predominately found in the Middle East and genotype 6 in Asia. To improve the patient's rate of sustaining virological response, it is prudent to encourage patients to be compliant with their medication regimens, and not miss any doses or discontinue the therapy without notifying their health care provider.

CASE SUMMARY

- The patient's comorbidities (coronary angioplasty with stents placed, psychiatric conditions, hypertension, hyperlipidemia) have been evaluated and cleared by specialists to initiate hepatitis C treatment.
- Treatment would include ribavirin and sofosbuvir. The patient would need to be monitored more frequently for DAA and ribavirin-induced anemia.
- Treatment response should be re-evaluated at week 4 to assess for HCV treatment response and adherence.

For more information on the care plan and facilitator's guide please visit http://www.mhpharmacotherapy.com

25 Acute Kidney Injury

Lena M. Maynor

PATIENT PRESENTATION

Chief Complaint

"My leg really hurts. I don't think the antibiotic is working at all."

History of Present Illness

Carol Parks is a 67-year-old Caucasian woman who was admitted to the hospital 3 days ago with complaints of redness, swelling, and discharge from a wound sustained when she fell down the stairs in her home 10 days ago. Upon admission, the medical resident noted that there was a significant laceration on the patient's right thigh, with purulent drainage. The area around the wound was indurated, red, and warm to touch. Antibiotic therapy was initiated, and while her initial fever has resolved, there has not been any significant change in the appearance of Ms. Parks' wound. Additionally, the patient has consistently complained of pain in her leg, which does not seem to be resolving. At home, the patient was taking ibuprofen 3 times daily consistently since she hurt her leg. During rounds this morning, the medical team notes that the patient's urine output over the last 24 hours has dropped significantly from the previous 2 days.

Past Medical History

Hypertension (HTN) (20 years)

Chronic kidney disease (8 years) (baseline Scr 1.8 mg/dL (159.12 μmol/L)

Family History

Father died of lung cancer at age 54. Mother with history of breast cancer at age 63 and is alive at age 71. Brother with HTN and type 2 diabetes mellitus (T2DM) and is alive at age 49.

Social History

Currently works as an accountant. Married for 32 years. Currently lives with husband.

Tobacco/Alcohol/Substance Use

(−) alcohol, tobacco, or illicit drug use

Allergies/Intolerances/Adverse Drug Events

Sulfa medications (hives)

Medications (Prior to Admission)

Lisinopril-HCTZ 20/12.5 mg po q 24 h

Ibuprofen 200 mg po 3 times daily prn pain

Multivitamin po q 24 h

Medications (Current)

Lisinopril 20 mg po q 24 h

HCTZ 12.5 mg po q 24 h

Vancomycin 1000 mg IV q 12 h

Morphine 2 mg IV q 4 h prn pain 6-10/10

Enoxaparin 40 mg SC q 24 h

Review of Systems (Current)

Subjective fever prior to admission. Currently feels fatigued, generally not well.

Physical Exam (Current)

▶ *General*

Female in no apparent distress, appears fatigued

▶ *Vital Signs*

BP 132/82 mm Hg, P 72, RR 16, T 36.8°C

Weight 253 lb. (115 kg)

Height 68 in. (172.2 cm)

Pain 8/10 (leg wound)

▶ *HEENT*

Normocephalic, PERRLA

▶ *Chest*

Clear to auscultation bilaterally

▶ *Cardiovascular*

RRR

▶ *Abdomen*

Not tender/Not distended; (−) organomegaly

▶ *Neurology*

Alert and Oriented × 3

▶ *Genitourinary*

Exam deferred

▶ *Rectal*

Exam deferred

▶ *Skin*

Redness, swelling, and drainage around wound

Otherwise, dry appearing skin; (–) rashes

Laboratory Tests (Hospital Day 2)

	Conventional Units	SI Units
Na	138 mEq/L	138 mmol/L
K	4.5 mEq/L	4.5 mmol/L
Cl	97 mEq/L	97 mmol/L
CO_2	24 mEq/L	24 mmol/L
BUN	51 mg/dL	18.207 mmol/L
SCr	2.0 mg/dL	176.8 μmol/L
Glu	109 mg/dL	6.0495 mmol/L
Ca	8.5 mg/dL	2.125 mmol/L
Mg	2.0 mEq/L	1.0 mmol/L
Phosphate	4.3 mg/dL	1.3889 mmol/L
Hgb	13.9 g/dL	8.618 mmol/L
Hct	41.3%	0.413
Platelets	$422 \times 10^3/mm^3$	$422 \times 10^9/L$
WBC	$13 \times 10^3/mm^3$	$13 \times 10^9/L$
Albumin	3.2 g/dL	32 g/L
Vancomycin trough after 4th dose	8.1 μg/mL	5.589 μmol/L

Wound Culture

Staphylococcus aureus

Agent	Sensitivity Result
Amoxicillin/Clavulanate	Resistant
Cefazolin	Resistant
Ciprofloxacin	Sensitive
Clindamycin	Sensitive
Oxacillin	Resistant
Tetracycline	Sensitive
Trimethoprim/ sulfamethoxazole	Sensitive
Vancomycin	Sensitive

Labs (Today)

	Conventional Units	SI Units
Na	139 mEq/L	139 mmol/L
K	4.9 mEq/L	4.9 mmol/L
Cl	101 mEq/L	101 mmol/L
CO_2	25 mEq/L	25 mmol/L
BUN	70 mg/dL	24.99 mmol/L
SCr	3.2 mg/dL	282.88 μmol/L
Glu	112 mg/dL	6.216 mmol/L
Ca	8.6 mg/dL	2.15 mmol/L
Mg	2.2 mEq/L	1.1 mmol/L
Phosphate	4.6 mg/dL	1.4858 mmol/L
Hgb	14.1 g/dL	8.742 mmol/L
Hct	41.7%	0.417
Platelets	$420 \times 10^3/mm^3$	$420 \times 10^9/L$
WBC	$13.2 \times 10^3/mm^3$	$13.2 \times 10^9/L$
Albumin	3.2 g/dL	32 g/L
Urine osmolality	586 mOsm/kg	586 mmol/kg
Urine sodium	19 mEq/L	19 mmol/L
Urine creatinine	109 mg/dL	9935.613 μmol/L
Urinalysis		
Character	Cloudy	
Color	Yellow	
Specific gravity	1.015	
Glucose	Negative	
Bilirubin	Negative	
Ketones	10 mg/dL	1 mmol/L
Blood	Negative	
pH urine	5.5	
Protein	<30 mg/dL	<300 g/L
Urobilinogen	Normal	
Nitrite	Negative	
Leukocytes	Negative	
RBC	0/hpf	
WBC	1/hpf	
Bacteria	Occasional	
Squamous epithelial cells	Moderate	

Assessment

Sixty-seven-year-old woman with signs, symptoms, and laboratory tests consistent with acute kidney injury.

Student Work-Up

Missing Information/Inadequate Data

Evaluate: Patient database

Drug therapy problems

Care plan (by problem)

TARGETED QUESTIONS

1. How would this patient's acute kidney injury be classified?

   Hint: See Table 25-1 in PPP

2. Which of the patient's medications could be contributing to the acute kidney injury?

   Hint: See pp. 393-395 in PPP

3. Which methods of assessing kidney function can be useful in patients with acute kidney injury?

   Hint: See pp. 395-396 in PPP

4. What signs and symptoms of acute kidney injury does the patient have?

   Hint: See pp. 388-389 in PPP

5. What potential adverse effects could be caused by the patient's current medications, given the patient's acute kidney injury?

   Hint: Some medications are eliminated renally, and thus, may accumulate during acute kidney injury. This accumulation may make patients more susceptible to adverse effects from those particular agents. A review of each medication the patient is receiving should be performed to assess the need for dosing adjustment and potential adverse effects that may occur

FOLLOW-UP

One month after the resolution of Ms. Parks' acute kidney injury, the patient presents to the emergency department with complaints of abdominal pain and her physician orders an abdominal CT with contrast. The physician orders ascorbic acid 3 gm IV 2 hours prior to her scan and 2 gm IV q12h for 2 doses after her scan. Is this the most affective prevention regimen for prevention of contrast induced nephropathy? What other therapeutic options are available?

Hint: See p. 394 in PPP

GLOBAL PERSPECTIVE

It is estimated that the true incidence of acute kidney injury (AKI) is severely underreported in developing countries, due to lack of data reporting and a lack of awareness. Acute kidney injury is thought to differ between developed and developing countries in a number of ways. In developed countries or large urban areas of developing countries, hospital-acquired AKI predominates. Most of these patients are elderly and have multiple comorbidities that contribute to the development of AKI. Alternatively, patients that acquire AKI in rural developing areas are generally younger. Acute kidney injury in these patients is usually community acquired and associated with acute, severe volume loss related to a single comorbidity such as gastroenteritis, malaria, leptospirosis, or ingestion of traditional herbal remedies. Factors such as poor sanitation, lack of access to clean water, and lack of education contribute to the overall incidence in these areas. Reported mortality rates in these patients are generally lower than the reported mortality in developed countries, attributed to the younger age and lack of comorbidities in these patients. Further, the incidence of AKI associated with pregnancy is significantly higher in developing countries and is associated with maternal and fetal mortality. In the first trimester, AKI is commonly associated with gravidic vomiting and nonmedically performed septic abortions, while postpartum AKI is frequently caused by sepsis and thrombotic microangiopathy. Patients with AKI requiring hemodialysis in developing areas are at a definite disadvantage as access to dialysis is generally limited to only large, urban cities within these countries. Additionally, the expense of dialysis generally prohibits the use of dialysis as a treatment option.

CASE SUMMARY

- The patient's current clinical picture is consistent with acute kidney injury.

- Treatment of acute kidney injury is dependent on the etiology of the injury and whether it is prerenal, intrinsic, or postrenal acute kidney injury.

- It is important to evaluate current medications to assess for potential causes of acute kidney injury and to determine if any medications may be more likely to cause adverse effects due to decreased elimination.

For more information on the care plan and facilitator's guide please visit http://www.mhpharmacotherapy.com

26 Chronic Kidney Disease: Progression Prevention

Marcella Honkonen   Chioma Obih
Samah Alsherhi

PATIENT PRESENTATION

Chief Complaint

"I am here to establish care, and I need prescriptions for my inhalers."

History of Present Illness

VP is a 30-year-old male who presents to the clinic for his annual exam and refills for his prescriptions. He recently moved to your town, and has not been seen in your clinic before. He states he has not been to the doctor for several years, as his family physician typically just writes for his refills when his pharmacy asks for them. He says he has no general complaints, other than his weight gain over the past few years.

Past Medical History

Asthma

Family History

Mother: Diabetes

Father: Hypertension, CKD

Social/Work History

Works in information technology

Tobacco/Alcohol/Substance Use

Drinks alcohol only socially

Never smoked

Allergy/Intolerance/Adverse Event History

Seasonal allergies

NKDA

Medication History

Albuterol HFA inhaled as needed

Fluticasone HFA 1 puff inhaled twice daily

Fexofenadine 180 mg by mouth daily

Fluticasone Nasal Spray 1 spray each nostril at bedtime

Physical Examination

▶ *General*

The patient is a 30-year-old obese male in no acute distress.

▶ *Vital Signs*

BP 147/98, HR 98, RR 16

Height: 5'10" (177.8 cm)

Weight: 284.46 lb (129.3 kg)

▶ *Skin*

No rashes, lesions

▶ *HEENT*

EOMI, PERRLA

▶ *Neck and Lymph Nodes*

Nl JVD, thyroid normal

▶ *Chest*

Clear to A&P

▶ *Cardiovascular*

RRR, nl S_1 and S_2, no murmurs, rubs or gallops

▶ *Abdomen*

Large abdominal circumference, obesity; difficult to palpate liver and spleen; no fluid wave

▶ *Neurology*

OX3, DTRs nl

▶ **Extremities**

No edema or joint swelling

▶ **Genitourinary**

Deferred

▶ **Rectal**

Deferred

Laboratory Tests (Fasting)

	Conventional Units	SI Units
Sodium	137 mEq/L	137 mmol/L
Potassium	4.2 mEq/L	4.2 mmol/L
Chloride	101 mEq/L	101 mmol/L
Bicarbonate	27 mEq/L	27 mmol/L
BUN	13 mg/dL	4.6 mmol/L urea
Serum creatinine	1.4 mg/dL	123.7 μmol/L
Estimated CrCl	79.66 mL/min	1.3 mL/s
Glucose	137 mg/dL	7.6035 mmol/L
Total cholesterol	233 mg/dL	6.0 mmol/L
LDL cholesterol	182 mg/dL	4.7 mmol/L
HDL cholesterol	24 mg/dL	0.62 mmol/L
Triglycerides	140 mg/dL	1.5 mmol/L
Cholesterol/HDL ratio	4.0 mg²/dL²	4.0 mmol²/L²
Urine protein	present	present
Hemoglobin A1c	5.9 %	0.059

Assessment

A 30-year-old male with asthma, presents to establish care. The patient has had lack of adequate care for many years. Today he is found to be obese and have multiple risk factors for chronic kidney disease.

> ### Student Work-Up
>
> **Missing Information/Inadequate Data**
>
> **Evaluate:**   Patient database
>
> Drug therapy problems
>
> Care plan (by Problem)

TARGETED QUESTIONS

1. Identify VP's risk factors for developing CKD? Explain the mechanism by which these factors may progress VP's CKD?

   Hint: See pp. 399-401, Table 26-3 in PPP

2. Which stage of CKD would you classify VP's CKD, assuming that he has stable kidney function? What are the goals of therapy?

   Hint: See Table 26-1 in PPP

3. What is VP's blood pressure goal?

   Hint: See pp. 404-405 in PPP

4. List the nonpharmacological and pharmacological therapy that may help in slowing the progression of the CKD in VP.

   Hint: See pp. 403-406 in PPP

5. How would you monitor the efficacy and safety of ACE inhibitors in VP?

   Hint: See p. 406 in PPP

FOLLOW-UP

Two weeks later, VP presents to the clinic for a follow-up appointment after starting on lisinopril. His laboratory values are as follows:

	Conventional Units	SI Units
Serum Creatinine	1.6 mg/dL	141.44 micromol/L
Potassium	4.5 mEq/L	4.5 mmol/L
Blood Pressure	125/77 mm Hg	—

What is your recommendation at this point? Which education points should be provided to VP about lisinopril therapy?

Hint: See p. 404-406 in PPP

🌎 GLOBAL PERSPECTIVE

In 2014, the World Health Organization categorized more than 600 million people worldwide as obese. Obesity is a major yet modifiable risk factor associated with CKD. There are many plausible mechanisms that show adiposity is linked to mediators of progressive kidney disease. However, it is not well elucidated in the literature as to whether a reduction in weight reduces the mortality associated with CKD. As the 12th most common cause of death in the world, CKD creates burden to many countries thus numerous international guidelines have been aimed at outlining recommendations to improve care. Currently, lifestyle modifications should be recommended for patients with obesity with comorbid hypertension and/or diabetes in an effort to slow the progression of CKD; although, obesity reduction in later stages of CKD may lead to no benefit and may cause harm.

REFERENCES

1. Obesity and overweight fact sheets. World Health Organization Media center. www.who.int/mediacentre/factsheets/fs311/en/. Accessed May 15, 2015.

2. McClellan WM, Plantinga LC. A public health perspective on CKD and obesity. Nephrol Dial Transplant. 2013; 28(4):iv37-iv42. Doi: 10.1093/ndt/gft030.

CASE SUMMARY

- The patient presents with multiple risk factors for kidney disease.

- Pharmacologic and lifestyle interventions must take place early to combat the progression of kidney disease.

- Pharmacists can play a key role in early identification of risk factors by providing health screenings in the community.

For more information on the care plan and facilitator's guide please visit http://www.mhpharmacotherapy.com

27 Chronic Kidney Disease: End Stage Renal Disease

Marcella Honkonen   Wendy Gabriel

PATIENT PRESENTATION

Chief Complaint

"I'm just here for my kidneys, I guess."

History of Present Illness

MB is a 68-year-old female recently discharged from the hospital for altered mental status secondary to a missed hemodialysis session. She presents to nephrology clinic today because she was told she needed to be seen more regularly. She also has some questions about the new medications: calcium acetate, erythropoietin, and omeprazole.

Past Medical History

Type 2 diabetes mellitus (T2DM)

ESRD on hemodialysis three times weekly

Coronary artery disease s/p coronary artery bypass grafting
   × 3

Retinopathy

Family History

Unknown

Social/Work History

Retired secretary, lives alone

Tobacco/Alcohol/Substance Use

Never drinker, never smoker

Allergy/Intolerance/Adverse Event History

Penicillins—rash

Sulfa—rash

Medication History

Aspirin 81 mg by mouth daily

Calcium acetate 1334 mg by mouth three times daily with
   each meal

Clopidogrel 75 mg by mouth daily

Erythropoietin 6000 units subcutaneously three times weekly

Folic acid/Vitamin B complex vitamin by mouth daily

Insulin detemir 10 units subcutaneously at bedtime

Insulin lispro 2-4 units subcutaneously with each meal

Omeprazole 20 mg by mouth daily

Simvastatin 20 mg by mouth at bedtime

Physical Examination

▶ **General**

The patient is a 68-year-old female in no acute distress

▶ **Vital Signs**

BP 131/55, HR 84, RR 16

Height: 5'5″ (165.1 cm)

Weight: 140.14 lb. (63.7 kg)

Dry weight: 136.4 lb. (62 kg)

▶ **Skin**

No rashes

▶ **HEENT**

Normocephalic, oral mucosa moist

▶ **Neck and Lymph Nodes**

Supple

▶ **Chest**

Clear to auscultation bilaterally

▶ **Breasts**

Not examined

▶ **Cardiovascular**

RRR, no murmurs, rubs or gallops

▶ **Abdomen**

Soft, nontender

▶ **Neurology**

Normal and back to baseline

▶ **Extremities**

Mild bilateral leg edema

▶ **Genitourinary**

Deferred

▶ **Rectal**

Deferred

Laboratory Tests (Fasting)

	Conventional Units	SI Units
Sodium	135 mEq/L	135 mmol/L
Potassium	3.7 mEq/L	3.7 mmol/L
Chloride	102 mEq/L	102 mmol/L
Bicarbonate	23 mEq/L	23 mmol/L
BUN	22 mg/dL	7.854 mmol/L urea
Serum creatinine	3.3 mg/dL	291.7 µmol/L
Estimated GFR		
Glucose	215 mg/dL	11.9 mmol/L
Total cholesterol	151 mg/dL	3.9 mmol/L
LDL cholesterol	77 mg/dL	1.9 mmol/L
HDL cholesterol	59 mg/dL	1.5 mmol/L
Triglycerides	74 mg/dL	0.8362 mmol/L
Cholesterol/HDL ratio	2.6 mg^2/dL^2	2.6 mmol^2/L^2
Albumin	2.1 g/dL	21 g/L
AST	15 IU/L at 37°C	0.2 µkat/L
ALT	9 IU/L at 37°C	0.1 µkat/L
Tbili	0.3 mg/dL	5.1 µmol/L
Hemoglobin A1c	7.7 %	0.077
PTH	219 pg/mL	23.4 pmol/L
Phosphorus	5.3 mg/dL	1.7 mmol/L
Magnesium	2.6 mg/dL	1 mmol/L
Calcium	10.3 mg/dL	2.5 mmol/L
25-OH, Vitamin D	12 ng/mL	29.9 nmol/L
WBC	10.1 × 10^3/µL	10.1 × 10^9/L
Hemoglobin	7.5 g/dL	75 g/L
Hematocrit	23.3 %	0.233
Platelets	267 × 10^3/µL	267 × 10^9/L
Iron	15 µg/L	2.6 µmol/L
Ferritin	175 ng/mL	175 µg/L
TSAT	18 %	0.18

Assessment

MB is a 68-year-old female presenting to nephrology clinic for follow-up visit after a recent hospitalization. Her renal disease was evaluated and she is found to have multiple chronic complications related to her end stage renal disease.

Student Work-Up

Missing Information/Inadequate Data

Evaluate: Patient database
                      Drug therapy problems
                      Care plan (by problem)

TARGETED QUESTIONS

1. Why are patients with ESRD at risk of having anemia?
   Hint: See pp. 406-407 in PPP

2. What are some considerations to account for when IV iron is prescribed?
   Hint: See pp. 407-409 in PPP

3. Why are patients with ESRD at risk of having mineral and bone disorders?
   Hint: See pp. 410-411 in PPP

4. What is secondary hyperparathyroidism?
   Hint: See p. 411 in PPP

5. What are the complications of receiving chronic hemodialysis?
   Hint: See pp. 420-422 in PPP

FOLLOW-UP

The patient follows up with her nephrologist 4 weeks later. The day of her appointment, her laboratory tests reveal the following:

	Conventional Units	SI Units
Total Ca	7.8 mg/dL	1.9 mmol/L
25-OH, Vitamin D	12 ng/mL	29.9 nmol/L
PTH	576 pg/mL	61.6 pmol/L
Phosphorus	6.2 mg/dL	2.0 mmol/L
Albumin	2.1 g/dL	21 g/L

How should her CKD—Mineral bone disorder be treated?
   Hint: See pp. 411-415 in PPP

⊙ GLOBAL PERSPECTIVE

The primary treatment for end stage renal disease (ESRD) is renal replacement therapy (RRT) with either hemodialysis (HD) or peritoneal dialysis. HD is the most common RRT modality worldwide, however a larger percentage of patients in underdeveloped countries receive peritoneal dialysis when compared to developed countries.

It is difficult to know the prevalence of ESRD worldwide because many countries do not have access to RRT and therefore do not accurately report the number of people with ESRD. More than 80% of people receiving RRT are in developed and wealthier countries. This disparity is due to several factors including lack of awareness and detection of chronic kidney disease (CKD) in underdeveloped countries. The MDRD equation is used in developed nations to routinely check and detect CKD early, however it has been shown to overestimate GFR in China, Japan, and Thailand populations, which can delay diagnosis and lead to worse outcomes.

The underlying cause of CKD also differs throughout the world. Diabetes, obesity and hypertension are the top causes of CKD in Western nations. The primary cause of CKD in Asia and Africa is glomerulonephritis. In Africa and Asia, herbal medications are more widely used and have been associated with acute kidney injury, tubular dysfunction, and CKD. In addition, patients in Africa are at a higher risk of developing CKD secondary to HIV when compared to Asians and African-Americans. Other causes that affect those at a socioeconomic disadvantage are inaccessibility to clean water that can cause kidney disease either by dehydration or bacterial infection, and inaccessibility to adequate nutrition while pregnant, which causes a reduction in nephron development in children while in utero.

Once diagnosed with ESRD and RRT is needed, many people in the world do not have access to HD or PD modalities. In countries where HD is available, the cost of care can be prohibitive. One session of HD in Nigeria costs two times the minimum monthly wage. Several countries, including China and India, have started to develop insurance and free dialysis for poor citizens, however these services are limited in their scope and cannot help everyone.

REFERENCES

Vivekanand J, Guillermo GG, Kunitoshi I, et al. Chronic kidney disease: global dimension and perspectives. *Lancet* 2013;382:260-72.

Anand S, et al. "Global Perspective of Kidney Disease." *Nutrition in Kidney Disease, Second Edition.* Byham-Gray L. D. et al. (eds). New York. 2014. 11-23. Print

CASE SUMMARY

- The patient presents with complications consistent with ESRD.

- Pharmacologic interventions should be implemented in addition to dialysis for ESRD patients.

- Pharmacists can help to educate, counsel, and ultimately maximize pharmacotherapy for each complication associated with this complex disease state.

For more information on the care plan and facilitator's guide please visit http://www.mhpharmacotherapy.com

28 Euvolemic Hyponatremia

Lee Morrow   Brittany Suzuki
Mark Malesker

PATIENT PRESENTATION

Chief Complaint

Headache and confusion

History of Present Illness (HPI)

Phyllis Glass is a 77-year-old female who was admitted to a long-term care facility secondary to overall decline in health. She was previously living at home with her husband but has agreed to long-term care secondary to progressive limitations in mobility. The patient has an extensive history of rheumatoid arthritis (RA) over the last 20 years. The recent decline in her being able to care for herself resulted in signs and symptoms of depression. Her primary care provider started sertraline approximately 4 weeks ago. She had no specific complaints, however, upon physical exam, Phyllis admitted to recent headaches and intermittent confusion. This was confirmed by her husband. Phyllis also complains of increased episodes of shortness of breath (SOB). Reviews of records indicate a recent hospital discharge for chronic obstructive pulmonary disease (COPD) exacerbation.

Past Medical History

COPD
Rheumatoid arthritis
Atrial fibrillation
Depression

Family History

Father deceased, had emphysema and Alzheimer's disease. Mother deceased from ruptured aortic aneurysm. Brother alive with hypertension and emphysema.

Social/Work History

Worked as a bartender and restaurant hostess for the past 40 years, but retired 15 years ago. Husband is retired postal worker.

Tobacco/Alcohol/Substance Abuse

Former smoker who quit smoking 15 years ago. She denies use of alcohol and illicit drugs. Admits to 2 cups of caffeinated coffee every morning for breakfast.

Allergies

Penicillin–unknown

Sulfa–unknown

Paper tape–rash

Medication History

Fluticasone/salmeterol 250/50 mcg diskus inhaler – 1 inhalation by mouth every 12 hours

Albuterol 90 mcg HFA inhaler—2 puffs by mouth every 4-6 hours as needed

Levothyroxine 50 mcg—1 tablet po every morning

Sertraline 50 mg—1 tablet po every morning

Methotrexate 7.5 mg po once weekly

Famotidine 20 mg—1 tablct po twice a day

Loratidine 10 mg—1 tablet po as needed

Metoprolol tartrate—50 mg po twice daily

Diltiazem XL 180 mg—1 capsule po daily

Apixaban 5 mg—1 tablet po twice daily

Vitamin D 1000 units—1 tablet po daily

Calcium carbonate 500 mg—1 tablet PpoO twice daily

Infliximab 3 mg/kg—IV every 8 weeks

Fentanyl patch 12.5 mcg/hr—apply one patch every 72 hours as needed

Tramadol 25 mg—1 tablet po every 6 hours as needed

Fiber capsules—6 capsules po by mouth QHS

Polyethylene glycol 17 gm po daily as needed

Amoxicillin 500 mg po q 8 h

Review of Systems

As per HPI, otherwise reviewed and unremarkable

Physical Exam

▶ **General**

Awake, and alert with intermittent confusion. Frail female with some wasting.

▶ *Vital Signs*

BP 140/80, not orthostatic, P 84, RR 19, T 97.8°F (36.6°C); SpO_2 94% (0.94) on room air

Weight 127.6 lbs (58 kg)

Height 63 inches (160.02 cm)

Pain reported as 2/10

▶ *HEENT*

PERRLA, with slight nasal discharge secondary to allergies. Mucous membranes appear moist.

▶ *Skin*

Does have some superficial bruising

▶ *Neck and Lymph Nodes*

Supple, no carotid bruits noted; JVD nl

▶ *Chest*

Clear to auscultation bilaterally; mild wheezing noted on exhalation bilaterally

▶ *Breasts*

Tender to palpation, no lumps or enlarged lymph nodes bilaterally

▶ *Cardiovascular*

Tachycardic, RRR; no murmur, rubs or gallops

▶ *Abdomen*

Soft, tender and nondistended; positive bowel sounds noted

▶ *Neurology*

Cranial nerves II-XII are intact; patient is awake and alert with mild confusion at times

▶ *Extremities*

No signs of edema, clubbing or cyanosis; warm to touch; 2+ pulses noted bilaterally

▶ *Genitourinary*

No pain upon palpation; patient reports mild pain on urination and frequency

▶ *Rectal*

No signs of tears or hemorrhoids

Laboratory and Other Diagnostic Tests

Laboratory Tests

April 20 1200

	Conventional Units	SI Units
Na	123 mEq	123 mmol/L
K	4.0 mEq	4.0 mmol/L
Cl	98 mEq	98 mmol/L
CO_2/HCO_3	26 mEq	26 mmol/L
BUN	16 mg/dL	5.71 mmol/L
Serum Creatinine (adult)	1.1 mg/dL	97.24 μmol/L
Creatinine Clerance (adult)	39.2 mL/min	0.37 mL/s
Glucose (fasting)	90 mg/dL	4.99 mmol/L
Total ca		
Mg		
PO_4		
Hemoglobin		
Hematocrit		
MCV		
WBC		
WBC Differential	////	
Platelet		
Albumin		
Billirubin (total)		
Billirubin (direct)		
AST		
ALT		
ALK phos (adult)		
Serum osmolaltity	259 mOsm	259 mmol/kg
Urine osmolality	145 mOsm	145 mmol/kg
Urine sodium	<20 mEq	<20 mmol/L

March 15 0830

	Conventional Units	SI Units
Na	135 mEq	135 mmol/L
K	3.9 mEq	3.9 mmol/L
Cl	100 mEq	100 mmol/L
CO_2/HCO_3	24 mEq	24 mmol/L
BUN	15 mg/dL	5.35 mmol/L
Serum Creatinine (adult)	1.0 mg/dL	88.4 μmol/L
Creatinine Clerance (adult)	42.2 mL/min	0.41 mL/s
Glucose (fasting)	100 mg/dL	5.55 mmol/L
Total ca		
Mg		
PO_4		
Hemoglobin		
Hematocrit		
MCV		

WBC

WBC Differential   ////

Platelet

Albumin

Billirubin (total)

Billirubin (direct)

AST

ALT

ALK phos (adult)

Serum osmolaltity

Urine osmolality

Urine sodium

Urinalysis

Urine appears slightly cloudy

Nitrite: positive

White blood cells (mm^3): >100

Assessment

Seventy-seven-year-old female admitted for acute rehabilitation. The patient presented with euvolemic hyponatremia upon admission. Cultures are currently pending.

Student Work-Up

Missing Information/Inadequate Data

Evaluate: Patient database

                       Drug therapy problems

                       Care plan (by problem)

TARGETED QUESTIONS

1. What are the signs and symptoms of euvolemic hyponatremia present in this patient?

   Hint: See p. 432 in PPP

2. What are the potential causes of euvolemic hyponatremia?

   Hint: See p. 432 in PPP

3. Which medications could have contributed to the euvolemic hyponatremia in this patient?

   Hint: See p. 432 in PPP

4. What are the treatment options for the management of euvolemic hyponatremia?

   Hint: See pp. 432-433 in PPP

5. After the patient recovers from her acute problems, what therapeutic options exist if she has chronic euvolemic hyponatremia?

   Hint: See p. 433 in PPP

⊙ GLOBAL PERSPECTIVE

Euvolemic hyponatremia is an electrolyte disorder commonly caused by the syndrome of inappropriate antidiuretic hormone (SIADH). Specific causes of euvolemic hyponatremia include carcinomas (lung and pancreas), pulmonary disorders (pneumonia, tuberculosis), CNS disorders (meningitis, strokes, tumors, and trauma) and medications. Recognized medication causes of SIADH include chlorpropamide, carbamazepine, chemotherapy, barbiturates, morphine, antipsychotics, TCAs, SSRIs, NSAIDs, nicotine, and PPIs. The relative frequency of the different etiologies may differ around the world due to different patterns of disease and availability of medications.

CASE SUMMARY

- Seventy-seven-year-old female with euvolemic hyponatremia and UTI.

- Possible causes of euvolemic hyponatremia include head trauma, pulmonary disorders, and medications.

- The euvolemic hyponatremia was managed with SSRI discontinuation and fluid restriction.

For more information on the care plan and facilitator's guide please visit http://www.mhpharmacotherapy.com

29 Hypovolemic Hyponatremia

John Kelly Wachira   Lee Morrow

Mark Malesker

PATIENT PRESENTATION

Chief Complaint

"I am dizzy since I got a stomach bug."

History of Present Illness (HPI)

Bennie Drill is 24-year-old African-American professional athlete who presents to the emergency department with dizziness, general malaise, and lethargy. The patient is on the practice squad for an NFL team. He admits that over the last several hours he has been practicing and running drills outdoors for an upcoming football game. Reported temperatures throughout the day have been above 95°F. The patient also states that over the last few days, he and other teammates have been experiencing a "stomach bug" associated with nausea and vomiting. He denies any known food poisoning, fever, chills, abdominal pain or diarrhea. BD is otherwise alert, oriented to place, time and person.

Past Medical History

Anxiety

Depression

Hypertension

BD just had team physical two weeks ago and all vaccines are up to date.

Family History

Hypertension in both parents

History of depression on his mother's side of family

Social/Work History

Recent college graduate with economics degree. Local celebrity in his home town. Professional athlete currently practicing with NFL team. Loves to spend time in the gym and has been nicknamed "the freak" due to his vigorous working out habits. BD has three younger siblings. He is single and in monogamous relationship with his girlfriend of 3 years.

Tobacco/Alcohol/Substance Use

Occasional alcohol use. Denies tobacco or other recreational drug use. Regular intake of sports drinks for energy and hydration following practice.

Allergy/Intolerance/Adverse Event History

Amitriptyline (according to the patient he developed "dry mouth and a low blood electrolyte")

Medication History

▶ Current Medications

HCTZ 25 mg po q day

Citalopram 20 mg po q day

Ibuprofen 600 mg po q 6 hrs prn (usually takes after practice sessions)

Review of Systems

As per HPI otherwise reviewed and unremarkable

Physical Exam

▶ General

Mildly distressed young male with "vomit-bag" in hand

▶ Vital Signs

BP 92/60 mm Hg (sitting), BP 80/50 (standing), P 70, RR 12, T 98.6°F (37°C) SpO$_2$ 96% on RA

Weight 235 lb. (106 kg)

Height 78 in. (196 cm)

Pain reported as 0/10

▶ Skin

Dry with poor skin turgor

▶ HEENT

Dry mucous membranes. No scleral icterus. Posterior oropharynx without erythema or exudate.

▶ Neck and Lymph Nodes

No thyromegaly or anterior cervical lymphadenopathy.

▶ Chest

Clear to auscultation with no wheezing or crackles. No use of accessory muscle.

▶ Cardiovascular

RRR, nl S$_1$, S$_2$, tachycardic, no JVD.

▶ *Abdomen*

Soft, nontender, and nondistended. Normal bowel sounds.

▶ *Musculoskeletal*

5/5 strength bilaterally in upper and lower extremities

▶ *Neurology*

Cranial nerves all are intact.

▶ *Extremities*

No lower extremity redness, swelling or edema

▶ *Genitourinary*

Deferred

▶ *Rectal*

Deferred

Laboratory and Other Diagnostic Tests

Laboratory Tests

	Conventional Units	SI Units
Na	123 mEq/L	123 mmol/L
K	4 mEq/L	4 mmol/L
Cl	95 mEq/L	95 mmol/L
CO_2/HCO_3	25 mEq/L	25 mmol/L
BUN	50 mg/dL	17.85 mmol/L
SCr	2 mg/dL	176.8 μmol/L
Cr Clearance	86 mL/min	0.82 mL/s
Glu	125 mg/dL	6.93 mmol/L
Ca	10 mg/dL	2.5 mmol/L
Mg	2 mEq/L	1 mmol/L
PO_4	3 mEq/L	0.97 mmol/L
Hgb	15 g/dL	150 g/L
Hct	45%	0.45
MCV	90 μm³	90 fL
WBC	$8 \times 10^3/mm^3$	$8 \times 10^9/L$
WBC Differential	////	
Platelets	$350 \times 10^3/mm^3$	$350 \times 10^9/L$
Albumin	4 g/dL	40 g/L
Total bilirubin	2 mg/dL	34.2 μmol/L
Bilirubin (direct)	0.2 mg/dL	3.42 μmol/L
AST	30 IU/L	0.50 μkat/L
ALT	31 IU/L	0.51 μkat/L
Alkaline phosphatase	100 IU/L	1.67 μkat/L
Serum Osmolality	270 mOsm/kg	270 mmol/kg

ECG: Sinus tachycardia

Assessment

Twenty-four-year-old male with new onset signs and symptoms consistent with hypovolemic hyponatremia.

Student Work-Up

Missing Information/Inadequate Data

Evaluate:	Patient database
	Drug therapy problems
	Care plan (by problem)

TARGETED QUESTIONS

1. What are the signs and symptoms of hypovolemic hyponatremia?

   Hint: See p. 428 in PPP

2. What are potential etiologies of hypovolemic hyponatremia?

   Hint: See p. 433 in PPP

3. Which medications could have exacerbated hypovolemic hyponatremia in this patient?

   Hint: See p. 432 in PPP

4. What are the treatment options for the management of hypovolemic hyponatremia in this patient?

   Hint: See p. 433 in PPP

5. What medication alternatives can be used in this patient to avoid future development of hyponatremia?

   Hint: See Hypertension chapter in PPP

FOLLOW-UP

Twenty-four-year-old male who was found to have hypovolemic hyponatremia likely multifactorial from dehydration (excessive sweating from exercise, vomiting) with hypotonic fluid replacement and exacerbated by chronic medications (HCTZ, citalopram, and ibuprofen).

⊙ GLOBAL PERSPECTIVE

Hypovolemic hyponatremia is an electrolyte disorder that occurs classically from overt dehydration. It can be exacerbated by chronic illness and some common medications. Intravenous fluid resuscitation is a standard of care and readily available for severe volume depletion and shock in developed countries. Patients in developing countries may not have access to health care facilities, and if they do, those facilities may not have sterile IV access equipment or solutions. Oral rehydration therapy is more readily available in these settings and considered the treatment of choice, particularly for diarrheal illnesses such as rotavirus and cholera. The World Health Organization[1] recommends that oral rehydration solutions be comprise of:

Total osmolality 200-310 mmol/L

Equimolar concentration of sodium and glucose

Na concentration 60-90 mEq/L (60-90 mmol/L)

K concentration 15-25 mEq/L (15-25 mmol/L)

Citrate concentration 8-12 mmol/L

Chloride concentration 50-80 mEq/L (50-80 mmol/L)

Such products are widely available commercially, but similar formulations can be made with household ingredients (assuming clean water is available). Oral rehydration therapy has had a major beneficial impact on childhood mortality in diarrheal illness[2] and it appears to be as effective as intravenous therapy.

REFERENCES

1. World Health Organization. Oral Rehydration Salts. Available at: http://apps.who.int/iris/bitstream/10665/69227/1/WHO_FCH_CAH_06.1.pdf?ua=1&ua=1 (Accessed on April 27, 2015).

2. Victora CG, Bryce J, Fontaine O, Monasch R. Reducing deaths from diarrhea through oral rehydration therapy. Bull World Health Organ. 2000;78:1246.

CASE SUMMARY

- Twenty-four-year-old male professional athlete with dehydration and hypovolemic hyponatremia.
- Thiazides, citalopram, and ibuprofen (NSAIDS) can all cause and/or exacerbate hyponatremia.
- Appropriate monitoring and treatment of hypovolemic hyponatremia often requires emergency department visit or hospitalization.

For more information on the care plan and facilitator's guide please visit http://www.mhpharmacotherapy.com

30 Hyperkalemia

Daniel Hershberger   Lee Morrow

Mark Malesker

PATIENT PRESENTATION

Chief Complaint

"My legs feel like jelly."

History of Present Illness (HPI)

SI is a 72-year-old female who presents to the Medicine Clinic to follow-up her increased lower extremity edema that started 1 month ago. Her primary physician prescribed furosemide and a low sodium diet 2 weeks ago. Two days ago she phoned the office with complaints of dysuria and the nurse sent an antibiotic order to her pharmacy. The lower extremity edema has improved but, now she feels weak. She notes no shortness of breath or chest pain. She does have an occasional palpitation. Her food tastes terrible without salt so she has been using a salt substitute that Dr. Oz recommended on TV.

Past Medical History

Hypertension
Hyperlipidemia
Osteoarthritis
Morbid obesity, BMI 45
Urinary tract infection, recurrent
Obstructive sleep apnea

Family History

Coronary artery disease

Social/Work History

Housewife. Widow for many years. Obesity limits social interactions but she attends garage sales several days a week. Three adult children, alive and well living in other states.

Tobacco/Alcohol/Substance Use

No alcohol use. Never used tobacco. Denies any recreational drugs.

Allergy/Intolerance/Adverse Event History

Lisinopril—cough

Medication History

► *Current Medications*

Albuterol HFA 2 puffs every 4-6 hours as needed

Carvedilol 6.25 mg po bid

Furosemide 40 mg po daily, started 2 weeks ago

Losartan 50 mg po daily

Naproxen 500 mg po bid

Simvastatin 20 mg po daily

Trimethoprim/Sulfamethoxazole 160/800 mg po bid, started 2 days ago

Review of Systems

As per HPI. Otherwise reviewed and unremarkable.

Physical Exam

► *General*

Fatigued appearing elderly female in no apparent distress

► *Vital Signs*

BP 110/70 mm Hg, P 65, RR 12, T 98.2°F (36.2°C)

Weight 265 lb. (120 kg)

Height 64 in. (162 cm)

Pain reported as 4/10

► *Skin*

Warm, dry skin without apparent rashes or breakdown

► *HEENT*

No scleral icterus. Posterior oropharynx without erythema or exudate. Poor dentition.

► *Neck and Lymph Nodes*

No thyromegaly. No anterior cervical lymphadenopathy.

► *Chest*

No wheezing or crackles. No accessory muscle use

► *Breasts*

Obese. Soft, no masses detected

► **Cardiovascular**

Regular rate and rhythm. No JVD.

► **Abdomen**

Obese. Soft, nontender, nondistended. No tympany. Normal bowel sounds.

► **Musculoskeletal**

5/5 strength bilaterally in upper and lower extremities.

► **Neurology**

Normal gait. Sensation intact.

► **Extremities**

Bilateral 2+ lower extremity edema.

► **Genitourinary**

Deferred

► **Rectal**

Deferred

Laboratory and Other Diagnostic Tests
Laboratory Tests
Laboratory Data, and Diagnostic Test Results

	Conventional Units	SI Units
Na	137 mEq/L	137 mmol/L
K	6.5 mEq/L	6.5 mmol/L
Cl	106 mEq/L	106 mmol/L
CO_2/HCO_3	22 mEql/L	22 mmol/L
BUN	40 mg/dL	14 mmol/L
Serum Cretinine (adult)	1.9 mg/dL	168 µmol/L
Creatinine Clerance (adult)	51 mL/min	0.49 mL/s
Glucose (fasting)	100 mg/dL	5.6 mmol/L
Total Ca	10 mg/dL	2.5 mmol/L
Mg	1.6 mEq/L	0.8 mmol/L
PO_4		
Hemoglobin		
Hematocrit		
MCV		
WBC		
WBC Differential		////
Platelet		
Albumin		
Bilirubin (total)		

ECG: Peaked T waves and 1st degree heart block (PR length 220 ms)

► **Imaging studies**

None

Assessment

Seventy-two-year-old female with hyperkalemia and acute kidney injury (AKI). She will be sent to the emergency department for assessment.

Student Work-Up

Missing Information/Inadequate Data

Evaluate: Patient database

Drug therapy problems

Care plan (by problem)

TARGETED QUESTIONS

1. What are the signs and symptoms of hyperkalemia in this patient?

   Hint: See p. 435 in PPP

2. What are the most likely causes of this patient's hyperkalemia?

   Hint: See p. 435 in PPP

3. Which medications could have contributed to the hyperkalemia and acute kidney injury in this patient?

   Hint: See p. 435 in PPP

4. What are the treatment options for the management of hyperkalemia?

   Hint: See p. 435 in PPP

CASE SUMMARY

- Seventy-two-year-old female with AKI and hyperkalemia.
- Hyperkalemia may be related to AKI, salt substitutes, and several medications.
- Appropriate monitoring and treatment of hyperkalemia often requires hospitalization, especially in the face of renal dysfunction.

For more information on the care plan and facilitator's guide please visit http://www.mhpharmacotherapy.com

31 Metabolic Alkalosis

Mark Malesker   Daniel Hershberger
Lee Morrow

PATIENT PRESENTATION

Chief Complaint

Fatigue, shortness of breath.

History of Present Illness (HPI)

Frank Secretion is a 68-year-old-man who presents to the hospital with complaints of worsening shortness of breath, increased weight gain, and peripheral edema over the last few weeks. He attributes these symptoms to his congestive heart failure (CHF). He receives 2 L/min of oxygen at home and has two pillow orthopnea. He has been hospitalized three times in the last year for exacerbations of chronic obstructive pulmonary disease (COPD) or CHF. Patient says he is compliant with medications but his wife says otherwise.

Past Medical History

Heart failure (HF)

COPD

Persistent atrial fibrillation

Family History

Diabetes mellitus, coronary disease, hypothyroidism

Social/Work History

Worked as librarian for 40 years, but retired last year. Married for 36 years. Spouse is also retired. No recent travel activity.

Tobacco/Alcohol/Substance Use

Former smoker but quit 15 years ago. Drinks socially, only on his birthday.

Allergy/Intolerance/Adverse Event History

Lidocaine—rash

Morphine—rash

Penicillin—unknown

Medication History

▸ Current Inpatient Medications

Albuterol HFA 2 puffs q 4 h prn or albuterol solution (2.5 mg) inhaled q 4 h prn

Apixaban 5 mg po bid

Budesonide/formoterol MDI (160 mcg/4.6 mcg) 2 puffs twice daily

Furosemide 40 mg IV bid × 2 doses

Heparin 5000 units SC q8h

Lisinopril 20 mg po daily

Metoprolol XL 50 mg po bid

Pantoprazole 40 mg po daily

Spironolactone 50 mg po bid

Tiotropium Respimat 2 inhalations daily

▸ Prior Medications (Home Medications)

Albuterol HFA 2 puffs q 4 h prn

Apixaban 5 mg po bid

Budesonide/formoterol MDI (160 mcg/4.6 mcg) 2 puffs twice daily

Lisinopril 20 mg po daily

Metoprolol XL 50 mg po bid

Pantoprazole 40 mg po daily

Spironolactone 50 mg po bid

Tiotropium Respimat 2 inhalations daily

Review of Systems

As per HPI

Physical Exam

▸ General

Awake and alert. Oriented × 3. Elderly male with moderate respiratory distress.

▸ Vital Signs

BP 150/100 mm Hg, P 90 beats/min, RR 29, T 99°F (37.2°C); SpO$_2$ 90% (0.9) on 2 L via nasal cannulae

Weight 180 lb. (81 Kg)

Height 70 in. (178 cm)

Pain reported as 2/10

▶ **Skin**

Warm, dry skin without apparent rashes or breakdown.

▶ **HEENT**

Wears glasses. No lid lag, no proptosis.

▶ **Neck and Lymph Nodes**

Thyroid not enlarged. No nodules palpable. No bruits.

▶ **Chest**

Symmetric thoracic movement and resonance to percussion; Wheezing bilaterally.

▶ **Cardiovascular**

Tachycardia; irregularly irregular with normal S_1 and S_2.

▶ **Abdomen**

Bowel sounds present. Soft, nontender.

▶ **Neurology**

Moves all four extremities with intent when stimulated; DTRs nl.

▶ **Extremities**

Bilateral 1+ pedal edema.

▶ **Genitourinary**

Unremarkable; urinary catheter placed for planned diuresis.

▶ **Rectal**

Deferred

Laboratory and Other Diagnostic Tests

Laboratory Tests

Day 1

Date March 14 0800

	Conventional Units	SI Units
Na	139 mEq/L	139 mmol/L
K	4.0 mEq/L	4.0 mmo/L
Cl	100 mEq/L	100 mmol/L
CO_2/HCO_3	28 mEq/L	28 mmol/L
BUN	38 mg/dL	13.56 mmol/L
Serum Creatinine (adult)	1.3 mg/dL	114.92 μmol/L
Creatinine Clearance (adult)	62.3 mL/min	0.59 mL/s
Glucose (fasting)	124 mg/dL	6.88 mmol/L
Total Ca	9 mg/dL	2.25 mmol/L
Mg	2.1 mEq/L	0.86 mmol/L
PO_4	4.0 mg/dL	1.29 mmol/L
Hemoglobin	12 g/dL	120 g/L
Hematocrit	42%	0.42%
MCV		
WBC	$14 \times 10^3/mm^3$	
WBC Differential	////	
Platelet	$286 \times 10^3/mm^3$	
Albumin	4.0	
Bilirubin (total)		
Bilirubin (direct)		
AST	40I U/L	0.68 μkat/L
ALT	35 IU/L	0.58 μkat/L
Alk phos (adult)		
Arterial pH	7.4	
Arterial PCO_2	40 mm Hg	5.32 kPa
Arterial PO_2		
C reactive protein	.03 mg/dL	
BNP	6284 pg/mL	741 pmol/L

Day 2

Date March 15 0630

	Conventional Units	SI Units
Na	136 mEq/L	136 mmol/L
K	3.1 mEq/L	3.1 mmol/L
Cl	91 mEq/L	91 mmol/L
CO_2/HCO_3	33 mEq/L	33 mmol/L
BUN	40 mg/dL	14.28 mmol/L
SCr	1.6 mg/dL	141.44 μmol/L
Cr Clearance	48 mL/min	0.46 mL/s
Glu	124 mg/dL	6.88 mmol/L
Ca	8.9 mg/dL	2.25 mmol/L
Mg		
PO_4		
Hgb	13.7 g/dL	137 g/L
Hct	44%	0.44
MCV		
WBC	$13 \times 10^3/mm^3$	$13 \times 10^9/L$
WBC Differential	////	////
Platelets		
Albumin		
Total bilirubin		
Bilirubin (direct)		
AST		

ALT

Alkaline phosphatase

Arterial pH   7.48

Arterial PCO$_2$ 42 mm Hg   5.58 kPa

Arterial PO$_2$

C reactive protein

BNP

▶ *Imaging Studies*

CXR with right lower and middle lobe opacities suggestive of pneumonia.

Assessment

Sixty-eight-year-old male who presents with worsening shortness of breath and edema secondary to HF exacerbation. Medication noncompliance is a contributing factor.

Student Work-Up

Missing Information/Inadequate Data

Evaluate: Patient database

Drug therapy problems

Care plan (by problem)

TARGETED QUESTIONS

1. What acid-base disorder(s) do you recognize?
   Hint: See pp. 442-443, Figure 28-1 in PPP
2. What factors may have contributed to this disorder?
   Hint: See p. 447 in PPP
3. What is the management for this acid-base disorder?
   Hint: See p. 447 in PPP
4. What electrolyte disorder(s) do you recognize?
   Hint: See p. 434 in PPP
5. Describe your treatment plan to correct the patient's electrolyte abnormalities?
   Hint: See pp. 434-435 in PPP

CASE SUMMARY

- Patient with metabolic alkalosis (contraction alkalosis) and hypokalemia as a consequence of diuretic therapy.
- Hypokalemia must be carefully corrected to resolve the acid-base disturbance.

For more information on the care plan and facilitator's guide please visit http://www.mhpharmacotherapy.com

32 Epilepsy: Chronic Management

Timothy Welty

PATIENT INFORMATION

Chief Complaint

"I had a grand mal seizure yesterday."

History of Present Illness

Mary Jones is a 21-year-old woman who is a college student. She comes to the student health center saying she had a major seizure yesterday after partying with her friends the previous night following a big mid-term examination. She visited the clinic 6 months ago to renew her prescription for oral contraceptives. During the clinic visits she explains that she had not slept well for a couple of days due to several exams happening at the same time. She also admits to being fairly drunk after the party. For about a year she has experienced full body jerks several times a week, just prior to getting up. There are also episodes when she loses track of a conversation or material she is reading. Otherwise, she is in good health and does well in her course work.

Past Medical History

Occasional headaches, about 1 "bad" headache every 6 months
Seasonal allergies

Family History

Her father is 51 and is in good health. Mother is 50 and has mild depression. She has 1 sibling in good health. She thinks there is a paternal aunt who has seizures.

Social History

She is a college senior, and works a part time job in the university's student affairs office.

Tobacco/Alcohol/Substance Use

Will binge drink about once a month. No tobacco use. Admits to smoking marijuana about once month.

Allergies

None

Medications (Current)

Ethinyl estradiol and drospirenone (Yaz 28®) po daily

Cetirizine 5 mg po as needed for allergies

Naproxen 220 mg po as needed for headache

Physical Examination

▶ **General**

WDWN, white female in no acute distress

▶ **Vital Signs**

BP 105/65 mm Hg, P 68, RR 10, T 37°C

Weight 120 lb. (54.5 kg)

Height 68 in. (173 cm)

Denies pain

▶ **Skin**

Normal color and turgor; (–) rashes or lesions

▶ **HEENT**

PERRLA, EOMI

▶ **Neck and Lymph Nodes**

Normal thyroid; (–) lymphadenopathy; (–) carotid bruits

▶ **Chest**

Clear to auscultation

▶ **Cardiovascular**

RRR; (–) murmurs or gallops

▶ **Neurologic**

A&O × 3; CN II-XII intact; DTR 3+ and normal; (–) Romberg; (–) plantar reflex: strength 5/5 throughout; normal gait; able to tandem walk; finger to nose intact; normal sensation to touch, pin prick, cold, and vibration.

Laboratory Tests

Fasting, Obtained the Next Day

	Conventional Units	SI Units
Na	137 mEq/L	137 mmol/L
K	3.9 mEq/L	3.9 mmol/L
CL	106 mEq/L	106 mmol/L
CO_2	24 mEq/L	24 mmol/L
BUN	7 mg/dL	2.499 mmol/L urea
SCr	0.6 mg/dL	53.04 µmol/L
Glu	75 mg/dL	4.1625 mmol/L
Ca	9.8 mg/dL	2.45 mmol/L
Mg	1.7 mEq/L	0.85 mmol/L
Phos	4.0 mg/dL	1.292 mmol/L
Albumin	4.1 g/dL	41 g/L
AST	38 IU/L	0.63346 µkat/L
ALT	33 IU/L	0.55011 µkat/L
INR	1.1	1.1
GGT	22 IU/L	3.68407 µkat/L
Hgb	13.1 g/dL	8.122 mmol/L
Hct	39.1%	0.391
WBC	$5.4 \times 10^3/mm^3$	$5.4 \times 10^9/L$
Platelets	$350 \times 10^3/\mu L$	$350 \times 10^9/L$

Student Work-Up

Missing Information/Inadequate Data

Evaluate: Patient database

Drug therapy problems

Care plan (by problem)

TARGETED QUESTIONS

1. What signs and symptoms of seizures does this patient have?

   Hint: See pp. 478-480 in PPP

2. What additional information is needed prior to making decisions about pharmacotherapy?

   Hint: See pp. 479-480 in PPP

3. Should an antiepileptic drug be started in this patient and what are the options for this patient?

   Hint: See pp. 480-484 in PPP

4. Which medication is the best selection for this patient and how should it be started?

   Hint: See pp. 483-492 in PPP

5. What are the common adverse effects and what additional items should be discussed with the patient?

   Hint: See pp. 484-492 in PPP

FOLLOW-UP

Three weeks later, she comes clinic having completed a MRI scan of the head and an EEG. The MRI is read as normal. The EEG showed bursts of 3-4 Hertz of generalized EEG activity, consistent with a generalized epilepsy. Combined with the clinical description of her seizures, what epilepsy syndrome is most likely? Should long term antiepileptic drug therapy be used? What actions, if any, should be taken at this point?

Hint: See pp. 478-480 in PPP

A year later, she returns to clinic. Her seizures are well controlled on levetiracetam 1500 mg twice daily, with only a few "jerks" a month. Other than some mild depression, she is tolerating the medication well. During the visit, she mentions that a pregnancy test last week was positive. What should she be told about the teratogenicity risk with pregnancy levetiracetam? What plan should be implemented to manage her levetiracetam dosing during her pregnancy?

Hint: See pp. 491-492 in PPP

☉ GLOBAL PERSPECTIVE

The World Health Organization estimates that there are 40 to 50 million people with epilepsy throughout the world. The annual incidence in third-world nations is twice that of the United States (2/100 compared to 1/100). In many countries the condition remains a stigmatizing condition surrounded with mystical beliefs and social taboos. On a global basis, an astonishing three-fourths of people with epilepsy receive no treatment for their seizures. Such lack of treatment is related to the above-mentioned social stigma as well as lack of access to medical care and medications. Patients may be treated with local traditional remedies in lieu of standard AED therapy. Also, the array of antiepileptic medications available in developing countries is more limited, so patients with seizures who do not respond to older first-line agents may have few options.

CASE SUMMARY

- Twenty-one-year old woman appears to have a newly diagnosed seizure disorder.

- The diagnosis was confirmed by EEG, and intracranial lesions were ruled out by MRI.

- The patient currently received a hormonal contraceptive and may use alcohol or other substances to excess.

For more information on the care plan and facilitator's guide please visit http://www.mhpharmacotherapy.com

33 Status Epilepticus

Eljim P. Tesoro　　　Gretchen M. Brophy

PATIENT PRESENTATION

Chief Complaint

"My head hurts."

History of Present Illness

Susan Lee is a 45-year-old Asian woman who is brought into the emergency room after being in a motor vehicle accident (MVA). She was an unrestrained driver who crashed her car into a telephone pole. She has multiple facial injuries and lacerations and she smells strongly of alcohol. She is suddenly noted to have rhythmic jerking of her arms and legs that lasts for 5 minutes after which she remains unresponsive to questions. Her brother is identified as an emergency contact and is called to get further information.

Past Medical History

Hypertension (20 years)

Diabetes type 2 (5 years)

Anxiety/depression (10 years)

Family History

Noncontributory

Social/Work History

She lives with her brother and his family; she has been divorced 10 years; works as a website developer

Tobacco/Alcohol/Substance Use

Does not smoke; drinks heavily on weekends; occasional cocaine use

Allergy/Intolerance/Adverse Event History

Alprazolam (drowsiness)

Lisinopril (hives)

Medication History

HCTZ 25 mg po daily

Metformin 500 mg po twice daily

Paroxetine 20 mg po daily

Review of Systems

Deferred (patient is now unresponsive)

▶ **Physical Exam**

Thin, middle-aged female with continuous convulsions of the extremities

▶ **Vital Signs**

BP 165/98 mm Hg, P 118, RR 22, T 38.2°C

Weight 110 lb. (50 kg)

Height 65 in. (165 cm)

Unable to evaluate pain

▶ **Skin**

Sweaty skin and scalp; (+) facial lacerations (+) bruising

▶ **HEENT**

Persistent upward gaze

▶ **Neck and Lymph Nodes**

Neck in cervical collar until spinal injury is ruled out

▶ **Chest**

Deferred

▶ **Breasts**

Deferred

▶ **Cardiovascular**

Tachycardic, RRR, normal S_1, S_2; (–) S_3 or S_4

▶ **Abdomen**

Not tender/not distended; (–) organomegaly

▶ **Neurology**

Unresponsive; unarousable; GCS 3

▶ **Extremities**

Actively convulsing, no LE edema

▶ **Genitourinary**

Incontinent of stool and urine, exam otherwise deferred

▸ *Rectal*

Deferred

Laboratory and Other Diagnostic Tests

Pending

FSBG in ED 164 mg/dL (9.1 mmol/L)

Assessment

Forty-five-year-old Asian woman with acute head trauma s/p motor vehicle accident with signs of status epilepticus.

Student Work-Up

Missing Information/Inadequate Data

Evaluate:
Patient database
Drug therapy problems
Care plan (by problem)

TARGETED QUESTIONS

1. What signs of status epilepticus does this patient have?

   Hint: See p. 498 in PPP

2. What are some possible causes of status epilepticus in this patient?

   Hint: See p. 497 in PPP

3. What medication(s) would you recommend to stop this patient's status epilepticus?

   Hint: See pp. 499-501 in PPP

4. What medication(s) would you recommend for preventing future seizures in this patient?

   Hint: See pp. 500-501 in PPP

5. What drug recommendations would you give for emergent and urgent therapy if intravenous access was not available in this patient?

   Hint: See pp. 499-500 in PPP

FOLLOW-UP

An endotracheal tube was placed for mechanical ventilation since the patient was unresponsive.

A CT scan revealed multiple facial fractures and an acute subdural hematoma. She was quickly sent to the operating room for emergency surgery and, afterward, the patient was admitted to the intensive care unit. The convulsions have stopped but the patient has not awakened as expected.

What further tests or interventions can be recommended at this time?

Hint: See pp. 501-502 in PPP

⊙ GLOBAL PERSPECTIVE

The incidence of seizures is greater in developing countries compared to the United States, and a large proportion of patients receive no treatment due to social taboos and lack of access to care. Given the higher incidence of seizure disorders and lack of access to therapy in many patients, it is likely there is a higher incidence of status epilepticus in developing countries. Although the overall therapeutic approach would be the same, patients in developing countries may have poor access to emergency medical care. While first-line medications, such as benzodiazepines, phenytoin, and valproic acid, may be available, newer intravenous medications may not be available for refractory status epilepticus.

CASE SUMMARY

- Status epilepticus is a medical emergency and should be assessed and treated immediately.
- Intravenous benzodiazepines are considered emergent therapy for status epilepticus.
- Intravenous anticonvulsants are considered urgent therapy to prevent future seizures.
- Electroencephalography can identify patients in nonconvulsive status epilepticus.

For more information on the care plan and facilitator's guide please visit http://www.mhpharmacotherapy.com

34 Parkinson's Disease

Jack J. Chen

PATIENT PRESENTATION

Chief Complaint

"My movement has gotten worse and my Parkinson's medications do not seem to be as effective anymore."

History of Present Illness

James Park is a 75-year-old, right-handed man who comes in for a routine follow-up visit at the movement disorders clinic. The patient is accompanied by his wife. The patient reports that his movements are much worse. He has more difficulty arising out of bed, getting dressed, and feels unsteady while walking. But he has not fallen. His wife confirms that walking and performing activities of daily living seem to be more difficult for him. He requires more assistance when arising out of a chair or the car. He notices that his Parkinson's medications improve his movement but this only lasts about 2 hours for each dose of carbidopa/levodopa. This leaves him in an "off" state for several hours in between doses. Additionally, he is very "slow and stiff" upon awakening in the morning. He also reports feeling very sleepy during the daytime. His wife asks to speak with the neurologist privately and reports that the patient has developed a gambling habit over that past 6 weeks and seems to be "obsessed" about any form of gambling but lottery tickets in particular. On weekdays, he demands that she drive him to the grocery store to purchase lottery tickets and on weekends, he will take a cab to the local casino and spend the whole day there. They have lost a substantial portion of their savings from his gambling activity. Additionally, he seems to be depressed, more forgetful, and is increasingly confused about the date and time. She is very concerned about these new developments.

Past Medical History

BPH (8 years)

Hyperlipidemia (10 years)

Hypertension (10 years)

Parkinson's disease (5 years)

Family History

He has an older sister; alive and well. His father died of lung cancer. Mother had Alzheimer's disease and died of complications related to pneumonia.

Social History

He has a college education. He is married and lives with his wife of 50 years, and has three children aged 40, 43, and 48. He is a retired plumber.

Tobacco/Alcohol/Substance Use

(–) Alcohol, tobacco, or illicit drug use

Allergies/Intolerances/Adverse Drug Events

Amantadine (livedo reticularis)

Medications (Current)

Atorvastatin 40 mg po q 24 h

Carbidopa/Levodopa 25/100 mg po three times daily (0800 – 1400 – 2000)

Pramipexole ER 3 mg po q 24 h

Rasagiline 1 mg po q 24 h

Diphenhydramine 25 mg po prn seasonal allergies (recently takes approximately 1-2 doses per day)

Doxazosin 8 mg po q 24 h (was increased 8 weeks ago from 4 mg to 8 mg)

HCTZ 12.5 mg po q 24 h

Multivitamin one tablet po q 24 h

Review of Systems

(–) Cancer, loss of consciousness, respiratory disease, pain, seizures, stroke, or vertigo. Reports depressed mood and dizziness.

Physical Examination

▶ *General*

WDWN Caucasian man in no acute distress. Oriented to person and place but not time. Affect appropriate. Masked facies. Hypophonic, slurred speech, palilalia. Shuffling, unsteady gait; right foot drags; reduced arm swing bilaterally. No dyskinesias or dystonic postures.

▶ *Vital Signs*

Supine BP 140/76 mm Hg; Standing BP 100/56 mm Hg

P 76, RR 16, T 36.4°C

Weight 180 lb. (81.8 kg)

Height 71 in. (180 cm)

▶ HEENT

Cranial nerves

II: Normal visual acuity, visual fields, fundi

III, IV, VI: PERRL, EOMI, (–) nystagmus, (–) gaze palsy

V: Facial sensation intact

VII: Normal facial asymmetry and strength

VIII: Whisper test normal

IX: Uvula midline with "Ah"

XI: Shoulder shrug strength normal

XII: Tongue midline with protrusion

▶ Neck and Lymph Nodes

Neck supple; (–) adenopathy

▶ Chest

Clear to auscultation

▶ Cardiovascular

Deferred

▶ Abdomen

Deferred

▶ Extremities

(–) Pedal edema

Pedal pulses are 2+ and equal

DTRs normal

Positive micrographia (Fig. 34-1)

▶ Skin

Warm and dry; (–) rashes or lesions

▶ MDS UPDRS Part III (Motor) Examination ("on")

UPDRS Part III (motor) = 36 while "on" (2 months ago)

▶ Today's Ratings

Speech = 2

Facial expression = 3

Rigidity: Neck = 2; RUE = 3; LUE = 1; RLE = 1; LLE = 1

Finger tapping: Right = 3, Left = 2

Hand movements: Right = 3, Left = 2

Hand pronation – supination: Right = 3, Left = 2

Toe tapping: Right = 1, Left = 1

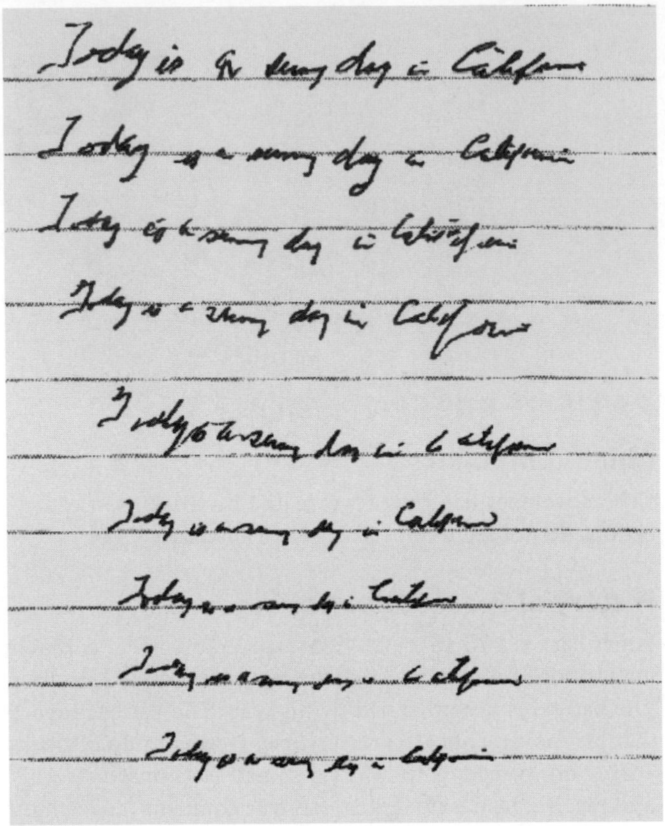

FIGURE 34-1. Micrographia. (Reprinted with permission from Jack J. Chen, PharmD, Loma Linda University Movement Disorders Center, Loma Linda, CA.)

Leg agility: Right = 2, Left = 1

Arising from a chair = 2

Gait = 2

Freezing of gait = 1

Postural stability = 2

Posture = 3

Global spontaneity of movement (body bradykinesia) = 3

Postural tremor of hands: Right = 0, Left = 0

Kinetic tremor of hands: Right = 0, Left = 0

Resting tremor amplitude: RUE = 2; LUE = 1; RLE = 0; LLE = 0; lip/jaw = 1

Constancy of rest tremor: 2

▶ Genitourinary

Deferred

▶ Rectal

Deferred

Other Rating Scales

Mini Mental Status Exam (MMSE) = 25/30 (today)

Mini Mental Status Exam (MMSE) = 28/30 (8 weeks ago)

Laboratory Tests

	Conventional Units	SI Units
Na	140 mEq/L	140 mmol/L
K	3.8 mEq/L	3.8 mmol/L
Cl	101 mEq/L	101 mmol/L
CO_2/HCO_3	23 mEq/L	23 mmol/L
BUN	16 mg/dL	5.7 mmol/L
SCr	1 mg/dL	88.4 μmol/L
Cr Clearance		
Glu	98 mg/dL	5.44 mmol/L
Ca	8.8 mg/dL	2.2 mmol/L
Mg		
PO_4		
Hgb	16 g/dL	160g/L
Hct	46%	0.46
MCV	92.1 μm³	92.1 fL
WBC	6.5×10^3/mm³	6.5×10^9/L
WBC Differential	////	
Platelets	240×10^3/mm³	240×10^9/L
Albumin	4.1 g/dL	41 g/L
Total bilirubin	0.8 mg/dL	13.7 μmol/L
Bilirubin (direct)	0.1 mg/dL	1.4 μmol/L
AST	36 IU/L	0.6 μkat/L
ALT	40 IU/L	0.67 μkat/L
Alkaline phosphatase	64 IU/L	1.1 μkat/L

Assessment

Seventy-five-old man with moderate-to-advanced stage idiopathic PD experiencing motor fluctuations including early-morning off time, orthostatic hypotension, daytime sleepiness, depressed mood, worsening cognition, and impulse control disorder.

Student Work-Up

Missing Information/Inadequate Data

Evaluate:
Patient database
Drug therapy problems
Care plan (by problem)

TARGETED QUESTIONS

1. Which signs and symptoms are associated with PD and what is your assessment of the severity of his motor signs and symptoms as rated by the neurologist?
   Hint: See pp. 508-509 in PPP

2. Based on the subjective and objective information, what do you think are this patient's most significant medical problems?
   Hint: See pp. 508-509 in PPP

3. Are any of the patient's current medications contributing to some of the problems? If so, what are they?
   Hint: See pp. 511-515 in PPP

4. What are the treatment goals and treatment options for this patient?
   Hint: See pp. 510-518 in PPP

FOLLOW-UP

Eight weeks later, the patient returns for follow-up. He states his motor fluctuations have improved with the new regimen. His MDS UPDRS Part III (motor) examination ("on") score is 40 and his MMSE is 25. The patient is tolerating the new regimen. His dizziness and drowsiness have resolved. On examination, his tremor, rigidity, and bradykinesia are still present, but improved. His wife reports that the gambling behavior has resolved. However, patient still has memory problems and is depressed. The patient confirms that he has lost interest in activities that he previously enjoyed such as oil painting, going on walks and socializing with family friends.

Given this new information, identify the treatment goals and treatment options for this patient and create a care plan for each problem.

Hint: See p. 515 in PPP

🌐 GLOBAL PERSPECTIVE

PD affects individuals worldwide and the signs and symptoms are not different for any ethnic or cultural group. Although there are isolated clusters of PD linked to genetic and/or environmental causes, the majority of PD cases worldwide are not attributable to an identifiable genetic or environmental element. Epidemiologic studies indicate there are differences in both incidence and prevalence among world regions but these differences are probably due to factors that may be demographic (variations in life expectancy across countries) and health care related (improper diagnosis, variations in access to health care), together with methodological differences in conducting the epidemiologic studies. Current medications used to treat PD appear to be similar in effect regardless of ethnicity and currently there is very little evidence to indicate that pharmacogenomic variations substantively affect PD medication response. Therefore, the application of PD treatment and medication guidelines are considered universal and not affected by ethnicity. However, when developing a care plan, it is important to consider the patient's desired outcomes and goals of treatment. As an example, for some individuals, a mild tremor or mild dyskinesia may not be perceived as sufficiently troublesome and, thus, a low priority therapeutic goal. However, for other individuals, a mild tremor may have a substantial negative impact on their quality of life and would rank symptomatic control as a high priority goal. Overall, the patient's and family's desired goals (which can vary among cultures) should be incorporated into the care plan to help guide therapy.

CASE SUMMARY

- This older patient with PD is experiencing motor fluctuations that are interfering with his quality of life. Motor fluctuations are common in moderate-to-advanced PD and occur due to a combination of disease progression (ongoing neurodegeneration) and the short half-life of carbidopa/levodopa.

- There are several pharmacotherapy options for management of motor fluctuations. The care plan should incorporate the most appropriate option based on the patient's medical history and current drug therapy.

- Patients with PD often present with several clinical problems that are uncovered during a visit. This patient is experiencing several additional problems that are related to his PD and/or medications. Once identified, the care plan should prioritize these problems and incorporate the appropriate recommendations or interventions.

- These additional problems include nonmotor symptoms of PD and known side effects of his current PD medications.

REFERENCES

1. Fox SH, Katzenschlager R, Lim SY, Ravina B, Seppi K, Coelho M, et al. The Movement Disorder Society Evidence-Based Medicine Review Update: Treatments for the motor symptoms of Parkinson's disease. Mov Disord. 2011 Oct;26 Suppl 3:S2-41.

2. Seppi K, Weintraub D, Coelho M, Perez-Lloret S, Fox SH, Katzenschlager R, et al. The Movement Disorder Society Evidence-Based Medicine Review Update: Treatments for the non-motor symptoms of Parkinson's disease. Mov Disord. 2011 Oct;26 Suppl 3:S42-80.

3. Refer http://www.movementdisorders.org/MDS-Files1/PDFs/Rating-Scales/MDS-UPDRSfinal_Update.pdf

For more information on the care plan and facilitator's guide please visit http://www.mhpharmacotherapy.com

35 Acute Pain Management

Asad E. Patanwala

PATIENT PRESENTATION

Chief Complaint

"The pain medication you are giving me is not working."

History of Present Illness

Mai Payne is a 51-year-old female who presented to the emergency department (ED) with acute abdominal pain that started 2 days ago. Her diffuse abdominal pain has been increasing in intensity over the last week during which time she has had no bowel movements. Also, she has had very little oral intake along with some nausea and vomiting. In the ED, she was given morphine 4 mg intravenously and 2 L of normal saline. The surgical team was consulted and she was taken to the operating room for surgical resection of intra-abdominal abscesses. She is currently on the general surgical ward after her surgery yesterday. Today she is tolerating clear liquids and is able to take oral medications.

Past Medical History

Depression (10 years)

Hypertension (15 years)

Appendectomy (3 months ago)

Family History

Father died at age 75 from myocardial infarction (MI); mother is alive; she has no siblings.

Social History

She is married; works at the local airport in baggage claims

Tobacco/Alcohol/Substance Use

Does not drink alcohol, smoke cigarettes, or use illicit substances

Allergies/Intolerances/Adverse Drug Events

Meperidine resulted in a seizure

Medications (Taken at Home)

Oxycodone/acetaminophen (5/325 mg) po 1-2 tablets q 6 h prn

Amlodipine 10 mg po daily

HCTZ 25 mg po daily

Celecoxib 200 mg po daily

Fluoxetine 20 mg po daily

Multivitamin 1 tablet po daily

Medications (Current during Hospitalization)

Ondansetron 4 mg IV q 6 h prn

Tramadol 100 mg po q 4-6 h prn

Acetaminophen 500 mg po 1-2 tablets q 6 h prn

Famotidine 20 mg po q 12 h

Metoprolol 5 mg IV q 6 h prn

Hydralazine 10 mg IV q 6 h prn

Fluoxetine 20 mg po daily

Docusate 100 mg po bid

Heparin 5000 units SC q 12 h

Insulin lispro per sliding scale (2-10 units q 6 h prn; 20 units used in last 24 hours)

Review of Systems

+ abdominal pain and distension that is not relieved by current therapy; + nausea

Physical Exam

▶ *General*

Well-developed, overweight, middle-aged, Caucasian female who appears to be grimacing in pain

▶ *Vital Signs*

BP 153/102 mm Hg, P 105, RR 15, T 37.1°C, Pain 8/10

Weight 176 lb. (80 kg)

Height 66 in. (168 cm)

▶ *Skin*

Normal skin turgor; dry abdominal incision

▶ *HEENT*

PERRLA, EOMI; TMs appear normal

► **Neck and Lymph Nodes**

Supple, (−) bruits, (−) thyromegaly, (−) lymphadenopathy

► **Chest**

Clear breath sounds bilaterally, (−) crackles

► **Breasts**

(−) Abnormalities

► **Cardiovascular**

Tachycardic, regular rhythm, normal S_1, S_2; (−) S_3 or S_4

► **Abdomen**

Soft, tender, distended, (−) bowel sounds, (−) masses, (−) hepatomegaly

► **Neurology**

Grossly intact, DTRs normal

► **Extremities**

(−) edema, (−) clubbing, (−) cyanosis

► **Genitourinary**

No abnormalities

► **Rectal**

(+) rectal tone, (−) gross blood

Laboratory Tests (Obtained This Morning)

	Conventional Units	SI Units
Na	143 mEq/L	143 mmol/L
K	4.5 mEq/L	4.5 mmol/L
Cl	102 mEq/L	102 mmol/L
CO_2	24 mEq/L	24 mmol/L
BUN	15 mg/dL	5.3 mmol/L
SCr	1.1 mg/dL	83.9 μmol/L
Glu	206 mg/dL	11.4 mmol/L
Ca	8.8 mg/dL	2.2 mmol/L
Mg	2.1 mEq/L	1.05 mmol/L
Phosphate	3.6 mg/dL	1.16 mmol/L
Hgb	14.5 g/dL	9.0 mmol/L
Hct	43.5%	0.435 fraction
WBC	$13.3 \times 10^3/mm^3$	$10.3 \times 10^9/L$
Platelets	$260 \times 10^3/mm^3$	$260 \times 10^9/L$
Albumin	3.8 g/dL	38 g/L
Total bilirubin	1.2 mg/dL	20.5 μmol/L
Direct bilirubin	0.3 mg/dL	5.1 μmol/L

AST	29 IU/L	0.48 μkat/L
ALT	22 IU/L	0.37 μkat/L
Alk phos	98 IU/L	1.6 μkat/L

Assessment

This is a 51-year old female with signs and symptoms of severe acute post-operative pain. She has a concurrent intra-abdominal infection.

Student Work-Up

Missing Information/Inadequate Data

Evaluate: Patient database

Drug therapy problems

Care plan (by problem)

TARGETED QUESTIONS

1. What signs and symptoms of this patient are consistent with poor pain control?

   Hint: See p. 523 in PPP

2. Why is intravenous opioid analgesia the treatment of choice for most patients with severe acute pain in the hospital setting?

   Hint: See pp. 527-528 in PPP

3. How does the potency of commonly used opioids differ?

   Hint: See Table 34-2 in PPP

4. What risks and adverse effects of opioid therapy would you discuss with the patient?

   Hint: See pp. 528-529 in PPP

5. Is this patient a candidate for patient controlled analgesia? Discuss typical components of a PCA order.

   Hint: See p. 528 in PPP

FOLLOW-UP

Three days after surgery, the patient is being discharged from the hospital. While in the hospital, she was only treated with intravenous opioids. She now needs to be switched to an oral medication for pain control. What are some of the pertinent pieces of information that you would need to create a regimen that this patient can take at home? What counseling and adjunctive therapy may be required if this patient is sent home with prescriptions for oral opioid analgesia?

   Hint: See pp. 527-529, 531 in PPP

☉ GLOBAL PERSPECTIVE

Pain is universal throughout the globe and the optimal management of acute pain is both humane and necessary. Regardless of age, race, ethnicity, gender, culture, or religion, all humans feel pain. However, response to pain may be expressed differently, and expectations for pain relief may vary based on these demographics. Thus it is important to understand each patient's expectations and goals related to pain control. There is no physiological or laboratory parameter for accurate pain assessment. Hence providers must rely on the patient's self-reported pain to make treatment decisions. Some patients may withhold expressing severe pain to health care providers in a stoic manner, while others are very expressive and communicative even for mild discomfort. Also, there is evidence that patients from ethnic minorities or cultures that are different from the health care provider are more likely to receive inadequate analgesia. All of this must be incorporated in the decision making process with regard to pain assessment and treatment.

CASE SUMMARY

- Her clinical picture is consistent with severe acute post-operative pain.
- She is currently on analgesics that are suboptimal for optimal pain control and with the potential for adverse effects due to drug interactions.
- She is experiencing constipation, which is likely to be exacerbated by opioids. Thus, a stimulant or osmotic laxatives should be provided.

For more information on the care plan and facilitator's guide please visit http://www.mhpharmacotherapy.com

36 Chronic Pain Management

Echo Fallon   Michael D. Katz

PATIENT PRESENTATION

Chief Complaint

"I don't know if I can keep living with this pain. My opioids used to help but they aren't working at this dose anymore—do we need to increase them again?"

History of Present Illness

Chevy Jones is a 24-year-old male with a 3-year history of chronic low back pain who presents anxiously to the pain management clinic. His pain began after a sports-related back injury. He is almost out of his prescriptions. He was originally started on opioids to treat severe pain following a failed nerve ablation procedural which was performed out of state. He then found a local prescriber, who just lost his medical license due to his opioid prescribing practices. Chevy is now seeking to establish care with a pain specialist and obtain his prescriptions. He reports that OTC pain medications and gabapentin have not worked for his pain in the past. He describes the pain as constant aching with occasional sharp, stabbing sensations. His pain is worse in the mornings at 9/10. He also describes sensations of "numbness and pinpricks" that travel down the back of his legs bilaterally. He reports trouble sleeping every night as well—usually he lays in bed watching TV until around 03:00 AM when he finally falls asleep.

Past Medical History

Seasonal allergies (16 years)

Past Surgical History

Appendicitis with periappendiceal abscess and appendectomy (2000)

Family History

Father with history of depression and hypertension, untreated. Mother and sister with a history of untreated anxiety but no other significant medical history.

Social History

Single. Living with his parents who are his caretakers. The pain has decreased his functioning to the point that he no longer attends school nor can he work consistently.

Tobacco/Alcohol/Substance Use

No tobacco, occasional alcohol (3 drinks/week), no illicit drug use

Allergies/Intolerances/Adverse Drug Events

Gabapentin—confusion, sedation

Medications (Current)

Oxycodone 10 mg po every 4 hours prn pain

MS Contin 30 mg po four times daily

Docusate 100 mg po TID prn

L-glutamine

Review of Systems

(+) chronic low back pain, previously relieved with current dose of opioids; nausea; (+) pinprick sensation bilaterally down the back of the legs; (+) constipation since starting opioids not relieved with OTC medications

Physical Examination

General

WDWN anxious-appearing young man in seemingly acute distress

▶ *Vital Signs*

BP 131/79 mm Hg, P 70, RR 16, T 37.1°C

Weight 200 lb. (90.9 kg)

Height 72 in. (182.8 cm)

Low back pain and radiating pinprick sensation down back of legs bilaterally

▶ *Skin*

Warm and dry

▶ *HEENT*

PERRLA, EOMI; TMs clear bilaterally

▶ *Neck and Lymph Nodes*

No lymphadenopathy; no cervical spine tenderness

▶ **Chest**

Clear to auscultation

▶ **Cardiovascular**

RRR, nl S_1 and S_2

▶ **Abdomen**

Distended; hard palpable stool on exam; + bowel sounds; no organomegaly

▶ **Neurology**

Cranial nerves II-XII grossly intact; normal DTRs; decreased pinprick sensation on posterior thighs bilaterally

▶ **Genitourinary**

Examination deferred

▶ **Rectal**

Examination deferred

▶ **Imaging Results**

Lumbar and sacral MRI – no significant findings

Lumbar and sacral CT – no significant findings

Laboratory Tests

	Conventional Units	SI Units
Na	140 mEq/L	140 mmol/L
K	3.5 mEq/L	3.5 mmol/L
Cl	100 mEq/L	100 mmol/L
CO_2	24 mEq/L	24 mmol/L
BUN	22 mg/dL	22 mmol/L
SCr	12 mg/dL	4.3 μmol/L
Glu	70 mg/dL	3.9 mmol/L
Ca	9 mg/dL	2.25 mmol/L
Mg	2.2 mg/dL	1.1 mmol/L
Phosphate	3.2 mg/dL	1.0 mmol/L
Hgb	17.1 mg/dL	10.6 mmol/L
Hct	50.1%	0.5
WBC	$5 \times 10^3/mm^3$	$5 \times 10^9/L$
MCV	$85 \ \mu m^3$	85 fL
PLT	$173 \times 10^3/mm^3$	$173 \times 10^9/L$
Albumin	4 g/dL	40 g/L
Alk Phos	96 U/L	1.6 μkat/L
AST	44 U/L	0.7 μkat/L
ALT	55 U/L	0.9 μkat/L
Total bilirubin	0.9 mg/dL	15.4 μmol/L

Urine toxicology screen + only for opiate

Assessment

Twenty-four-year-old man with chronic low back pain of unknown etiology and neuropathic pain.

Student Work-Up

Missing Information/Inadequate Data

Evaluate: Patient database

Drug therapy problems

Care plan (by problem)

TARGETED QUESTIONS

1. What other information would be useful in characterizing, assessing, and treating this patient's pain?

   Hint: See pp. 523-524 in PPP

2. What symptoms of neuropathic pain does the patient describe, and how is this type of pain treated differently than other types of chronic pain?

   Hint: See p. 523 in PPP

3. Why are both scheduled and prn pain medications used for chronic pain?

   Hint: See pp. 527-528 in PPP

4. What concepts would be helpful to use to make reasonable changes to this patient's opioid regimen?

   Hint: See pp. 523, and 526-530 in PPP

5. What nonpharmacologic therapies may be useful for this patient?

   Hint: See pp. 526, 53-531 in PPP

FOLLOW-UP

One month later, the patient returns for a follow-up pain appointment. He reports improved pain relief, mood, functionality, and sleep with the regimen you implemented on his first visit. He continues to experience nausea and constipation from the opioids, however, and expresses willingness to do "whatever it takes" to help these symptoms. What changes would you make to his current regimen? Is the total morphine daily equivalent dose this patient is taking considered safe?

   Hint: See Table 34-3 in PPP

⊙ GLOBAL PERSPECTIVE

International health authorities agreed more than 20 years ago that most cancer-related pain could be relieved with opioid analgesics and that every national government should implement pain relief programs. Pain management, particularly in the setting of palliative care, is often not possible without the potent analgesia that opioids provide.

Many national and state regulations, however, are overly strict in preventing access to opioids.[1] This occurs partly because drug control, rather than provision of appropriate care, can be the focus of government legislation. Concern among regulatory agencies and international health authorities has increased due to large discrepancies in national opioid consumption, prompting them to ask governments to address such barriers to opioids. Almost 90% of the world's morphine supply is consumed by only 15% of the world's population. The United States (U.S.) population, for example, is less than 5% of the world population, but uses approximately half of the global supply of morphine. Most other countries are therefore left with only low quantities of opioids for use.

This large use of opioids in the U.S. has increased during the past 20 years as more opioid prescriptions are written to treat patients with chronic, noncancer pain. During this time, however, prescription opioid misuse and overdose have also increased in both adults and adolescents.[2] This has been referred to as an opioid "epidemic" and includes public health issues of abuse, diversion, and addiction that are currently prompting changes toward tighter control of opioid prescribing practices.[3] Additionally, there is a sparsity of scientific evidence that opioids effectively and safely control noncancer pain, and reports of adverse effects of chronic opioid use such as respiratory depression, opioid endocrinopathy, and opioid-induced hyperalgesia are increasing. Therefore, the tide of opioid prescribing patterns in the U.S. are shifting, and it will be interesting to see if and how this impacts opioid use throughout the rest of the world.

REFERENCES

1. Joranson DE, Ryan KM. Ensuring opioid availability: Methods and resources. *J Pain Sympt Manage.* 2007;33:527-32.
2. Chou R, Fanciullo GJ, Fine PG, et al. Opioid Treatment Guidelines—Clinical Guidelines for the Use of Chronic Opioid Therapy in Chronic Noncancer Pain. *The Journal of Pain.* 2009;10(2):113-30.
3. Lee-Iannotti J, Parish JM. The Epidemic of Opioid Use: Implications for the Sleep Physician. *J Clin Sleep Med.* 2014;10(6):645-6.

CASE SUMMARY

- His clinical picture is consistent with chronic noncancer pain secondary to injury.
- His current regimen is not providing sufficient pain relief and he is experiencing adverse effects from opioids.
- He would benefit from a regimen that addresses both his somatic and neuropathic pain. His opioid regimen should include both prn and scheduled medication as well as a bowel regimen to help alleviate and prevent recurrence of opioid-related adverse effects.

For more information on the care plan and facilitator's guide please visit http://www.mhpharmacotherapy.com

37 Headache

James J. Pitcock   Leigh Ann Ross

PATIENT PRESENTATION

Chief Compliant

"My headaches just keep getting worse no matter what I try. I had to miss class again yesterday, which was the second time in the past 3 weeks. I just need some relief from the pounding or I might fail out of school."

History of Present Illness

BH is a 27-year-old Caucasian male that presents to the outpatient neurology clinic associated with an academic medical institution. He was referred to the clinic by his local primary care physician (PCP) due to worsening of the intensity and frequency of his headaches. He is seeing Dr. Brown, one of the neurology fellows in the clinic this morning. BH states his headaches previously were "not be that bad," occurring about every 4 to 5 months, and were generally treated them with "one Goody's powder along with some peace and quiet." However in the past 6 months, the headaches have increased in both frequency and severity to the point that they are now interfering with his research and schoolwork. He reports the pain is usually "just on one side of my head," grows steadily over a span of a few hours, and typically lasts most of the day despite treatment. He describes the pain as pulsating in nature and generally associated with nausea and vomiting. "Almost any kind of stress" can bring on a headache and the pain makes it hard for him to study and sleep, which further leads to more stress and anxiety over passing his classes and getting his research completed. Bright lights can make the pain worse, but he denies experiencing any neurological deficits prior to or during an attack. He has had headaches since his teenage years, but they were easily treated with OTC analgesics and stress avoidance. Reports that his blood pressure has not been under the best control since starting graduate school, so his PCP started him on a new blood pressure medication a few months ago. States that his other medical conditions are stable.

Past Medical History

Hypertension (HTN) (5 years)

Dyslipidemia (5 years)

GERD (10 years)

"Headaches" (10 years) (reports having 2-3 yearly in the past, but now has had 4 in the past 6 months)

Seasonal allergic rhinitis "his whole life"

Family History

Mother and father are both living. Mother aged 52 years has diabetes and suffers from migraine HAs. Father aged 54 years has dyslipidemia and HTN. Has one older and one younger sibling: one sister is aged 30 and one brother aged 25. Both siblings are healthy.

Social/Work History

He has been married for 7 years. Has one daughter aged 2 years. Currently a biochemistry graduate student at a local public university. Wife works as a nurse. Has health and prescription insurance through wife's employer.

Tobacco/Alcohol/Substance Use

He admits to smoking ½-1 ppd cigarettes. He drinks an occasional beer on the weekends. He drinks 5-6 caffeinated beverages per day. No current or history of illicit drug use.

Allergies/Intolerances/Adverse Drug Events

Sulfa (rash)

Propranolol (erectile dysfunction)

Medications (Current)

Nifedipine extended release 30 mg 1 tablet po daily (started 8 months ago)

Simvastatin 10 mg 1 tablet po daily (started 5 years ago)

Benazepril/HCTZ 10mg/12.5 mg 1 tablet po daily (started 5 years ago)

Ranitidine 150 mg 1 tablet po bid (started 10 years ago)

Loratadine 10 mg 1 tablet po prn allergy symptoms

Goody's Extra Strength powder 1 packet po prn pain (recently increased to 5-6 packets per HA)

An unknown herbal supplement to help improve memory that his wife recommended. He doesn't remember the name.

Medications (Previous)

Propranolol 40 mg 1 tablet po twice daily (prescribed 5 years ago for HTN, but stopped after a few months due to erectile dysfunction)

Review of Systems

(+) Rhinorrhea reported in spring and autumn, (−) chest pain, palpitations, lower extremity edema, and dyspnea. (+) "Smoker's cough" in the morning, but denies sputum production. (+) frequent heartburn and reflux symptoms currently controlled with medication. (+) nausea and vomiting associated with headaches. (−) dizziness or vertigo reported with HAs, however does report minor photophobia with HAs.

Physical Examination

▶ General

Anxious, well-developed, well-nourished Caucasian male in no acute distress

▶ Vital Signs

BP 122/81 mm Hg, HR 73, RR 18, T 37°C

Weight 180 lb. (82 kg), Height 70 in. (178 cm)

Pain 4/10 currently (reports pain was 8/10 yesterday)

▶ HEENT

PERRLA, EOMI, fundoscopic examination benign, (−) mucopurulent nasal discharge, external auditory canals and TMs clear, oropharynx without erythema, (−) temporal artery tenderness, occipital prominences tender bilaterally, without referred pain

▶ Chest

Clear to auscultation bilaterally

▶ Cardiovascular

RRR, (−) murmur or gallop, (−) carotid bruit, (−) JVP elevation

▶ Abdomen

Nontender, (−) organomegaly; normal bowel sounds

▶ Neurology

Appears nervous, but not agitated. Alert and fully oriented. Cranial nerves intact. Motor and sensory examinations without focality. No cerebellar abnormalities. Speech and thought appropriate to situation.

Laboratory and Other Diagnostic Tests
(Nonfasting Labs Obtained at PCP Office 2 weeks Previously)

	Conventional Units	SI Units
Na	141 mEq/L	141 mmol/L
K	4.0 mEq/L	4.0 mmol/L
Cl	101 mEq/L	101 mmol/L
CO_2	25 mEq/L	25 mmol/L
BUN	12 mg/dL	4.3 mmol/L
SCr	0.8 mg/dL	71 mmol/L

	Conventional Units	SI Units
Glu	93 mg/dL	5.2 mmol/L
Hgb	14.4 g/dL	144 g/L; 8.94 mmol/L
Hct	45.4%	0.454
TSH	3.0 µU/mL	3.0 mU/L
Urine toxicology	(+) cotinine	

Assessment

Migraine without aura complicated by potential medication adverse effect and/or analgesic medication overuse headache (MOH).

Student Work-Up

Missing Information/Inadequate Data

Evaluate: Patient database

Drug therapy problems

Care plan (by problem)

TARGETED QUESTIONS

1. What signs and symptoms allow the practitioner to differentiate this as migraine HA without aura from others, such as migraine HA with aura or cluster headache?

   Hint: See pp. 836-837 in PPP

2. What lifestyle issues, medical comorbidities, or medication therapies may be contributing to the development and/or perpetuation of HA symptoms, as well as potentially complicate therapy in this patient?

   Hint: See pp. 537-538 and Table 35-2 in PPP

3. What nonpharmacologic measures or complementary and alternative medicine (CAM) therapies might be recommended to reduce the number of HAs, as well as provide pain relief during an acute HA?

   Hint: See pp. 537-538 in PPP

4. What would you recommend for acute pharmacological therapy, as well as, prophylactic treatment, if applicable?

   Hint: See pp. 538-541 in PPP

5. How will the practitioner assess the outcome of the interventions, assess the need for alterations and/or additions in the chosen treatment regimen?

   Hint: See p. 542 in PPP

6. What risks are assumed with the concurrent use of triptans in patients with hypertension? How would one counsel a patient to monitor and appropriately react to unwanted adverse effects?

   Hint: See p. 539 in PPP

⊙ GLOBAL PERSPECTIVE

Headache is the most common condition seen by neurologists, with tension-type HAs (TTH) being the most common primary HA disorder. Despite its higher prevalence, the societal impact of TTH is much less than that of migraines. Unlike in cluster HAs, females predominate in chronic TTH and migraine cohorts compared to males. The peak incidence of all three HA types occurs in the middle-aged, with some data suggesting that attacks diminish with age. Complementary and alternative medicine (CAM) approaches to HA treatment and prevention are more commonly employed in non-Western societies, with acupuncture demonstrating benefit in limiting headache frequency in clinical trials. Multiple herbal remedies are purported to have analgesic, antispasmodic, and anxiolytic properties that might be beneficial for sufferers of tension-type HAs: feverfew, valerian, and chamomile are frequently mentioned. Herbal therapies must be used cautiously when prescription drugs are employed, so as to avoid adverse pharmacokinetic or pharmacodynamic interactions, such as the serotonin interactions with the concurrent use of St. John's Wort and triptans or the increased bleeding risk of OTC NSAIDs and ginko.

CASE SUMMARY

- The clinical presentation is most consistent with migraine without aura: unilateral, pulsating, moderate-to-severe pain accompanied with N/V and photophobia. There is no discernable transient focal neurological symptoms, thus the patient does not an associated aura. The presence of the HAs prior to initiation of nifedipine and overuse of OTC analgesics further supports this diagnosis.

- The daily use of analgesic agents may be complicating definitive diagnostic classification, as unrestrained pain medication use lead to the so-called MOH. Analgesic withdrawal may be difficult and protracted in MOH cases. The recent addition of a medication known to cause HAs (nifedipine) only further complicates the definitive diagnosis.

- The patient's comorbidities and current medication use may complicate the choice of therapeutic options to limit HA frequency and severity, his HTN and need for multiple HTN medications for instance. But they may also serve to direct drug and nonpharmacologic choices, so that the targeted HA therapies chosen benefit the other conditions as well, such as the use of a different antihypertensive for his HTN or stress-reducing massage therapy for his self-reported anxiety.

- An accurate and up-to-date medication reconciliation, including OTC, herbal, and other nonprescription therapies, is vitally important to minimize the risk of potential drug-drug, drug-disease, and drug-food interactions.

For more information on the care plan and facilitator's guide please visit http://www.mhpharmacotherapy.com

38 Alzheimer's Disease

Megan J. Ehret   Kevin W. Chamberlin

PATIENT PRESENTATION

Chief Complaint

"I want out of here."

History of Present Illness

John Smith is a 75-year-old widowed man who presents to the emergency department (ED) from his skilled nursing facility. He does not have any other information when brought to the ED except that he wants out of here and wants to return home to his mother. The skilled nursing facility staff who presents with Mr. Smith states that Mr. Smith has been a resident of the skilled nursing facility for the past 5 years. He has Alzheimer's disease, for which he has been treated with donepezil and memantine. The staff has noticed that recently Mr. Smith has become more aggressive, physically assaulting a staff member earlier in the day while the staff member was trying to bathe Mr. Smith. Mr. Smith has been verbally assaultive as well, constantly yelling at the staff to take him home and let him out of this place. He appears to spend more time pacing around the facility as well.

Past Medical History

Alzheimer's disease (5 years ago)

HTN (16 years)

Depression (10 years)

GERD (12 years)

Urinary incontinence (2 years)

Unsteady gait (with history of two falls in last year)

Osteoporosis (with rib fracture history from fall)

Osteoarthritis, diagnosed at age 62

BPH, diagnosed at age 59

Hearing loss (left ear worse than right)

Vitamin B12 deficiency, diagnosed at age 67

Family History

Unable to obtain from patient

Social/Work History

Has two children who live in the area who visit the patient on a weekly basis according to the skilled nursing staff member

Tobacco/Alcohol/Substance Use

Denies smoking and alcohol use

Allergy/Intolerance/Adverse Event History

Rivastigmine Patch 4.6 mg/day: red, itchy rash from the patch adhesive

Medication History

▶ Current Medications at Skilled Nursing Facility

Donepezil 10 mg po once daily

Memantine 20 mg po twice daily

Mirtazapine 7.5 mg po once daily

Pantoprazole 40 mg po once daily

Amlodipine 10 mg po once daily

Tamsulosin 0.8 mg po once daily

Senna-S 2 tablets po daily at bedtime

Calcium carbonate 500 mg po twice daily

Tolterodine LA 4 mg po once daily

Acetaminophen 650 mg po every 6 hours

Cyanocobalamin 1000 mcg IM injection each month

Finasteride 5 mg po once daily

▶ Medications Administered in the ED

Haloperidol 2.5 mg po once

▶ Prior Medication Use

Rivastigmine patch 4.6 mg/day × 2 weeks; discontinued due to rash

Review of Systems

Appears angry and unable to answer many questions regarding why he was brought to the ED. (−) history of seizures, head injuries, or loss of consciousness, (+) symptoms of dementia

Physical Exam

▶ General

Moderately disheveled Caucasian male who is angry

▶ *Vital Signs*

BP 163/72, P 92, RR 22, T 36.5°C

▶ *Skin*

Moist skin; (–) rashes or lesions

▶ *HEENT*

PERRLA, EMOI; (–) sinus tenderness, ear examination deferred

▶ *Neck and Lymph Nodes*

Normal

▶ *Chest*

Clear to auscultation

▶ *Breast*

Examination deferred

▶ *Cardiovascular*

RRR, normal S_1, S_2, (–) S_3 or S_4

▶ *Abdomen*

Examination deferred

▶ *Neurology*

Folstein Mini-Mental State Examination score (MMSE) 17/30; unable to state the date and day of the week, unable to state hospital name and location in the hospital, unable to recall 3 items, unable to completely spell word backward, unable to complete the paper task, and unable to copy the picture.

▶ *Extremities*

Examination deferred

▶ *Genitourinary*

Examination deferred; patient had odor of urine-saturated clothes

▶ *Rectal*

Examination deferred

Laboratory and Other Diagnostic Tests

	Conventional Units	SI Units
Na	140 mEq/L	140 mmol/L
K	4.2 mEq/L	4.2 mmol/L
Cl	100 mEq/L	100 mmol/L
CO_2	24 mEq/L	24 mmol/L
BUN	13 mg/dL	2.9 mmol/L
SCr	0.9 mg/dL	80 μmol/L
Glu	140 mg/dL	8.3 mmol/L
Vitamin B_{12}	600 pg/mL	443 pmol/L
ALT	20 IU/L	0.33 μkat/L
AST	18 IU/L	0.30 μkat/L
TSH	3.1 μIU/mL	3.1 mIU/L
Free T_4	1.1 ng/dL	14.2 pmol/L

Assessment:

Seventy-five-year-old man with s/s consistent with behavioral disturbances associated with dementia of the Alzheimer's type.

Student Work-Up

Missing Information/Inadequate Data

Evaluate: Patient database

Drug therapy problems

Care plan (by problem)

TARGETED QUESTIONS

1. What signs and symptoms of Alzheimer's disease does the patient have?

   Hint: See pp. 452-453 in PPP

2. Would an increase to 23 mg/day on the donepezil dose be an appropriate choice for this patient?

   Hint: See p. 454 in PPP

3. What are the nonpharmacological treatment options for the behavioral symptoms this patient is experiencing?

   Hint: See p. 454 in PPP

4. What are the pharmacological treatment options for the behavioral symptoms this patient is experiencing?

   Hint: See p. 457 in PPP

5. What are the risks and adverse effects of the pharmacological treatment of the behavioral symptoms you would discuss with the caregivers?

   Hint: See p. 457 in PPP

🌏 GLOBAL PERSPECTIVE

Minorities tend to be underrepresented in many clinical trials of Alzheimer's disease. Many times this can be due to exclusion criteria including high levels of comorbidity among minorities and the inability to speak English. Additionally, past research including the Tuskegee Syphilis Study have left many not wanting to participate in research trials. Some barriers to participation include child- and elder-care costs and travel expenses to and from the research site. Factors to consider when attempting to increase the diversity of a trial include choice of the study site and the proximity of the research location to places where minorities live and work. Additionally, recruitment materials should be altered to increase participation from those underrepresented. Information on the trial should be included in direct invitations to minority populations.

CASE SUMMARY

- JS's current clinical picture is consistent with behavioral disturbances due to dementia of the Alzheimer's type.

- Nonpharmacological treatment should be considered first line at aid in the treatment of these symptoms.
- Antipsychotics can be considered if needed to help treat these neuropsychiatric symptoms.

For more information on the care plan and facilitator's guide please visit http://www.mhpharmacotherapy.com

39 Alcohol Withdrawal

Krina H. Patel

PATIENT PRESENTATION

Chief Complaint

"I'm going through withdrawal and I need help!"

History of Present Illness

Bill Smith is a 41-year-old male who has a history of alcoholism. Bill has been struggling with alcoholism since the age of 20. Bill has been through periods in his life where he was able to maintain abstinence from alcohol, however has also had periods where he has relapsed. Bill has maintained sobriety for the past 2 years however relapsed about 3 months ago. Yesterday morning, Bill's wife and children decided to leave him due to his alcoholism. Right after his family left, Bill drank heavily for several hours. He also found a bottle of his wife's hydrocodone/ibuprofen tablets, and he decided to take a couple pills of along with the alcohol. Bill then came to realization that he needs to change his life to have a relationship with his family and has not had a drink since yesterday evening.

Past Medical History

Alcohol dependence (21 years)

Depression (15 years)

HTN (5 months)

GERD (6 years)

Family History

Maternal grandmother had a history of depression. Mother is 72 and has a diagnosis of dyslipidemia, osteoporosis, and was recently diagnosed with breast cancer. His father left his family at the age of 4. He has a brother who committed suicide due to depression 5 years ago. Has a younger sister who has a diagnosis of hypothyroidism.

Social History

History of alcohol dependence for 21 years. During his 21 years of alcoholism, the patient has had numerous relapses. Patient was sober for the past two years until about 3 months ago. His wife of 10 years along with his 9-year-old son and 7-year-old daughter left him yesterday. He remains to live in his home by himself. Currently, he works as a car salesman, however he has missed a substantial amount of work over the past few months.

Tobacco/Alcohol/Substance Use

Denies tobacco use; drinks a half bottle of whiskey along with 1-2 bottles of red wine daily; denies use of recreational drugs; denies abuse of prescription medications with the exception of the one-time episode of taking his wife's hydrocodone/ibuprofen.

Allergies/Intolerances/Adverse Drug Events

Penicillin

Medications (Prior to Admission)

Sertraline 300 mg po daily

Atenolol 50 mg po daily

Omeprazole 20 mg po daily

Review of Systems

(−) chest pain, (+) tachycardia, (+) nausea, (−) vomiting, (+) tremors, (−) seizures, (−) hallucinations, (−) delusions, (−) headache, (−) insomnia, (+) increased depression, (+) decreased energy, (−) appetite changes, (−) suicidal ideations

Physical Exam

▶ **General**

Forty-one-year-old Caucasian male appears disheveled and moderately distressed.

▶ **Vital Signs**

BP 146/96 mm Hg, P 110, RR 18, T 36.7°C

Weight 145 lb. (65.8 kg)

Height 67 in. (170 cm)

Denies Pain

▶ **Skin**

(−) rash or lesions

▶ **HEENT**

PERRLA, EOMI

▶ **Neck and Lymph Nodes**

(−) lymphadenopathy

► **Chest**

Lung clear to auscultation

► **Cardiovascular**

Tachycardia, RRR, (–) murmurs, rubs or gallops

► **Abdomen**

Normal bowel sounds, (+) hepatosplenomegaly, (–) abdominal pain

► **Neurology**

(+) tremors, (–) seizure, (–) hallucinations, (–) delirium, A&O × 3

► **Genitourinary**

Exam deferred

► **Rectal**

Exam deferred

Laboratory Tests

	Conventional Units	SI Units
Na	136 mEq/L	136 mmol/L
K	3.6 mEq/L	3.6 mmol/L
Cl	105 mEq/L	105 mmol/L
CO_2	23 mEq/L	23 mmol/L
BUN	10 mg/dL	3.6 mmol/L
SCr	0.8 mg/dL	70.7 µmol/L
CrCl	110 mL/min	1.06 mL/s/m²
Glu	98 mg/dL	5.4 mmol/L
Ca	9.0 mg/dL	2.25 mmol/L
Mg	2.1 mEq/L	1.05 mmol/L
Phosphate	4.3 mg/dL	1.39 mmol/L
Albumin	3.5 g/dL	35 g/L
PT	12.0 sec	
Platelet	220 × 10³/mm³	220 × 10³/mm³
GGT	110 IU/L	1.8 µkat/L
LDH	200 IU/L	3.3 µkat/L
AST	250 IU/L	4.17 µkat/L
ALT	123 IU/L	2.05 µkat/L
Alk phos	128 IU/L	2.1 µkat/L
Total bilirubin	0.7 mg/dL	11.97 µmol/L
Direct bilirubin	0.2 mg/L	3.42 µmol/L
Ammonia	30 mcg/dL	17.62 µmol/L

Assessment

Forty-one-year-old male with current signs, symptoms and laboratory tests consistent with alcohol withdrawal. His current CIWA-Ar score is 22.

TARGETED QUESTIONS

1. What signs and symptoms of alcohol withdrawal is Bill currently experiencing?

    Hint: See Table 36-4 in PPP

2. What are the treatment goals for alcohol withdrawal?

    Hint: See pp. 552-553 in PPP

3. What is the CIWA-Ar and how can it be utilized for this patient?

    Hint: See Table 36-2 in PPP

4. What is the treatment of choice for the management of alcohol withdrawal?

    Hint: See pp. 552-553 in PPP

5. Does this patient require treatment for opioid intoxication or withdrawal? What measures should be taken with regards to the opioid intoxication/withdrawal?

    Hint: See p. 549 in PPP

FOLLOW-UP

It is a few days later and Bill is ready to be discharged from the hospital and go back to his home. Bill is no longer experiencing any withdrawal symptoms and is doing much better. During his stay at the hospital, Bill realized that he needs to remain abstinent to improve his relationship with his family and to maintain a job. Bill understands the importance of abstinence, however he knows that once he returns home he will most likely experiencing the urge to drink. He states his intention is not to drink, however he is not sure if can abstain from alcohol.

What nonpharmacologic and pharmacologic treatment options for alcohol abstinence are available for Bill?

Hint: See pp. 555-557 in PPP

⟳ GLOBAL PERSPECTIVE

Alcohol consumption is not only a concern in the United States but it is also concern across the globe. According to the World Health Organization's Global Status Report on Alcohol[1], there were 3.3 million deaths or 5.9% of global deaths were alcohol related in 2012. The incidence of alcohol use does vary depending on the country and other factors. For example, countries with greater economic wealth had higher rates of alcohol consumption and lower rates of abstinence. Other environmental factors also can have an influence on alcohol consumption such as culture, availability of alcohol, and the effectiveness of alcohol policies. Globally, consequences associated with alcohol use are a concern. Alcohol use is not only associated with health problems such as liver cirrhosis, cancers, and cardiovascular diseases, but can also lead to mental and behavioral disorders. In addition, violence and motor vehicle accidents are also concerning consequences associated with alcohol consumption. Overall, it is important to keep in mind that the use of alcohol is not only a major concern within the United States, but also is a challenge globally.

CASE SUMMARY

- The patient requires treatment for alcohol withdrawal since he exhibitis signs and symptoms of withdrawal.

- Benzodiazepine treatment should be initiated for alcohol withdrawal. In addition, this patient should also receive thiamine supplementation.
- The patient should be evaluated for medication adherence to his current medications.
- Consider treatment options for abstinence once the patient has gone through the withdrawal phase.

KEY REFERENCE/READING

1. World Health Organization. Global Status Report on Alcohol and Health 2014. Geneva: WHO, 2014.

For more information on the care plan and facilitator's guide please visit http://www.mhpharmacotherapy.com

40 Schizophrenia

Heidi J. Wehring   Deanna L. Kelly

PATIENT PRESENTATION

Chief Complaint

"I don't belong here. I didn't bother anyone."

History of Present Illness

Jerry Chase is a 33-year-old man who was brought to the emergency department (ED) overnight by police. He lives in a group home, but hasn't gone back there for 6 days because "my roommate is a demon and he put a curse on my pillow to take my thoughts." Jerry was arrested for trespassing when he wouldn't leave a shed where he'd been squatting for about a week. Prior to his visit to the shed, he had been on his way to a doctor's appointment when a voice spoke to him at the bus stop, telling him to "go, go, get away now." He wandered across the city and found an unlocked shed. Jerry is afraid that his roommate wants to harm him, and became so agitated when the police tried to drop him off at the group home that he was brought to the hospital. He spent all the money he had in his pockets on food the first couple of days while staying in the shed, and presents to the hospital as unkempt, malodorous, and hungry. He is upset about being hospitalized. When contacted, the group home supervisor stated that Jerry's roommate is a mild-mannered older gentleman and there have been no behavioral or interpersonal complaints about him from any staff or other residents.

Past Medical History

Jerry was diagnosed with schizophrenia at the age of 24 while attempting to join the U.S. Army. His symptoms resulted in his first psychiatric hospitalization before he could start basic training. He has been hospitalized 6 times since this first hospitalization for recurrent symptoms of schizophrenia. The last hospitalization was for a period of 7 months, after which he was accepted into the group home approximately 5 months ago. Per the hospital report, Jerry had responded well to asenapine and his symptoms were greatly diminished, however, he has not been doing well since a few weeks after the discharge. He continues to have a prescription for asenapine, but has also had taken quetiapine and haloperidol in the past. Prior to leaving the group home, staff members state that Jerry had been adherent to the asenapine, stating "He always pops it right in his mouth and swallows it right away with a big gulp of orange juice. I wish all our clients took their meds that easy!"

Family History

Jerry reports no known family history of mental illness; however, he is estranged from his parents so they are unavailable for collection of family history. Jerry is allegedly an only child.

Social/Work History

Jerry is a single, never-married man who lives in a group home. He reports being a good student up through middle school before "going a different way" in high school. He started having difficulty with schoolwork, and had trouble getting along with his parents. He eventually saw a school psychologist due to parental concerns. He reports a past history of a having a girlfriend in his early 20's, but they broke up during his first episode of psychotic symptoms and he reports no subsequent romantic relationships. This doesn't seem to bother him. Jerry has not been employed in a paid position since he was first hospitalized at age 24, but volunteers at a local library through a program related to his group home.

Tobacco/Alcohol/Substance Use

Jerry denies any current alcohol use; smokes cigarettes and/or marijuana "when I can afford it."

Allergies/Intolerances/Adverse Drug Events

He reports an "allergy" to haloperidol, but states, "I don't want to talk about it."

Medication History

Current: Asenapine 10 mg bid

Prior: Quetiapine and haloperidol, duration and response unknown

Review of Systems

(−) History of head injury or loss of consciousness; (−) tinnitus, vertigo, or infections; (−) history of seizures or syncope

Physical Examination

▶ *General*

Disheveled and unkempt, appears older than stated age, somewhat agitated but in no physical distress

▶ *Vital Signs*

BP 150/84 mm Hg, P 74, RR 14, T 36.8°C

Weight 167 lb. (75.8 kg)

Height 67 in. (170.2 cm)

Denies pain

▶ *Skin*

Oily-appearing skin and scalp; (–) rashes or lesions

▶ *HEENT*

PERRLA, EOMI

▶ *Neck and Lymph Nodes*

(–) Thyroid nodules; (–) lymphadenopathy; (–) carotid bruits

▶ *Chest*

Clear to auscultation

▶ *Cardiovascular*

RRR, normal S_1, S_2

▶ *Abdomen*

Not tender, not distended; (–) organomegaly

▶ *Neurology*

Grossly intact; DTRs normal

▶ *Genitourinary*

Examination deferred

▶ *Rectal*

Examination deferred

Laboratory Tests

Fasting, Obtained STAT in ED

	Conventional Units	SI Units
Na	146 mEq/L	146 mmol/L
K	4.8 mEq/L	4.8 mmol/L
Cl	102 mEq/L	102 mmol/L
CO_2	24 mEq/L	24 mmol/L
BUN	9 mg/dL	3.2 mmol/L
SCr	0.9 mg/dL	80 μmol/L
Glu	98 mg/dL	5.4 mmol/L
Ca	9.6 mg/dL	2.40 mmol/L
Mg	1.6 mEq/L	0.66 mmol/L
Phosphate	4.1 mg/dL	1.32 mmol/L
Hgb	13.7 g/dL (127 g/L)	7.88 mmol/L
Hct	40.6%	0.403

WBC	5.6×10^3/mm³	5.6×10^9/L
MCV	80 μm³	80 fL
Albumin	4.3 g/dL	43 g/L
Total cholesterol	195 mg/dL	5.04 mmol/L

Mental Status Examination

Jerry is a 33-year-old male of average build, appearing older than stated age, disheveled, unkempt, malodorous, and wearing inappropriately layered clothes. He is somewhat guarded in conversation, but will answer some questions when asked. He frequently states that he doesn't need to be in the hospital and that he doesn't want to talk about certain topics. He makes intermittent eye contact but spends the majority of the interview time looking around the room. When asked, he states this is because he is worried that there may be devices hidden that would record and broadcast what he says back to his roommate. Jerry describes his mood as "just fine." His range of affect is somewhat blunted but he appears worried and somewhat agitated. He is alert and oriented to person, place, and time. Intellectual functioning appears average, although, at times, it is difficult to assess due to his tendency to become distracted during the interview. Thought processes are coherent and goal directed; however, his conclusions that his roommate has planted listening devices in the interview room and that his thoughts are being broadcast are not logical. Prominent delusions are apparent, including his beliefs about his roommate. Jerry endorses periodic command auditory hallucinations. He denies suicidal or homicidal ideation. His insight and judgment are poor.

Assessment

Thirty-three-year old man with signs and symptoms consistent with schizophrenia.

Student Work-Up

Missing Information/Inadequate Data

Evaluate: Patient database

Drug therapy problems

Care plan (by problem)

TARGETED QUESTIONS

1. What signs and symptoms of schizophrenia does the patient have?

   Hint: See pp. 564-565 pp. 54-55 in PPP

2. What types of information would you want to have in order to make decisions about pharmacologic treatment options?

   Hint: See pp. 565-566, Figure 37-1 in PPP

3. What pharmacologic options are available for the treatment of Jerry's symptoms of psychosis? What changes, if any, would you consider making to his medication regimen?

   Hint: See pp. 565-570, Table 37-2, Table 37-4 in PPP

4. Which of the options from above would you recommend for Jerry, including titration schedule and monitoring plan, and why?

   Hint: See Tables 37-2, 37-4, pp. 565-570 in PPP

5. What risks and adverse effects of therapy would you discuss with the patient?

   Hint: See pp. 576-570 and Tables 37-3, 37-6 in PPP

FOLLOW-UP

Two years later, you happen to see Jerry at an outpatient clinic where you work. He is sitting in a chair, with a grimacing look on his face and rhythmically pursing his lips. His body seems to be swaying slightly back and forth. Later in the day, you are brought in to consult on Jerry's clinical case. You discover that after being discharged from your hospital 2 years prior, he was placed on fluphenzaine. His doctors have been trying to decrease his fluphenazine dose the past 6 months due to side effects, but his delusions are getting worse and they are trying to find alternative options. You learn that his history has been documented as treatment failures on aripiprazole, asenapine, haloperidol (side effects), olanzapine, and ziprasidone.

Given Jerry's history of symptoms, side effects, and past treatment options, what pharmacotherapy changes would you recommend, if any?

   Hint: See pp. 575-576 PPP

☉ GLOBAL PERSPECTIVE

Schizophrenia is present worldwide. However, when assessing for the signs and symptoms of schizophrenia (delusions, hallucinations, etc.), it is important to take cultural and religious beliefs into consideration as what is considered within the norm for a certain ethnic group may not be considered within normal limits for another. Differences in response to antipsychotic treatment may exist due to differences in genetic makeup of persons with schizophrenia, from both an efficacy and adverse effect standpoint, although information is limited. Antipsychotic medications are the treatment of choice for schizophrenia; however, the particular agents available in various countries may differ. In addition, the treatment algorithms may differ widely depending on the location of treatment.

CASE SUMMARY

- Jerry's current clinical picture is consistent with the symptoms of schizophrenia and warrants continued treatment with antipsychotic medication.

- Current and past medication trials, as well as patient-specific variables, will contribute to the pharmacotherapy plan for this patient.

- Upon his presentation to the clinic 2 years later, with the knowledge of side effects, decompensation, and treatment failure of several antipsychotic medications, a change in treatment may be warranted.

For more information on the care plan and facilitator's guide please visit http://www.mhpharmacotherapy.com

41 Depression

Cherry W. Jackson   Nicole Slater

PATIENT PRESENTATION

Chief Complaint

"Everyone in my life would be better off if I weren't around anymore."

History of Present Illness

Mr. Jones is a 61-year-old white male who presents to the primary care clinic for an annual follow-up. His main complaint is that he "doesn't want to be around anymore." He was diagnosed with depression several years ago after he lost his job and had to move out of his home. Lately, he has been feeling "on edge," and has started drinking more alcohol to help him feel relaxed. Over the last 6 weeks he's experienced crying spells, insomnia, loss of appetite, isolative behaviors, and he feels like he is a burden to everyone in his life. He was diagnosed with depression 3 years ago that was controlled on citalopram. He was initiated on treatment for atrial fibrillation about 2 months ago and was told to follow-up with his primary care doctor for further evaluation of his depression and current medications, but he was unable to keep his appointments.

Past Medical History

Atrial fibrillation (diagnosed 4 months ago)
Hypothyroidism (diagnosed 7 years ago)
Hypertension (diagnosed 15 years ago)
Depression (diagnosed 3 years ago)

Family History

Mother suffered from depression and alcohol abuse, she passed away at age 69 from end stage liver disease. Father has hypertension, diabetes and bipolar disorder.

Social History

Patient is divorced. He has 3 daughters and 6 grandchildren. He is a retired college professor. He currently lives alone.

Tobacco/Alcohol/Substance Abuse

Patient does not smoke cigarettes; however he does have a history of marijuana abuse. He drinks 5-6 beers per day and has 3-4 shots of vodka every evening.

Allergies/Intolerances/Adverse Drug Events

HCTZ (rash)

Medications (Current)

Amlodipine 10 mg po daily
Rivaroxaban 20 mg po daily
Flecanide 100 mg po q 12 hours
Levothyroxine 125 mcg po daily
Tramadol 50 mg po as needed up to 4 times daily
Ibuprofen 600 mg po 4 times daily

Prior Medication Use

Venlafaxine 150 mg daily (discontinued due to uncontrolled blood pressure)

Review of Systems

▶ **Cardiovascular**

Denies chest pain, pressure or discomfort. No edema or palpitations.

▶ **Gastrointestinal**

No anorexia, nausea, vomiting, diarrhea, denies abdominal pain. History of GI bleed approximately 2.5 years ago

▶ **Musculoskeletal**

Denies muscle, back pain, joint pain or stiffness

▶ **Psychiatric**

Chronic depressed mood, poor sleep, minimal appetite, isolative behaviors, suicidal ideation, anxiety.

▶ **Endocrine**

Cold intolerance, dry skin, fatigue, constipation

Physical Exam

▶ **Vital Signs**

BP 118/78 mm Hg, P 70, RR 17, T 36.3°C
Weight 205 lb. (92.9 kg)
Height 66.93 in. (173 cm)
BMI 32.1

Mental Status Examination

Appearance

Patient appears to be older than stated age wearing dirty clothes and smells strongly of aftershave and alcohol. He does not make direct eye contact and is tearful during the discussion.

▶ Movement/Behavior

Appears anxious, rubbing hands together, responds and moves slowly.

▶ Speech

Speech is very slow, monotone, and responds with minimal explanation to questions.

▶ Mood and Affect

The patient is sad and pessimistic, with anxiety and a flat affect

▶ Thought Content

Denies paranoia, hallucinations, delusions, compulsions, obsessions, phobias, or homicidal ideations. He often thinks of dying to put fewer burdens on his family and states "my wife moved on without me, I don't have anything to live for." He reports having a passive death wish, but he does not have a plan to commit suicide at this time.

▶ Cognition

A&O × 3. The patient has poor concentration, and is tearful and distracted throughout the interview, but he could perform serial 7's. His memory is intact. Difficulty with abstract reasoning, evidenced by the meaning of the question "people in glass houses shouldn't throw stones" he stated that if you throw rocks at a glass house it will probably break.

▶ Judgement/Insight

The patient has poor insight and judgment. He states that although he currently has no plan for suicide, at some point "suicide may be the only way out."

Laboratory Tests

	Conventional units	SI Units
Na	140 mEq/L	140 mmol/L
K	3.8 mEq/L	3.8 mmol/L
Cl	103 mEq/L	103 mmol/L
CO_2	25 mEq/L	25 mmol/L
BUN	10 mg/dL	3.57 mmol/L
SCr	0.78 mg/dL	69 μmol/L
Glu	102 mg/dL	5.66 mmol/L
Ca	8.8 mg/dL	2.2 mmol/L
Mg	1.9 mg/dL	0.78 mmol/L
PO_4	2.8 mg/dL	0.9 mmol/L
Hgb	14.4 g/dL	8.9 mmol/L
Hct	43.2%	0.432
MCV	6.2 um³	6.2 fL
WBC	$6.2 \times 10^3/mm^3$	$6.2 \times 10^9/L$
Albumin	4.6 g/dL	46 g/L
Bili (total)	0.6 mg/dL	10.26 μmol/L
Bili (direct)	0.1 mg/dL	1.71 μmol/L
AST	25 U/L	0.42 μkat/L
ALT	17 U/L	0.28 μkat/L
Alk Phos	42 IU/L	0.7 u/kat/L
Total cholesterol	236 mg/dL	6.1 mmol/L
LDL cholesterol	152 mg/dL	3.93 mmol/L
HDL cholesterol	42 mg/dL	1.1 mmol/L
Triglycerides	209 mg/dL	2.36 mmol/L
TSH	7.9 uU/mL	7.9 mU/L

Assessment

Sixty-one-year old man with symptoms indicative of major depressive disorder (MDD).

Student Work-Up

Missing Information/Inadequate Data

Evaluate: Patient database

Drug therapy problems

Care plan (by problem)

TARGETED QUESTIONS

1. What symptoms and clinical features of MDD does the patient have?

   Hint: See Table 38-1, p. 584 in PPP

2. What real or potential drug therapy problems has this patient experienced?

   Hint: See Table 38-3, pp. 587-589 in PPP

3. What questions do you have about the patient's depression treatment? How would you treat his depression now?

   Hint: See Figure 38-1, pp. 589-593 in PPP

4. How do you treat partial response to an antidepressant?

   Hint: See pp. 589-593 in PPP

5. What is the time course of response for antidepressant therapy and what is the response rate with antidepressants?

   Hint: See p. 589 in PPP

6. What if the patient was initiated on Robitussin DM for cough?

Hint: See p. 589 in PPP

🌐 GLOBAL PERSPECTIVE

Depression is a common mental disorder that presents with a depressed mood, loss of interest or pleasure, feelings of guilt, low self-esteem, sleep and appetite disturbances, low energy, and poor concentration. These problems become chronic and recurrent, and may lead to substantial impairment in an individual's ability to care for his or her daily responsibilities. At its worst, depression can lead to suicide, with the loss of about 850,000 lives every year.

Depression in the year 2000 was the leading cause of disability worldwide as measured by years lived with disability (YLD) and the fourth leading contributor to the global burden of disease on the basis of disability adjusted life—years (DALY's).[1] By the year 2020, depression is projected to reach second place of the rankings of DALYs calculated for all ages, and both sexes. Today, depression is already the second cause of DALYs worldwide in the age category 15-44 years for both sexes combines. According to the World Health Organization, fewer than 25% of depressed patients have access to care and in some countries the rate is less than 10%. Barriers to effective care include lack of resources and trained providers, and the social stigma associated with mental disorders, including depression.

REFERENCE

1. World Health Organization. http://apps.who.int/gb/ebwha/pdf_files/WHA65/A65_R4-en.pdf. Accessed May 1, 2015.

CASE SUMMARY

- The patient's clinical picture is consistent with MDD, and an antidepressant medication should be used.
- The patient's adherence with current antidepressant therapy needs to be assessed.
- His NSAID use must be reassessed since he is anticoagulated.

For more information on the care plan and facilitator's guide please visit http://www.mhpharmacotherapy.com

42 Bipolar Disorder

Brian L. Crabtree

PATIENT PRESENTATION

Chief Complaint

"My mind's going too fast."

History of Present Illness

Leon N. is a 28-year-old man who has been admitted to the psychiatric service of a community hospital. He has been sleeping little, some nights staying up all night, yelling and saying he is communicating with God. He is accompanied by his girlfriend who says Leon has been "hyper" over the past few weeks, speaks rapidly, and changes the subject of conversation constantly. He has been irritable, talks about "seeing into the future" and other special powers. Leon admits, "I have trouble with my nerves and I don't sleep."

Past Medical History

Leon had all of the usual childhood illnesses. He has a history of psychiatric illness with two previous hospitalizations dating to 2006, but this is the first admission to this hospital and none of the previous records are immediately available. He says he sometimes attends a clinic at a community mental health center where he sees a nurse practitioner or physician.

He has a history of hypertension (HTN) but denies other health problems.

Family History

Father healthy, except HTN, well controlled on medication. Mother has depression, takes paroxetine. Leon has 3 siblings, 2 brothers and 1 sister. One brother is alcoholic.

Social History

He lives with a girlfriend, never married, and has no children. Unemployed; worked previously as a salesman as a shoe store, but has not worked in the past 6 months. Says, "God will provide." High school graduate, but has difficulty with reading and writing. Receives Medicaid coverage. No pending legal problems. No special diet. No regular exercise program.

Tobacco/Alcohol/Substance Use

Occasional binge-drinking episodes. Smokes 1 ppd with approximately 12 pack-year history. Denies illicit substances. Drinks several cups of caffeinated coffee daily.

Allergies/Intolerances/Adverse Drug Events

Diazepam (nausea and vomiting after injection) during a previous hospitalization

Divalproex (claims his hair became thin and changed color)

Medications

Citalopram 20 mg po daily × 6 months, started during a previous hospitalization

Clonazepam 0.5 mg po 3 times daily × 1 month, started during an outpatient clinic visit

HCTZ 25 mg po daily × 4 years

Acetaminophen 500 mg po as needed, about twice weekly

Previously treated with olanzapine 20 mg po at bedtime, divalproex 750 mg po twice daily, stopped when last hospitalized 7 months ago. Denies other prescription and nonprescription medication

Denies herbal or other complementary and alternative therapies

Review of Systems

The patient says he feels "alive and on fire" and is impatient with people who do not listen to his ideas. (–) Headaches or dizziness, but states dizziness was a problem when he took divalproex in the past. No history of asthma or other lung disease. Says he had a TB skin test recently, but does not know results. (–) Chest pain, palpitations, or heart disease other than HTN. Appetite has been less lately. "I don't need to eat. I have natural energy." Denies weight loss. (–) Genitourinary complaints. Says some of the medications interfere with his sexual ability, which is bothersome to him. (–) History of sexually transmitted diseases. (–) Neuromuscular complaints. Says "strength is getting better every day."

Physical Examination

▶ General

Well-developed, well-nourished Caucasian male in no acute distress; appears stated age, disheveled, mildly obese

▶ Vital Signs

BP 154/105 mm Hg sitting, P 102, RR 22, T 97.9°F (36.6°C)

Weight 197 lb. (89.5 kg)

Height 66 in. (168 cm)

Denies pain

► **Skin**

Unremarkable

► **HEENT**

PERRLA, EOMI; discs sharp, AV nicking noted; TMs normal, normal hearing to conversational volume; a few missing teeth

► **Neck and Lymph Nodes**

Supple; (–) thyromegaly, JVD, or lymphadenopathy

► **Chest**

Clear to auscultation

► **Breasts**

Unremarkable

► **Cardiovascular**

Tachycardia, RRR, no murmurs, rubs, or gallops

► **Abdomen**

Nontender, nondistended, (+) bowel sounds, (–) hepatosplenomegaly

► **Neurology**

Mental status—mood is elevated, slightly irritable, affect is animated; speech is loud and pushed; thoughts indicate flight of ideas, looseness of associations, ideas of reference, delusions; reports he feels he possesses special powers of healing and predicting the future; says he receives special messages from God through radio or television; denies auditory and visual hallucinations; denies suicidal and homicidal ideas; alert and oriented to person, year, not place; mild deficits in long- and short-term memory; concentration poor; judgment poor; insight poor.

Cranial nerves II to XII grossly intact; normal gait; (–) nystagmus, facial weakness, tremor; DTRs normal.

► **Genitourinary**

Deferred

► **Rectal**

Deferred

Laboratory Tests

Urine for toxicology collected the day of hospital admission; ECG and blood obtained fasting at 6:30 AM day after admission.

	Conventional Units	SI Units
Na	137 mEq/L	137 mmol/L
K	3.5 mEq/L	3.5 mmol/L
Cl	100 mEq/L	100 mmol/L
CO_2/HCO_3	24 mEq/L	24 mmol/L
BUN	12 mg/dL	4.3 mmol/L
SCr	0.9 mg/dL	80 μmol/L
Cr Clearance	123 mL/min	2.05 mL/s
Glu	108 mg/dL	6.0 mmol/L
Ca	10.2 mg/dL	2.55 mmol/L
Mg	1.6 mEq/L	0.8 mmol/L
PO_4	3.8 mg/dL	1.23 mmol/L
Hgb	15.9 g/dL	159 g/L; 9.87 mmol/L
Hct	46.7%	0.467
MCV	88 μm³	88 fL
WBC	$9.7 \times 10^3/mm^3$	$9.7 \times 109/L$
WBC Differential	65/1/1/25/8	
Platelets	$283 \times 10^3/mm^3$	$283 \times 109/L$
Albumin	4.2 g/dL	42 g/L
Total bilirubin	1.0 mg/dL	17.1 μmol/L
Bilirubin (direct)	0.1 mg/dL	1.71 μmol/L
AST	48 IU/L	0.8 μkat/L
ALT	54 IU/L	0.9 μkat/L
Alkaline phosphatase	57 IU/L	0.95 μkat/L
TSH	0.97 μIU/mL	
Urine toxicology	(+) benzo, cotinine	

Assessment

Bipolar I disorder, most recent episode was manic, with psychotic features; hx of HTN.

Student Work-Up

Missing Information/Inadequate Data

Evaluate: Patient database

Drug therapy problems

Care plan (by problem)

TARGETED QUESTIONS

1. What signs and symptoms of bipolar disorder does this patient have?

   Hint: See pp. 600-603 in PPP

2. What prescribed or nonprescribed drugs could be exacerbating this patient's illness?

   Hint: See Table 39-3 in PPP

3. What is the purpose of the laboratory examination?

   Hint: See Table 39-1 and p. 603 in PPP

4. Should drug therapy be initiated with mood-stabilizing monotherapy, antipsychotic drug monotherapy, or mood-stabilizing and antipsychotic drug combination therapy?

    Hint: See Table 39-2 in PPP

5. What risks of drug therapy would you discuss with this patient when he is appropriate for patient education?

    Hint: See Table 39-4 and p. 615 in PPP

FOLLOW-UP

Drug therapy is initiated with the combination of a mood stabilizer, antipsychotic and antianxiety agent. He responded well to this regimen and his hospital discharge drug therapy regimen was included the antipsychotic and mood stabilizer. He was counseled to moderate caffeine intake. The length of stay in the hospital was 17 days. After 6 months, still feeling well with a generally euthymic mood state, he says he would like to stop medication. He doesn't like having to take it every day and complains he has gained a few pounds. How should he be advised about this issue?

Hint: See p. 615 in PPP

For more information on the care plan and facilitator's guide please visit http://www.mhpharmacotherapy.com

43 Anxiety

Sheila R. Botts

PATIENT PRESENTATION

Chief Complaint

"I'm really stressed and feel like I'm losing it. I'm so tense that I am having trouble sleeping and feel like I'm a time bomb about to explode."

History of Present Illness

Janis Azi is a 24-year-old female who presents to the primary clinic with complaints of nausea, restlessness, fatigue, poor sleep, and headaches. She states that since starting her graduate school program approximately 6 months ago, she has been on edge and worries about everything. She worries about her school performance, paying for her tuition, her father's health, and even her younger brother, who is a freshmen undergraduate at Colorado State University. She states her mother reassures her that everything is "OK" with her dad and brother but she worries about them anyway. She was offered a summer internship program with a pharmaceutical company and is considering not taking it as she feels overwhelmed and is not sure she can manage moving to the east coast for the summer. She reports having a couple of "episodes" while at home studying, where her heart races, she feels shaky, and has difficulty concentrating on her work. This prompted her to seek treatment at an urgent care clinic last month and she was provided a prescription for quetiapine. "They said it would help me sleep and feel less anxious." She also describes being easily startled when someone taps her on the shoulder. This happened in class and she was embarrassed by her response. Janis states she has taken a friend's medication for anxiety a couple of times and that it "calms her immediately." She also reports seeing a therapist for several sessions a couple of months ago with little improvement, so she stopped.

Past Medical History (PMH)

Knee surgery (age 16, ACL tear while playing soccer)

Mild traumatic brain injury (TBI) (age 19 from motor vehicle accident (MVA). Treated with levetiracetam for 1 year)

Mild depression (age 21, resolved with counseling)

Family History

Father has coronary artery disease (CAD) and had myocardial infarction (MI) 3 months ago at age 52. Mother with depression, treated with venlafaxine. Paternal grandfather with alcoholism and a maternal aunt who died at age 60 of suicide.

Social/Work History

Ms. Azi is a graduate student in biomedical engineering at the University of Colorado. She lives alone in a condominium and works part-time as a research assistant in the College of Medicine.

Tobacco/Alcohol/Substance Use

Nonsmoker, ETOH 2-3 drinks daily

Allergy/Intolerance/Adverse Event History

NKDA

Medication History

Levetiracetam 500 mg bid × 12 months for seizure prophylaxis 8 years ago

Quetiapine 25 mg orally twice daily as needed–received 30 days supply from urgent care physician last week

Ibuprofen 400 mg po prn

Review of Systems

Frequent tension headaches relieved by ibuprofen; muscle ache in shoulders; nausea and intermittent loose stools

Physical Examination

▶ **General**

Anxious-appearing 24-year-old woman in no acute distress

▶ **Vital Signs**

BP 130/76 mm Hg, P 88, RR 18, T 37.3°C

Weight 169 lb. (65.9 kg)

Height 65 in. (165 cm)

Denies pain

▶ **Skin**

(–) rashes or lesions

▶ **HEENT**

PERRLA, EOMI; normal fundi; TMs appear normal

▶ **Neck and Lymph Nodes**

Supple, thyroid normal size without nodules; (–) adenopathy

▶ **Chest**

Clear to auscultation

▶ **Breasts**

Exam deferred

▶ **Cardiovascular**

Tachycardia, normal S_1, S_2

▶ **Abdomen**

Not tender/Not distended; (–) organomegaly

▶ **Neurology**

Grossly intact; mild tremor in hands; DTRs normal

▶ **Genitourinary**

Examination deferred

▶ **Rectal**

Examination deferred

Mental Status Examination

A 24-year-old cooperative, casually dressed, well-groomed female. Appears dysphoric and moderately anxious. Speech is normal in rate and volume. Mood is "irritable" and "sometimes down," affect congruent to mood. No apparent delusions or hallucinations. Denies suicidal or homicidal ideation. She appears to have good attention and concentration.

Laboratory Tests

	Conventional Units	SI Units
Na	142 mEq/L	142 mmol/L
K	4.1 mEq/L	4.1 mmol/L
Cl	100 mEq/L	100 mmol/L
CO_2	24 mEq/L	24 mmol/L
BUN	10 mEq/L	3.6 mmol/L
SCr	0.7 mg/dL	62 µmol/L
Glu	98 mg/dL	5.4 mmol/L
AST	55 IU/L	0.91 mkat/L
ALT	28 U/L	0.47 mkat/L
Alk phos	40 IU/L	0.67 mkat/L
Hgb	14.5 g/dL	9.00 mmol/L
Hct	42%	0.42
WBC	$6.8 \times 10^3/\mu L$	$6.8 \times 10^9/L$
Albumin	3.8 g/dL	38 g/L
TSH	1.2 µU/mL	1.2 mU/L

Total Cholesterol	178 mg/dL	4.60 mmol/L
LDL	89 mg/dL	2.30 mmol/L
HDL	36 mg/dL	0.93 mmol/L

Urine pregnancy test (–)

Urine drug screen (+) benzodiazepine

▶ **ECG**

QTc 442 ms

Assessment

▶ **Generalized Anxiety Disorder (GAD)**

Student Work-Up

Missing Information/Inadequate Data

Evaluate: Patient database

Drug therapy problems

Care plan (by problem)

TARGETED QUESTIONS

1. What signs and symptoms of GAD does the patient have?

   Hint: See p. 619 in PPP

2. What nonpharmacological interventions might be useful for this patient?

   Hint: See p. 620 in PPP

3. Why is an antidepressant the drug therapy of choice for GAD?

   Hint: See pp. 620-624 in PPP

4. What adverse effects of therapy would you discuss with this patient?

   Hint: See p. 621 in PPP

5. What if the patient fails the first choice of antidepressant treatment?

   Hint: See Figure 40-2 in PPP

FOLLOW-UP

The patient returns 6 weeks later and reports a minor improvement in anxiety symptoms. She reports continuing to struggle with her coursework. She requests to be treated with diazepam as she thinks it will help her feel better immediately.

What are the risks of treating GAD with benzodiazepines?

   Hint: See pp. 621-623 in PPP

⊙ GLOBAL PERSPECTIVE

Generalized Anxiety Disorder may occur more frequently in individuals of European descent than individuals of non-European descent (i.e., Asian, African, Native American, and Pacific Islander). Likewise, it's reported that individuals from developed countries are more likely to report experiencing symptoms that meet criteria for GAD in their lifetime, than individuals from undeveloped countries. There may also be cultural differences in the presentation of GAD. Some cultures are more likely to express cognitive symptoms, whereas others may express predominantly somatic symptoms. It's important to consider cultural context when evaluating whether worries are excessive. Treatment guidelines for GAD are similar worldwide.

CASE SUMMARY

- Patient presents with excessive worry, restlessness and poor sleep, fatigue, irritability, and GI symptoms over a six-month period resulting in functional impairment and should be treated.

- SSRI/SNRI antidepressants reduce cognitive and somatic symptoms of anxiety, with or without comorbid depression. Patients better tolerate a lower initial dose than used for depression, but targeted daily doses are similar. Treatment should be continued for 1 year.

- Benzodiazepines should be limited to acute therapy for rapid reduction of disabling anxiety symptoms and may be overlapped with antidepressant initiation when appropriate.

For more information on the care plan and facilitator's guide please visit http://www.mhpharmacotherapy.com

Sleep

Kristen E. Ellis

PATIENT PRESENTATION

Chief Complaint

"I need a sleep medication that won't give him dementia."

History of Present Illness

Gerald Garza is an 85-year-old male brought by his daughter to your geriatric clinic today. Despite having no history of cognitive dysfunction, he has been increasingly confused over the past week. His daughter also indicates that he has had trouble sleeping for months. She has been giving him diphenhydramine, which helps him intermittently. When that does not work, he takes an herbal medication for insomnia that his family sends him from Mexico. A week ago, his primary care physician prescribed him temazepam. Mr. Garza says that he "doesn't like the way the medication makes him feel." Despite these efforts, he continues to take an hour or more to fall asleep each night. Mr. Garza denies nightmares, pain, loud noises or other disturbances at night, caffeine late in the day, or exercise before bed. His daughter said that she does often find him napping in front of the television during the day, and says that he does not snore.

Past Medical History

Insomnia

HTN (diagnosed 30 years ago)

GERD (diagnosed four years ago)

BPH (diagnosed 15 years ago)

Past Surgical History

ORIF (open reduction internal fixation) 6 months ago following hip fracture

Family History

Daughter has HTN and depression. Mother died giving birth at age 30, father lived until age 72. Brother is 82, has HTN, COPD and is s/p CABG (coronary artery bypass graft) 5 years ago. No family history of cancer.

Social/Work History

Mr. Garza is a retired Army veteran. He was an airplane mechanic during the Korean War, and retired as a Sergeant Major in 1989. He has full benefits through the VA. He is a widower (his wife passed away 10 years ago), and has 1 daughter, who lives next door to him. Up until this week, patient did all activities of daily living (ADLs) and Instrumental ADLs with no/little assistance. He remains very active in the community, and volunteers at the hospital three or four times per week, with the exception of the past week.

Tobacco/Alcohol/Substance Use

Denies ever using tobacco or illicit substances. He admits to using alcohol "every once in a while" before bed to help with sleep.

Allergies/Intolerances/Adverse Drug Events

Penicillin—he does not remember what the allergy was, occurred when he was a child

Medication History (Current)

Temazepam 15 mg po q hs prn insomnia

Unknown herbal supplement po q hs prn insomnia

Diphenhydramine 50 mg po q hs prn insomnia

Propranolol 80 mg po bid

HCTZ 25 mg po q am

Famotidine 20 mg po bid

Tamsulosin 0.4 mg po daily

Pravastatin 40 mg po q hs

Aspirin 81 mg po daily

Review of Systems

Complains of acute confusion, persistent difficulty falling asleep; (+) urinary retention, (−) nocturia, incontinence; (−) depressed mood; (+) agitation, (+) falls, unsteady gait; (−) heartburn, reflux; (−) history of seizures, syncope, stroke

Physical Examination

▶ **General**

Well-developed, well-groomed elderly man in mild distress. Entered the room using a walker with unsteady gait. Becomes irritated easily.

▶ **Vital Signs**

BP 140/82 mm Hg, P 101, RR 17, T 36.9°C

Weight 140.8 lb. (64 kg)

Height 66 in. (167.6 cm)

Denies pain

▶ Skin

Skin warm and dry; (–) rashes or lesions; (+) bruising on left arm, right shin

▶ HEENT

PERRLA; EOMI; dry mucous membranes

▶ Neck and Lymph Nodes

(–) Thyromegaly; (–) lymphadenopathy; (–) carotid bruits; pulses 2+ bilaterally, (–) JVD

▶ Chest

Lungs clear to auscultation

▶ Cardiovascular

Sinus tachycardia; normal S_1, S_2; no murmurs, rubs, or gallops

▶ Abdomen

Not tender, not distended; normoactive bowel sounds; (–) organomegaly

▶ Neurology

DTRs normal; cranial nerves II-XII grossly intact; 5/5 strength in all extremities bilaterally; extremity sensation intact; denies numbness/tingling; face symmetric, (–) mouth droop; unsteady gait, (–) foot drop

▶ Extremities

(–) cyanosis, clubbing, or edema

▶ Genitourinary

Examination deferred

▶ Rectal

Examination deferred

▶ Mental Status Examination

A&O × 3; denies depression; became agitated and refuses to answer further questions

Laboratory Tests
Nonfasting

	Conventional Units	SI Units
Na	148 mEq/L	148 mmol/L
K	4.2 mEq/L	4.2 mmol/L
Cl	102 mEq/L	102 mmol/L
CO$_2$	23 mEq/L	23 mmol/L
BUN	21 mg/dL	7.5 mmol/L
SCr	1.0 mg/dL	88.4 µmol/L
Glu	89 mg/dL	4.9 mmol/L
Ca	9.1 mg/dL	2.28 mmol/L
Hgb	16.6 g/dL	10.29 mmol/L
Hct	49.8%	0.498 (fraction)
WBC	$7.6 \times 10^3/\mu L$	$7.6 \times 10^9/L$
MCV	83 µm^3	83 fL
Plt	$410 \times 10^3/\mu L$	$410 \times 10^9/L$
Albumin	3.9 g/dL	39 g/L
TSH	1.0 µU/mL	1.0 mU/L
Urinalysis	(–) Nitrite; 1 WBC; 0 RBC; No bacteria	

Assessment

Eighty-five-year-old male with insomnia as well as delirium likely secondary to medication use.

Student Work-Up

Missing Information/Inadequate Data

Evaluate: Patient database

Drug therapy problems

Care plan (by problem)

TARGETED QUESTIONS

1. Which medications are most likely contributing to Mr. Garza's confusion?

    Hint: See pp. 634-635 in PPP

2. What factors could be causing or exacerbating Mr. Garza's insomnia?

    Hint: See pp. 631-632, 638-639 in PPP

3. What pharmacologic options are available for the treatment of insomnia for Mr. Garza?

    Hint: See pp. 634-635, Figure 41-1, and Table 41-2 in PPP

4. What medication and/or lifestyle changes would you recommend to Mr. Garza and his daughter to treat his insomnia? Include a monitoring and follow-up plan.

    Hint: See pp. 634-635, Table 41-1, Figure 41-1, and Table 41-2 in PPP

FOLLOW-UP

Mr. Garza returns to your clinic 2 weeks later to follow up on your previous intervention. To his and his daughter's relief, his mental status is back to baseline. He has followed all of your recommendations, however, he continues to have trouble falling asleep. He indicates that he has stopped volunteering as much due to fatigue, and he feels that his quality of life has been affected. He would like to be prescribed a medication to help with sleep, but is very nervous about the side effects due to his previous experience.

Depending upon your previous recommendation, what pharmacologic therapy for insomnia would you recommend? How would you educate Mr. Garza and his family about this therapy?

Hint: See pp. 634-635, Figure 41-1, Table 41-2 in PPP

🌐 GLOBAL PERSPECTIVE

The use of natural remedies for insomnia is prevalent both in developed and developing countries. Common therapies include teas, aromatherapy, and herbal supplements. Some patients may feel more comfortable using natural remedies over prescription medications, especially due to familiarity, accessibility, price, and the stigma or fear associated with the addictive properties of some sleep medications. Patient history should include discussion about natural remedies and over the counter supplements. Unfortunately, the efficacy and safety of herbal medicines for sleep is not well-studied, and many herbal products have been associated with pharmacokinetic or pharmacodynamic interactions with drugs and/or toxicity. In addition, the active ingredient content of many herbal supplements is not well-regulated. It is important to discuss herbal remedies with patients, and to help them with researching the efficacy and safety of the product. In 2005, ramelteon, a melatonin receptor agonist, was approved by the FDA. This medication may be an option for patients who prefer herbal treatments or treatments with less abuse potential.

CASE SUMMARY

- The patient experienced delirium likely related to the use of multiple sedating and anticholinergic medications. These medications should be minimized and/or discontinued.

- Secondary insomnia related to medications, medical conditions, and poor sleep hygiene was likely for this patient. A complete history should be obtained. Alternatives for medications that could contribute to insomnia should be used, medical conditions should be treated, and the patient and his daughter should be educated about nonpharmacologic therapies for insomnia.

- Despite nonpharmacologic interventions, the patient experienced continued insomnia that affected his quality of life. Appropriate pharmacotherapy should be individualized based upon patient-specific factors.

For more information on the care plan and facilitator's guide please visit http://www.mhpharmacotherapy.com

45 Attention-Deficit Hyperactivity Disorder

John Erramouspe   Rebecca Hoover

PATIENT PRESENTATION

Chief Complaint

"School is still a struggle for me, I don't sleep well at night, and my skin is horrid."

History of Present Illness

Carol Lesnus (CL) is a white 13-year-4-month-old female who presents with her mother to the pediatrician's clinic office for a behavior/ADHD medication recheck. Strattera was added to her stimulant regimen 3 months ago but no subsequent improvement in attention or hyperactivity has been seen. She has been on 27 mg of Concerta and clonidine 0.1-0.2 mg for 15 months that she claims seems to wake her up but does not help her pay attention. She feels like it does not work as well as it used to. CL and her mother claim that she has never experienced any adverse effects with any of her past or currently prescribed medications for ADHD. Although school is a struggle, her grades have improved since she has been on Concerta. She now has some Bs, Cs but also Ds, and Fs. She has to do a lot of homework on weekdays and weekends to catch up. On certain days, teachers say she is fidgety and can't concentrate unless a teacher sits down right next to her and forces her to do her work. At times she can be all over the classroom disrupting other students, being destructive, stealing things from other kids, and not heeding her teachers' requests to stop. She knows that people are angry with her, which she resents and claims to make her cause more mistakes. CL and her mother moved from out of state to this community and her present school a little over 4 years ago. Since then, CL has experienced difficulties making friends, establishing relationships, and is described by her teachers as a more of a loner. Occasionally she has hit other girls out of anger at school. She claims that kids pick on her at school and don't want to play or "hang out" with her with the exception of one boy who is 3 years younger than her.

The clonidine takes 1½ hours to work at night and CL still wakes up in the middle of the night. Without it sometimes she stays up all night long. CL receives Benadryl at bedtime about 2 times a week but it hasn't seemed to help much. The pediatrician has considered but never prescribed trazodone to help with sleep. Mother is planning to test CL for learning disabilities next week with a clinical psychologist.

Has mild acne with pustules and comedones but currently is not taking anything. Bactrim has been very helpful in the past but was discontinued due to concerns of resistance from extended use. The acne has since come back.

Past Medical History

Attention Deficit Disorder (combined subtype) plus comorbid Oppositional Defiant Disorder and Mixed Development Disorder (7 years)

Insomnia (difficulty falling and staying asleep) (2½ years)

Constipation (about 1 year)

Acne (mild, pustular and comedonal) (2 years)

Family History

Biological parents are alive but divorced. Mother has since moved to new state while father remains in the original state. Mother has full custody of CL. Father has history bipolar disorder symptoms (though he will not "admit it" per mother) with extremes of happiness and then anger control issues. Father has had significant legal trouble including jail time after starting fights. Father has experienced addictions to alcohol and benzodiazepines. Paternal side of the family experiences lots of depression. Mother drank alcohol heavily during the first month of pregnancy with CL before she knew she was pregnant but claims to have stopped at that time due to guilt and presently does not drink. Maternal grandmother has depression and is on fluoxetine.

Social History

CL lives full-time with biological mother who is divorced and has no other children. Both are staying in the home of a friend of their family.

Tobacco/Alcohol/Substance Use

None

Allergies/Intolerances/Adverse Drug Events

None

Current Medications

Concerta 27 mg po q am (increased from 18 mg 15 months ago)

Strattera 40 mg po once daily (added 3 months ago)

Clonidine 0.1 mg, 1-2 po q hs (usually takes 2 tablets)

Benadryl 25 mg po q hs prn for sleep

Magnesium Citrate 30 mL po tid prn constipation (hates due to taste and frequency of administration, wants stool softener)

Prior Medication Use

Adderall 5 mg, 2 po q am × 1wk then 2 po q am & 1 pm × 1wk then 2 po bid (used temporarily when lacked third-party prescription coverage)

Benzoyl peroxide gel 5%, Apply sparingly to acne prone areas once daily (discontinued after 1 month of intermittent application to individual lesions due to lack of effect, switched to Bactrim DS)

Bactrim DS, 1 po once daily for acne (discontinued after 7 months despite good results due to concerns of resistance development from prolonged use)

Citalopram 10 mg, 1 po daily [at 9¼ years tried for suspected, albeit unproven, depression, anxiety, and posttraumatic stress disorder (PTSD), discontinued secondary to resolution of depression, anxiety, and PTSD since moving to new state]

Review of Systems

(–) weight loss; (–) poor appetite; (–) palpitations; (–) headaches; (–) vomiting; (–) depression; (–) anxiety; (+) inattention; (+) school difficulties; (+) possible learning difficulties; (+) poor sleep without medication; (+) acne

Physical Examination

▶ General

Well-appearing 13-year-4 month-old female, not very talkative/communicative, difficult to engage today due to blank looks, poor eye contact, and listless/blunted affect.

▶ Vital Signs

BP 113/79 mm Hg, P 86, RR 16, T 37°C

Weight 102 lb. (46.4 kg)

Height 66 in. (167.6 cm)

▶ Skin

Mild facial/forehead and back acne with blackheads and pustules

▶ HEENT

Normocephalic, atraumatic, tympanic membranes and oropharynx WNL, conjunctivae clear

▶ Neck and Lymph Nodes

Supple without lymphadenopathy

▶ Chest

Clear to auscultation bilaterally

▶ Cardiovascular

Heart: RRR without murmurs

Extremities: Normal pulses

▶ Abdomen

Soft, nontender, nondistended, without hepatosplenomegaly, positive bowel sounds

▶ Neurology

WNL

▶ Genitourinary

Examination deferred

▶ Rectal

Examination deferred

Laboratory and Other Diagnostic Tests

Laboratory Last Assessed 6 months ago at Age 12 years 10 months

	Conventional Units	SI Units
Na	139 mEq/L	139 mmol/L
K	3.9 mEq/L	3.9 mmol/L
Cl	106 mEq/L	106 mmol/L
CO_2/HCO_3	25 mEq/L	25 mmol/L
BUN	17 mg/dL	6.1 mmol/L
SCr	0.5 mg/dL	44.2 μmol/L
Cr Clearance		
Glu	92 mg/dL	5.1 mmol/L
Ca	10.2 mg/dL	2.55 mmol/L
Mg		
PO_4		
Hgb	13 g/dL	8.1 g/L
Hct	40.5%	0.405
MCV	91.9 μm³	91.9 fL
WBC	$5.3 \times 10^3/mm^3$	$5.3 \times 10^9/L$
WBC Differential	34.2///56.8/	
Platelets	$402 \times 10^3/mm^3$	$402 \times 10^9/L$
Albumin	4.5 g/dL	45 g/L
Total bilirubin	0.2 mg/dL	3.42 μmol/L

Bilirubin (direct)

AST	28 IU/L	0.47 μkat/L
ALT	19 IU/L	0.32 μkat/L
Alkaline phosphatase	213 IU/L	3.55 μkat/L

Psychological evaluation at age 9 years 3 months found no evidence of depression, anxiety, or psychosis. PTSD from possible mistreatment was explored but never proven.

Assessment

A 13-year-4 month-old female with suboptimal control of ADHD (who still struggles in school with inattention, hyperactivity/impulsivity, suboptimal grades, and bad behavior), insomnia (difficulty falling and staying asleep), constipation (laxative nonadherence), and currently untreated mild pustular and comedonal acne.

Student Work-Up

Missing Information/Inadequate Data

Evaluate: Patient database

Drug therapy problems

Care plan (by problem)

TARGETED QUESTIONS

1. What signs and symptoms of ADHD (plus comorbid Oppositional Defiant Disorder) has this patient manifested in the past, and which ones does she presently display that may respond to stimulant therapy?

   Hint: See pp. 641-642 in PPP

2. Why are stimulants the treatment of choice for most patients with ADHD?

   Hint: See pp. 642-643 in PPP

3. What adverse effects of stimulant therapy would you discuss with this patient and her parent(s) and what remedies would you offer to decrease them?

   Hint: See p. 643, Table 42-2 in PPP

4. Was the trial of Concerta adequate for this patient before a nonstimulant was added? If it was not adequate, what would you do now that atomoxetine has been added?

   Hint: See pp. 642-643 in PPP. (CL claims that she has never experienced any adverse effects with any of her past or currently prescribed medications for ADHD)

5. Is there a preferred medication for treating ADHD children who have difficulty falling and staying asleep despite proper adjustment of their sleep hygiene habits and stimulant and nonstimulant therapies?

   Hint: See Table 42-2, p. 645 in PPP, references 1-4

FOLLOW-UP

Strattera was discontinued in CL and her other medications were adjusted per your recommendations. At her next visit 1 month later, she still claimed that the current meds only help her wake up and that she does not notice any difference in her performance or behavior. However her mother and teachers did notice a change and say she does seem to have fewer mood swings and is more level-headed. Her teachers say she is better at attending during class to their directions and her assignments. Her grades have improved with all Bs and Cs except for one D. Her mother noticed that this occurred despite the fact she has less homework to do on the weekdays and weekends. Concurrent with CL's improvements of her ADHD symptoms, her sleep has also improved. She reduced her napping and television viewing during the weekdays, although she still likes to nap excessively during the day and views a lot of television on the weekends.

🌐 GLOBAL PERSPECTIVE

ADHD is a behavioral disorder that affects up to 12% of school-aged children in the United States. The predominance of American research into this disorder over the past 40 years has led to the impression that ADHD is largely an American disorder and much less prevalent elsewhere. This impression was reinforced by the perception that ADHD may stem from social and cultural factors that are most common in American society. However, another school of thought suggested that ADHD is a behavioral disorder common to children of many different races and societies worldwide, but that is not recognized by the medical community, perhaps due to confusion regarding its diagnosis and/or misconceptions regarding its adverse impact on children, their families, and society as a whole. Studies performed in U.S. and non-U.S. populations suggest that the prevalence of ADHD is at least as high in many non-U.S. children as in U.S. children, with the highest prevalence rates being seen when using DSM-V diagnostic criteria. Recognition that ADHD is not purely an American disorder and that the prevalence of this behavioral disorder in many countries is in the same range as that in the United States will have important implications for the psychiatric care of children. Although the treatment strategies and medication availability may differ among countries, most published ADHD treatment guidelines from Europe and other parts of the world show similar approaches to managing this disorder.[4]

CASE SUMMARY

- CL's stimulant dose titration with Concerta seemed inadequate before the nonstimulant atomoxetine was added since no adverse effects have ever been reported to any of her ADHD medications.

- CL's age and weight plus the dosing, tablet strengths, adverse effects, and cost of Concerta need to be considered when titrating CL's stimulant regimen to control her symptoms of ADHD.

- CL's sleep problems are common to ADHD patients and may respond to modification of sleep hygiene habits combined with pharmacological interventions involving stimulant, alpha$_2$-adrenergic agonist and selected hypnotic therapy shown effective for ADHD.

- CL displays medication adherence and educational deficit problems related to her present constipation and past acne treatments that needs to be addressed. Her laxative needs to be changed to a more palatable, less frequently administered preparation, and pharmacological treatment of mild acne should be initiated.

KEY REFERENCES/READINGS

1. PL Detail-Document, Management of ADHD: When a stimulant is not enough. Pharmacist's Letter/Prescriber's Letter. April 2015.
2. Gringras P. When to use drugs to help sleep. Arch Dis Child 2008 Nov93;(11):976-981.
3. Sweis D. The uses of melatonin. Arch Dis Child Educ Pract Ed 2005;90:ep74-ep77.
4. Faraone SV, Sergeant J, Gillberg C, Biederman J. The worldwide prevalence of ADHD: Is it an American condition? World Psychiatr 2003;2(2):104-113.

For more information on the care plan and facilitator's guide please visit http://www.mhpharmacotherapy.com

46 Substance-Related Disorders

Lisa W. Goldstone

PATIENT PRESENTATION

Case Components

Chief Complaint

"Someone broke into my car and stole my Adderall."

History of Present Illness

AR is a 20-year-old woman who presents to the clinic at student health services for a new prescription for dextroaphetamine/amphetamine as she claims someone broke into her car 3 days ago and stole the handbag she had placed under the seat of her car while she was working out at the gym. Per AR, her prescription stimulant medications were in the handbag that was stolen. AR states that since her medication was stolen, she has had an extremely difficult time concentrating and she is concerned this will adversely affect her grades and her chances of getting into pharmacy school. She also reports that on some nights she stays up very late studying and then cannot go to sleep at a reasonable time the following evening. She wonders if there is anything she can take to help her sleep.

Past Medical History

Attention-Deficit/Hyperactivity Disorder (ADHD) × (13 years)

Migraine headaches (3 years)

Family History

Father and older sister are healthy with no reported medical conditions. Mother suffered from major depressive disorder and died from suicide at age 42.

Social/Work History

The patient is a pre-pharmacy major at the state university. She is single and unemployed.

Tobacco/Alcohol/Substance Use

Denies alcohol and illicit substance use. Smokes ½ ppd cigarettes with approximately a 2 pack-year history. Drinks one grande Starbucks coffee per day but has a "few extra" when studying for exams.

Allergy Intolerance/Adverse event history

No known allergies

Medication History

▶ Home Medications

Dextroamphetamine/amphetamine XR 20 mg po daily

Amitriptyline 25 mg po daily

Aspirin 500 mg/acetaminophen 500 mg/caffeine 130 mg as needed for migraine headache

▶ Prior Medication Use

Methylphenidate (patient unable to recall dose)

Review of Systems

(+) migraines 2-3 times per month (−) chest pain (−) history or head injury or seizures (+) difficulty falling asleep some nights (+) decreased ability to concentrate since the beginning of the semester (+) anxiety (−) depressed mood

Physical Examination

▶ General

Patient is a thin, 20-year-old Caucasian female who appears to be stressed by her current academic standing and is at times, tearful.

▶ Vital Signs

BP 125/79 mm Hg, P 82, RR 14, T 38.2°C

Weight 109 lb. (49.4 kg)

Height 63 in. (160 cm)

▶ Chest

Clear to auscultation

▶ Cardiovascular

RRR, (−) murmurs, rubs, or gallops

▶ Neurology

Grossly intact

▶ *Mental Status Examination*

Patient is a thin, 21-year-old Caucasian female who appears her stated age. She is well-groomed and dressed in casual attire. Patient is cooperative but seems distracted and anxious with only fair eye contact. She is tearful when discussing her academic performance and concerns. She is alert and oriented to person, place, time, and situation. Speech is of normal rate and volume. Mood is predominantly euthymic and affect is mood congruent. Thought process is logical. No evidence of hallucinations, delusions, mania, or paranoia. Patient denies suicidal or homicidal ideation. Insight is fair. Judgment is poor. Patient understands the potential consequences of misusing prescription medication but misused her prescription medications and took another person's prescription medication without knowing what she was taking. Memory is intact. Patient appears to be of above average intelligence.

Laboratory and Other Diagnostic Tests

	Conventional Units	SI Units
Na	141 mEq/L	141 mmol/L
K	3.8 mEq/L	3.8 mmol/L
Cl	104 mEq/L	104 mmol/L
CO$_2$	28 mEq/L	28 mmol/L
BUN	12 mEq/L	4.28 mmol/L
SCr	0.6 mg/dL	45.8 μmol/L
Glu	78 mg/dL	4.33 mmol/L
Ca	9.6 mg/dL	2.40 mmol/L
Mg	1.6 mEq/L	0.8 mmol/L
Phos	3.6 mg/dL	1.16 mmol/L
Total Protein	6.1 g/dL	61 g/dL
Albumin	3.4 g/dL	34 g/dL
ALT	17 U/L	0.28 μkat/L
AST	23 U/L	0.38 μkat/L
Alk Phos	63 IU/L	1.05 μkat/L
T. Bili	0.5 mg/dL	8.55 μmol/L

ECG: Normal

Urine toxicology: (+) amphetamines (+) benzodiazepine

State Controlled Substances Prescription Monitoring Program

- Dextroamphetamine/amphetamine 20 mg po daily #30 capsules filled 2 weeks ago (written by Dr. Amphi)
- Dextroamphetamine/amphetamine 20 mg po daily #30 capsules filled 4 weeks ago (written by Dr. Dennison)

Assessment

Patient is a 20-year-old Caucasian female who presents with a claim that her prescription stimulant medication was stolen from her vehicle. After confronting the patient with the results of her urine toxicology screen and the information provided by the state controlled substances prescription monitoring program, she admits to misusing her prescription for dextroamphetamine/amphetamine. She reports feeling overwhelmed by her classes and struggling to keep up and feels her current dose is not adequate to allow her to concentrate when studying for exams. She states she will take an extra dose later in the afternoon when she needs to study for an exam so she can better concentrate. As a result she has trouble sleeping, which then interferes with her ability to wake up in time to attend her 9 AM class. One of her friends offered her an unknown pill to help her sleep a few nights ago that she found to be effective. No evidence to support that patient is misusing prescription medications for a euphoric or mind altering effect. Prescription medication misuse appears to be a result of inadequately treated ADHD.

Student Work-Up

Missing Information/Inadequate Data

Evaluate: Patient database

Drug therapy problems

Care plan (by problem)

TARGETED QUESTIONS

1. What are the signs and symptoms of stimulant withdrawal? Is the patient experiencing any of these?

   Hint: See Table 36-4 in PPP

2. Does the patient have sufficient criteria to warrant a diagnosis of stimulant use disorder or benzodiazepine use disorder?

   Hint: See Table 36-1 in PPP

3. What screening instrument(s) could be used to assess for the presence of a substance use disorder?

   Hint: See Table 36-2 in PPP

4. What nonpharmacological treatment options could be recommended for this patient?

   Hint: See p. 555 in PPP

5. What are the advantages and/or disadvantages of the various pharmacotherapeutic options that could be used to treat her tobacco use disorder?

   Hint: See Table 36-9 in PPP

FOLLOW-UP

What if the patient also tested positive for cocaine or marijuana on her urine toxicology screen? Would that have changed your approach to this case and if so, how?

⊙ GLOBAL PERSPECTIVE

Misuse of prescription stimulants is largely reported by countries in North and South America and to some extent, Indonesia. The prevalence of the misuse of prescription stimulants is reported to range from 0.1% (Argentina) to 3.28% (El Salvador). In most countries, males have higher rates of misuse of prescription stimulants. Typically, youth are more likely to misuse prescription stimulants. For example, in Costa Rica, the rate of misuse among the youth population is nearly 4 times greater than that seen in the general population. Although reports of prescription stimulant misuse are not available for other countries, it is important to keep in mind that lack of data does not indicate that prescription stimulant misuse does not occur in other parts of the world.

REFERENCE

1. United Nations Office on Drugs and Crime. World Drug Report 2014. (United Nations publication, Sales No. E.14.XI.7). www.unodc.org/documents/wdr2014/World_Drug_Report_2014_web.pdf. Accessed on May 21, 2015.

CASE SUMMARY

- The patient displays behaviors that may be indicative of a stimulant or benzodiazepine use disorder.

- However, the patient's misuse of prescription medications is more than likely related to inadequately treated ADHD.

- Regardless, the patient should be referred for a substance use disorder evaluation/screening to determine if additional treatment is necessary.

For more information on the care plan and facilitator's guide please visit http://www.mhpharmacotherapy.com

47 Type 1 Diabetes Mellitus: Diabetic Ketoacidosis

Alex C. Lopilato   Christopher Edwards
Hanna Phan

PATIENT PRESENTATION

Admitted October 1 from emergency department (ED).

Chief Complaint

"My stomach hurts and I'm nauseated."

History of Present Illness

John Bean is a 23-year-old male with a history of type 1 diabetes mellitus (T1DM) who presents to the ED with a 3-day history of abdominal pain and nausea. He states that prior to the abdominal pain and nausea, he was "extremely thirsty" and he had been urinating much more frequently compared to when he is in his usual state of health. Prior to the onset of these symptoms, he admits to having frequent headaches on a daily basis. He also admits to breathing fast and having what he thinks is a fast heartbeat. He denies altered mental status. He has lost several pounds in the last week or so. His medical history is significant for hypertension, stage 2 chronic kidney disease, and peripheral neuropathy. He currently does not have a primary care physician and has been relying on the ED to provide his medical care for the past several years.

Past Medical History

T1DM (since 8 years of age)

Hypertension (diagnosed at 15 years of age)

Chronic kidney disease (diagnosed at 15 years of age)

Peripheral neuropathy (diagnosed at 21 years of age)

Family History

Father is 48 years old with hypertension and dysipidemia, S/P NSTEMI with stenting, as well as T1DM requiring insulin therapy. Mother is 47 years old who has hypertension, dyslipidemia and depression.

Social History

John currently works at a grocery store as a cashier. However, given his recent worsening of "nerve pain," he has had to cut back his hours as he has difficulty bagging groceries.

Tobacco/Alcohol/Substance Use

He drinks alcohol several times a week and does not use recreational drugs.

Allergies/Intolerance/Adverse Drug Events

Lisinopril—he remembers taking it and having a dry cough within several days of starting it

Medication History

▶ **Medications Prior to Admission**

Insulin glargine 20 units subcutaneously nightly

Insulin lispro 7 units subcutaneously prior to meals

Gabapentin 900 mg po tid prn nerve pain

Ibuprofen 400 mg po tid prn nerve pain

Vitamin B complex (Nephrocap) 1 gel capsule po daily

Immunizations

Up to date with influenza given 2 weeks ago.

Review of Systems

General: (+) weight loss, (−) fevers, chills, or rigors

HEENT: (−) visual changes, diplopia, tinnitus, vertigo

Respiratory: (+) tachypnea; (−) SOB and cough

Cardiovascular: (+) rapid heartbeat or palpitations; (-) chest pain

Gastrointestinal: (+) polydipsia, nausea, and vomiting; (+) abdominal pain

Genitourinary: (+) urinary frequency, urgency, polyuria; (−) dysuria

Musculoskeletal: (−) joint or muscle pain

Neurological: (+) fatigue, numbness, HA

Physical Examination

▶ **General**

Underweight male who looks ill appearing. Fruity breath noted during examination.

▸ **Vital Signs**

BP 155/85, P 110, RR 25, T 37.4°C

Weight 145 lb. (66 kg)

Height 70 in. (173 cm)

Denies pain

▸ **Skin/Extremities**

Warm and dry. No rashes, petechiae, ecchymosis, or jaundice

▸ **HEENT**

Normocephalic; PERRLA, EOMI intact; TMs benign bilaterally; oropharynx benign; mucous membranes dry

▸ **Neck and Lymph Nodes**

Supple; no thyroid nodules, lymphadenopathy, or carotid bruits; neck veins flat (JVD 0)

▸ **Chest**

Breathing mildly labored; mild tachypnea; breath sounds equal bilaterally; no wheezes, crackles, or rhonchi

▸ **Cardiovascular**

RRR, normal S_1, S_2; no S_3 or S_4 detected

▸ **Abdomen**

Nontender, nondistended; no organomegaly; bowel sounds present

▸ **Neurology**

Grossly intact; DTRs normal; A&O × 4

▸ **Genitourinary**

Examination deferred

▸ **Rectal**

Examination deferred

Laboratory Tests

Fasting, Obtained on Admission

	Conventional Units	SI Units
Na	128 mEq/L	128 mmol/L
K	4.7 mEq/L	4.7 mmol/L
Cl	96 mEq/L	96 mmol/L
HCO3	12 mEq/L	12 mmol/L
Scr	2.2 mg/dL	194.5 μmol/L
Glu (fasting)	467 mg/dL	25.9 mmol/L
Ca	9.5 mg/dL	2.35 mmol/L
Mg	1.7 mEq/L	0.7 mmol/L
PO_4	4.2 mg/dL	1.36 mmol/L
Hgb A_{1C}	11%	0.11
WBC	$10.5 \times 10^3/mm^3$	$10.3 \times 10^9/L$

Platelets	$333 \times 10^3/mm^3$	$333 \times 10^9/L$
Hemoglobin	16 g/dL	160 g/L
Hematocrit	47.5%	0.45 fraction
MCV	92 μm³	92 fL

▸ **Venous Blood Gas**

pH	7.07	7.07
PCO_2	22 mm Hg	2.93 kPa
PO_2	61 mm Hg	6.53 kPa
Calculated HCO_3	8 mEq/L	8 mmol/L

▸ **Urinalysis**

pH 5

Specific gravity	1.013	
Nitrite	neg	
Glucose	555 mg/dL	30.8 mmol/L
Ketones	300 mg/dL	16.7 mmol/L
RBC	0	
Protein	100 mg	0.1 grams
WBC	0	

Assessment

Twenty-three-year-old male with signs, symptoms, and laboratory tests consistent with DKA with further workup required to determine an etiology. A peripheral IV catheter was just placed in the ED by his nurse and therapy is ready to be started.

Student Work-Up

Missing Information/Inadequate Data

Evaluate: Patient database

Drug therapy problems

Care plan (by problem)

TARGETED QUESTIONS

1. What signs and symptoms of DKA does the patient have?

   Hint: See p. 672 in PPP

2. What is the pathophysiologic mechanism for DKA onset and how does that manifest as signs and symptoms?

   Hint: See p. 672 in PPP

3. What electrolyte disturbances are you likely to see in a patient presenting with DKA?

   Hint: See pp. 672-673 in PPP

4. In appropriate order, which therapies should be provided to a given patient with DKA?

   Hint: See Table 43-11 in PPP

5. After starting continuous infusion insulin therapy, which criteria would you use to discontinue it?

   Hint: See Table 43-11 in PPP

FOLLOW-UP

John follows-up to your clinic 1 month later and due to his nerve pain is having difficulty drawing up his insulin and administering it to himself. What other treatment options are available that John is more likely to be adherent to?

   Hint: See Table 43-9 in PPP

⊙ GLOBAL PERSPECTIVE

Worldwide, 387 million people live with diabetes. Upward of 10% of which have T1DM, placing them at increased risk of DKA episodes with subsequent morbidity and mortality.[1,2] Approximately one-quarter of all children with T1DM live in the European region and another quarter in South-East Asia. In developing countries, mortality rates in patients with T1DM are significantly higher as evidenced by Sudan's mortality rate of 42.6 deaths per 100,000 children compared to 0.63 deaths per 100,000 children in the United States.[3] This disparity in mortality is likely attributable to lack of access to care, lack of education on signs and symptoms of diabetes, as well as lack of access to insulin. In newly diagnosed T1DM patients, it is sometimes difficult for families and patients to grasp their diagnosis and understand that this is a lifelong condition for which there will be lifelong treatment. In these situations, continual teaching and reinforcement of need for therapy and monitoring improve likelihood of adherence and decrease incidence of DKA. Internationally, the treatment for DKA in children and adults is guideline driven, generally universally agreed upon, and consists of three key aspects: fluid replacement, insulin therapy, and electrolyte correction.[4]

CASE SUMMARY

- The patient's current clinical picture is consistent with DKA and he should be given fluid replacement, placed on an insulin infusion, given dextrose containing fluids once hyperglycemia resolves, and electrolyte replacement as needed.

- Care should be taken to avoid rapid fluctuations in serum electrolyte levels when correcting the patient's serum glucose level.

- The patient will require extensive education on diabetes, the proper use of insulin, and the important of adherence with insulin therapy.

KEY REFERENCES/READINGS

1. IDF Diabetes Atlas: Sixth edition. http://www.idf.org/diabetesatlas/5e/Update2012. Accessed May 20th, 2015.
2. Type 1 Diabetes: quo vadis? *Diabetes Voice.* 2011;56:5.
3. Guaraguata L. Estimating the worldwide burden of type 1 diabetes. *Diabetes Voice.* 2011;56:6-8.
4. Kitabchi A, Umpierrez G, Miles J, Fisher J. Hyperglycemic crises in adult patients with diabetes. *Diabetes Care.* 2009;32:1335-1343.

For more information on the care plan and facilitator's guide please visit http://www.mhpharmacotherapy.com

48 Type 2 Diabetes Mellitus

Susan Cornell

PATIENT PRESENTATION

Chief Complaint

"My primary care provider told me I need to lose weight and control my sugar better. I'm feeling okay in general, but I am disgusted with gaining weight and being tired all the time."

History of Present Illness

JS is a 38-year-old woman who presents to the community pharmacy/clinic complaining about her weight and fatigue. She is adherent to her primary care provider (PCP) appointments every 3 months since she was diagnosed with T2DM 3 years ago. She is aware that her glucose and A_{1c} are not at goal and she needs to control her diabetes. She states that she takes her medications daily as prescribed and only misses an occasional dose (about 2-3 per month). She checks her fasting blood glucose almost every day. She tries to monitor the amount and type of food she eats, but occasionally "cheats," especially during holiday seasons. She walks 3 to 4 days per week for 20 to 30 minutes, depending on the weather. She mentions she is annoyed with her recent weight gain (in last 6 months), despite her efforts to eat healthy and exercise. She also comments on occasional feelings of dizziness, lightheadedness, and ringing in her ears.

Past Medical History

Dyslipidemia (3 years)

T2DM (3 years)

Obstructive sleep apnea (OSA) (4 years)

Recurrent yeast infections (4 years)

Obesity (10 years)

Family History

Father had T2DM, dyslipidemia, and HTN, and died from a MI at the age of 56. Mother is alive at age 68 and has T2DM, dyslipidemia, sleep apnea, and GERD. Brother is alive at age 42 and has T2DM and HTN. Sister is alive at age 35 and is healthy.

Social History

She is married for 14 years and lives with husband and two children aged 11 and 8. Works as an administrative assistant at a local community college.

Tobacco/Alcohol/Substance Use

Social drinker (1-2 glasses of wine 2-3 times per week); (–) tobacco or illicit drug use.

Allergies/Intolerances/Adverse Drug Events

No known drug or food allergies

Medications (Current)

Metformin 1000 mg po q day (with dinner) started 2 years ago, 1 year after diagnosis

Glimepiride 4 mg daily (with breakfast) started 7 months ago

Atorvastatin 20 mg po q day (at bedtime) started 3 years ago, upon diagnosis

Ortho Tri-Cyclen-28 po q day (at bedtime) started 15 years ago; stopped and restarted during planned pregnancies

Continuous positive airway pressure (CPAP) therapy while sleeping; started 1 year ago

Naproxen 500 mg po prn

Review of Systems

Occasional body aches and headaches relieved with naproxen. (–) Increased frequency and burning upon urination. (–) Vaginal discharge or dyspareunia; (+) tinnitus, (+) dizziness, lightheadedness, and fatigue. (+) Dry skin, minor bruises on left upper arm.

Physical Examination

▶ *General*

Well-appearing Caucasian woman in no acute distress

▶ *Vital Signs*

BP 136/78 mm Hg, P 68, RR 14, T 36.8°C

Weight 203.5 lb. (92.5 kg)

Height 66 in. (167.6 cm)

BMI 33.8 kg/m²

Waist circumference 35 in. (88.9 cm)

Denies any discomfort, except for fatigue, occasional dizziness and occasional ringing in her right ear.

▶ *Skin*

Dry appearing skin, two visible, minor bruises on left upper arm that patient states have been there for several weeks after "bumping into a door" at her office.

▶ *HEENT*

PERRLA, (–) sinus tenderness

▶ *Chest*

Clear to auscultation

▶ *Breast*

Examination deferred

▶ *Cardiovascular*

RRR, normal S_1, S_2, (–) S_3 or S_4

▶ *Abdomen*

Not tender/not distended; (–) organomegaly

▶ *Extremities*

No edema, (+) pedal pulses, (–) lesions or callus, (+) hair on first toe at the interphalangeal joint on both feet; normal monofilament examination bilaterally

▶ *Genitourinary*

Examination deferred

▶ *Rectal*

Examination deferred

Laboratory Tests
Fasting

	Conventional Units	SI Units
Na	137 mEq/L	137 mmol/L
K	4.7 mEq/L	4.7 mmol/L
Cl	101 mEq/L	101 mmol/L
CO_2	22 mEq/L	22 mmol/L
BUN	9 mg/dL	3.2 mmol/L
SCr	0.8 mg/dL	71 mmol/L
Glu	192 mg/dL	10.6 mmol/L
HbA_{1c}	8.7%	0.087
AST	22 U/L	0.37 μkat/L
ALT	44 U/L	0.73 μkat/L
Total cholesterol	180 mg/dL	4.65 mmol/L
LDL cholesterol	108 mg/dL	2.79 mmol/L
HDL cholesterol	32 mg/dL	0.83 mmol/L
Triglycerides	188 mg/dL	2.12 mmol/L
Hgb	13.5 g/dL	135 g/L; 8.38 mmol/L
Hct	37.7%	0.377
WBC	$11.2 \times 10^3/mm^3$	$4.47 \times 10^9/L$
Platelets	$172 \times 10^3/mm^3$	$172 \times 10^9/L$
Vitamin D	15 ng/mL	37.44 nmol/L

Urinalysis: Trace (–) protein, (–) heme, (–) nitrite

Assessment

Thirty-eight-year-old woman with fatigue, obesity, uncontrolled T2DM, dyslipidemia, tinnitus and OSA. She has signs and symptoms suggestive of uncontrolled diabetes, hypoglycemic episodes, and weight gain possibly due to current diabetes pharmacotherapy.

Student Work-Up

Missing Information/Inadequate Data

Evaluate: Patient database
Drug therapy problems
Care plan (by problem)

TARGETED QUESTIONS

1. What signs and symptoms is the patient experiencing that indicate her diabetes in not controlled?

   Hint: See p. 653 in PPP

2. What diabetes-related complications does the patient have?

   Hint: See pp. 673-674 in PPP

3. Which diabetes pharmacotherapy agent(s) is/are contributing to the patient's weight gain and hypoglycemia?

   Hint: See Table 43-7 in PPP

4. What are the therapeutic goals for this patient?

   Hint: See Table 43-6 in PPP

5. What modifications should be made to her drug therapy and diabetes self-management plans?

   Hint: See Figures 43-2, 43-3, Tables 43-7 in PPP

6. How should the patient's therapeutic plan be monitored?

   Hint: See p. 675 in PPP

⚙ GLOBAL PERSPECTIVE

T2DM is growing at an epidemic rate. Worldwide more than 387 million people have diabetes, and more than 4.9 million people die each year from diabetes-related problems. Every 7 seconds a person dies from diabetes. Almost 80% of deaths due to diabetes occur in low- to middle-income countries. As many developing countries adopt a Western diet and lifestyle, increased rates of obesity are associated with increased diabetes morbidity and mortality. The approach to T2DM is similar in all countries, including eating a healthy diet and exercise. However, low-income patients may have poor access to health care resources and may not be able to afford or have access to healthier foods and optimal medications.[1]

REFERENCE

1. http://www.idf.org/sites/default/files/Atlas-poster-2014_EN.pdf accessed May 1, 2015. http://www.cdc.gov/diabetes/data/statistics/2014statisticsreport.html accessed May 1, 2015.

CASE SUMMARY

- The patient needs diabetes self-management education. She is unaware of the relationship between her hypoglycemic episodes and medication, and the relationship between her delayed wound healing, fatigue, tinnitus, obstructive sleep apnea, and cardiovascular complications and her type 2 diabetes.

- Changing blood glucose-lowering agents may be warranted. Considerations regarding adverse effects and drug/disease interactions must be addressed.

- Lifestyle modifications must be aggressively addressed to achieve improved control of diabetes, cholesterol, and weight.

For more information on the care plan and facilitator's guide please visit http://www.mhpharmacotherapy.com

Diabetes and Pain

Amy K. Kennedy

PATIENT PRESENTATION

Chief Complaint

"I can't stand anything touching my feet at night and I cannot sleep."

History of Present Illness

Isabella Ramirez is a 67-year-old Mexican female with type 2 diabetes who presents to your ambulatory care clinic with allodynia in both feet. She reports that "nothing has helped, even the medication I take for sleeping." The pain has worsened over the past several months and is preventing her from falling asleep. Patient also says that in the last few months she has felt down and not herself.

Past Medical History (PMH)

Type 2 diabetes (diagnosed at age 57)

HTN (diagnosed at age 32)

Dyslipidemia (diagnosed at age 54)

Obesity (diagnosed at age 32)

Family History

Father had DM and died from a MI at age 57

Mother is alive at age 89 and has HTN and dyslipidemia

Brother is alive at age 64 with a history of HTN

Social/Work History

Widowed 3 months ago, lives with mother and is working as a secretary.

Tobacco/Alcohol/Substance use

(–) alcohol and (–) smoking

Allergy/Intolerance/Adverse event history

Sitagliptin: Rash

Medication History

▶ Current Medications

Aspirin 81 mg po daily

Amlodipine 10 mg po daily

Metformin 1000 mg po twice daily

Atorvastatin 40 mg po daily

Melatonin 5 mg po at bedtime as needed (has used over the past several days without relief)

▶ Prior Medication Use

Was on sitagliptin 2 years ago, but had a rash and has been on metformin only since.

Review of Systems

Feet: (–) paresthesia (burning, tingling) and (+) allodynia that is worse at night, (–) for ulcer, cuts, sores, or deformities, (–) dry skin. PHQ9 18, (+) for insomnia, (–) chest pain, SOB or dizziness.

Physical Exam

▶ General

The patient is a healthy-looking individual who is alert and oriented in severe distress due to her insomnia and mood.

▶ Vital Signs

BP 148/76 mm Hg, P 88 bpm, RR 18, T 36.8°C

Height 5'2" (157.48 cm)

Weight 189 lb. (85.729 kg)

Pain 6/10

▶ Skin

Dry, warm, intact

▶ HEENT

PERRLA

▶ Neck and Lymph Nodes

Thyroid not enlarged and without nodules. No lymphadenopathy

▶ Chest

(–) for pain, lungs are clear to auscultation without rhonchi, rales, or wheezing

▶ Breasts

Exam deferred

▶ **Cardiovascular**

RRR without S_3, S_4

▶ **Abdomen**

Nontender, normal BS

▶ **Neurology**

A&O, cranial nerves II-XII intact

▶ **Extremities**

Dry, intact skin. (+) pedal pulses, (+) allodynia, (−) paresthesia, (−) cuts, sores or lesions. Semmes–Weinstein 10 g monofilament exam normal except for decreased sensation on second and third metatarsal bilaterally.

▶ **Genitourinary**

Deferred

▶ **Rectal**

Deferred

Laboratory and Other Diagnostic Tests

	Conventional Units	SI units
Na	136 mEq/L	136 mmol/L
K	4.6 mEq/L	4.6 mmol/L
Cl	100 mEq/L	100 mmol/L
CO_2	24 mEq/L	24 mmol/L
BUN	18 mg/dL	6.4 mmol/L
SCr	1.3 mg/dL	114.92 μmol/L
Glu	257 mg/dL	14.3 mmol/L
Hgb	14.6 g/dL	9.052 mmol/L
Hct	46.2%	0.462
WBC	8.3×10^3/μL $103/mm^3$	8.3×10^9/L
Platelets	186×10^3/μL $103/mm^3$	186×10^9/L
Albumin	3.9 g/dL	39 g/L
AST	24 U/L	0.4 μkat/L
ALT	36 U/L	0.6 μkat/L
Alk Phos	124 U/L	2.07 μkat/L
HgbA1c	10.4%	0.104
Total cholesterol	215 mg/dL	5.56 mmol/L
Triglycerides	224 mg/dL	2.53 mmol/L
HDL cholesterol	52 mg/dL	1.34 mmol/L
LDL cholesterol	118 mg/dL	3.05 mmol/L
TSH	0.89 uIU/ml	0.89 mIU/ml

Assessment

Sixty-seven-year-old female with hypertension, dyslipidemia, and poorly controlled type 2 diabetes. She presents today with new onset painful diabetic peripheral neuropathy and possible depression/bereavement.

TARGETED QUESTIONS

1. What signs, symptoms, and physical exam data support the diagnosis of peripheral neuropathy?

   Hint: See pp. 522, 674 in PPP

2. What other diabetes-related neuropathies should be ruled out at this time?

   Hint: See p. 674 in PPP

3. What indicators are present for depression?

   Hint: See p. 584 in PPP

4. What are the treatment goals for this patient?

   Hint: See pp. 522, 674 in PPP

5. What would be the most appropriate course of treatment for this patient? Please address pharmacological and non-pharmacological aspects. For the pharmacological agent, please include dose, route, frequency and duration. Please explain your rationale. How would the presentation of peripheral neuropathy change in the setting of a sudden change in glycemic control?

   Hint: See pp. 522, 658-670, 674 in PPP

☻ GLOBAL PERSPECTIVE

Peripheral neuropathy is one of the most common diabetic complications with a prevalence of 30-50%. This prevalence increases in developing countries. Even in developed countries, peripheral neuropathies account for more hospitalizations than all other neuropathies combined and is a major risk factor for complications. Additionally, common prescribing patterns lag behind treatment guidelines. In one study, almost 40% of patients reported that they were never treated and 33% were treated with medications with no known efficacy for neuropathy.

CASE SUMMARY

- The patient's clinical presentation was consistent with peripheral diabetic neuropathy characterized by allodynia.
- Treatment for peripheral neuropathy is symptomatic in nature, with control of hyperglycemia the best mechanism for prevention of complications.

- When a patient presents with peripheral neuropathy, it is prudent to assess whether other neuropathies are present.

KEY REFERENCES/READINGS

1. Bril V, England J, Franklin GM, et al. Evidence-based guideline: treatment of painful diabetic neuropathy: report of the American Academy of Neurology, the American Association of Neuromuscular and Electrodiagnostic Medicine, and the American Academy of Physical Medicine. Neurology 2011;76:1758-1769.

2. Finnerup NB, Attal N, Haroutounian S, et al. Pharmacotherapy in neuropathic pain in adults: a systematic review and meta-analysis. Lancet Neurol. 2015;14(2):162-173.

For more information on the care plan and facilitator's guide please visit http://www.mhpharmacotherapy.com

50 Hyperthyroidism (Graves' Disease)

Michael P. Kane

PATIENT PRESENTATION

Chief Complaint

"I am here for evaluation of recently diagnosed Graves' thyroid disease."

History of Present Illness

The patient is a 31-year-old Caucasian female who was referred for further evaluation and management of newly diagnosed hyperthyroidism. She has experienced 4-6 months of progressive heat intolerance, diaphoresis, palpitations, weight loss, hyperactivity, hair thinning, tremulousness, and some anxiety with difficulty going to sleep. She has a thyroid stare and lid lag. Her primary care physician (PCP) made a diagnosis based on these symptoms and suppressed TSH and elevated free T_4 levels. She was started on beta-blocker therapy at that time and referred to this office.

The patient denies any difficulty with swallowing, expresses no concerns regarding her voice and has no shortness of breath. She reports no loose stools. The patient has no knowledge of prior exposure to external irradiation of the head, ears, neck, throat, or chest.

Past Medical History

HTN (2014)

GERD (2006)

Family History

Father—alive and well

Mother—alive and well

Brothers—2 alive and well

Sisters—0

Paternal grandmother, 2 aunts and 1 cousin with thyroid disease

Children 0 sons; 0 daughters

Social/Work History

Marital status: Married

Employment: Exam proctor

Caffeine: 1 cup per day

Physical Activity: exercises a few times a week

Tobacco/Alcohol/Substance Use

Tobacco: yes, 1 PPD

Alcohol: social drinker

Allergies/Intolerance/Adverse Drug Events

Amoxicillin (rash)

Medications

Lansoprazole 15 mg po daily

HCTZ 25 mg po daily

Triphasil 28 po daily

Propranolol 40 mg po twice daily (started 1 week ago)

Review of Systems

The patient denies chest pain, SOB, abdominal pain, hematochezia, dysuria, hematuria, changes in urinary frequency or urgency. She reports losing 35 pounds (15.9 kg) over the previous 6 months.

Physical Examination

▶ General

The patient is a well developed, well nourished Caucasian female. She is tremulous, hot, sweating, and cannot sit still. She has hair loss and her hands are very warm.

▶ Vital Signs

BP 142/70 mm Hg, P 105 bpm, RR 18 breaths/min

Weight 136 lb (61.8 kg)

Height 62 in. (157.5 cm)

BMI 24.9 kg/m²

The patient denies pain.

▶ Skin

Warm, moist skin; no rashes or dermopathy.

▶ HEENT

Sclerae are nonicteric. Conjunctivae are slightly injected. PERRLA. Fundi are not visualized. + bilateral proptosis.

▶ Neck and Lymph Nodes

Supple. The carotids are 2+ bilaterally. There is no JVD. The thyroid is diffusely enlarged, 3-4 times normal size. The lobes are equal by palpation. The texture is rubbery, the surface is globular, there are no distinct palpable nodules. An audible bruit is heard over the thyroid gland. There is no lymphadenopathy.

▶ Chest

Unremarkable.

Lung: There is a normal A-P diameter. Respiratory excursions are symmetrical. There is no abnormality to percussion or auscultation.

▶ Breast

Deferred

▶ Cardiovascular

Heart: S_1 and S_2 are normal in intensity. There are no murmurs, rubs or gallops noted.

She is tachycardic.

▶ Abdomen

+ BS NT/ND, no HSM

▶ Neurology

The CN II-XII are intact. Motor and sensory exams are normal. Cerebellar function is normal. There are no long tract signs. Reflexes are 2+ and symmetrical. She is DTRs 4+ with slow relaxation. (+) bilateral resting tremor.

▶ Extremities

The dorsalis pedis pulses are equal and 2+. There is some proximal muscle weakness; (–) Cyanosis, clubbing or edema. She has a bilateral hand tremor.

▶ Genitourinary/Rectal

Deferred

Laboratory/Diagnostic Tests

	Conventional Units	SI Units
Na	140 mEq/L	140 mmol/L
K	4.9 mEq/L	4.9 mmol/L
Cl	105 mEq/L	105 mmol/L
CO_2	25 mEq/L	25 mmol/L
BUN	13 mg/dL	4.6 mmol/L
SCr	0.36 mg/dL	31.8 μmol/L
Glu	100 mg/dL	5.55 mmol/L
Ca	9.7 mg/dL	2.43 mmol/L
Mg	2.2 mEq/L	1.1 mmol/L
Phosphate	3.4 mg/dL	1.1 mmol/L
ALP	135 IU/L	2.25 μkat/L
AST	22 IU/L	0.37 μkat/L
ALT	29 IU/L	0.48 μkat/L
WBC	$5.8 \times 10^3/mm^3$	$5.8 \times 10^9/L$
Neutrophils	64.7%	0.647
Hgb	13.4 g/dL	134 g/L; 8.31 mmol/L
Hct	40.4%	0.404
MCV	75 μm	75 fL
PLT	$215 \times 10^3/mm$	$215 \times 10^9/L$
Albumin	4.2 g/dL	42 g/L
Bilirubin	0.4 mg/dL	6.84 μmol/L
AST	22 IU/L	0.366 μkat/L
ALT	29 IU/L	0.48 μkat/L
Alk phos	135 IU/L	2.25 μkat/L
Anti-thyroid peroxidase (TPO) antibody	(+)	
Thyrotropin receptor (TSHR)-S antibody	(+)	
TSH	<0.005 μU/mL	<0.005 mU/L
T3	651 ng/dL	10.0 nmol/L
Free T4	7.77 ng/dL	100 pmol/L

EKG – sinus rhythm, tachycardia; 105 beats/min

RAIU – 65% at 24 hours

Assessment

This is a 31-year-old woman with signs, symptoms, and thyroid function test results consistent with severe Graves' disease. Thyrotropin receptor (TSHR)-S antibody level of 542 and RAIU test of 65% are consistent with autoimmune (Graves') etiology of her hyperthyroid symptoms. The patient is interested in starting a family in the near future so we will initiate drug therapy in plans for eventual thyroidectomy.

It was made very clear to the patient that weight gain often occurs with treatment of hyperthyroidism as her current metabolic rate will be slowed; dietary strategies were, therefore, discussed.

Student Work-Up

Missing Information/Inadequate Data

Evaluate: Patient database

Drug therapy problems

Care plan (by problem)

TARGETED QUESTIONS

1. What signs and symptoms of hyperthyroidism does the patient have?

   Hint: See p. 688 in PPP

2. What are the advantages and disadvantages of thionamide therapy, radioactive iodine (RAI), and surgery for Graves' disease treatment?

   Hint: See pp. 689-690 in PPP

3. What medications can cause hyperthyroidism?

   Hint: See Table 44-6 in PPP

4. What risks and adverse effects of thioanmide therapy would you discuss with the patient?

   Hint: See pp. 689-690 in PPP

5. What complications of hyperthyroidism is this patient experiencing or at risk for?

   Hint: See pp. 687-688 in PPP

FOLLOW-UP

The patient returns for follow up 4 weeks later. She continues to take the medications you recommended with no untoward side-effects. She is feeling much better; the diaphoresis and tremulousness have vastly improved, she feels much less anxious, she is sleeping better, and she has more energy. Her husband remarks that she appears close to back to her normal self. Her repeat TSH level today is still undetectable at <0.005 μIU/mL (<0.005 mIU/L); however, her total T3 and free T4 levels have significantly decreased, to 339 ng/dL (5.2 nmol/L) and 2.9 ng/dL (37.3 pmol/L), respectively.

At what point would you recheck thyroid function tests? When would you expect her to become euthyroid? Once a euthyroid state is achieved what, if any, dosage changes would you recommend in her thioamide therapy? At what point would she be ready for surgery? What medication changes should be considered prior to surgery? At what point can this patient consider starting a family?

◑ GLOBAL PERSPECTIVE

Iodine deficiency is a common cause of hypothyroid disease in developing countries. Percentages of hyperthyroid patients treated with RAI, surgery, or drug therapy vary among countries. Several drugs are associated with drug-induced thyroid disease.

CASE SUMMARY

- The patient's clinical status is consistent with Graves' disease and treatment is needed.

- Combination drug therapy should be initiated to manage symptoms acutely and chronically.

- Once symptoms are adequately managed, a discussion of the pros and cons of definitive treatment (RAI vs. surgery) should take place. RAI would delay attempts at pregnancy for a year.

- Since this patient has signs of Graves' ophthalmopathy, she should be referred to ophthalmology for evaluation. The patient should be encouraged to stop smoking as smoking tends to exacerbate Graves' eye disease.

KEY REFERENCE/READING

1. Marino M, Latrofa F, Menconi F, Chiovato L, Vitti P. An update on the medical treatment of Graves' hyperthyroidism. J Endocrinol Invest 2014; Sep 4.[Epub ahead of print]; doi:10.1007/s40618-014-0136-z.

For more information on the care plan and facilitator's guide please visit http://www.mhpharmacotherapy.com

51 Hypothyroidism

Mantiwee Nimworapan   Michael D. Katz

PATIENT PRESENTATION

Chief Complaint

"I still feel really bad. I have no energy and I can't take care of my baby."

History of Present Illness

HT is a 32-year-old Thai woman who was hospitalized 1 month ago for overt hypothyroidism. At that time, she was found in the park appearing confused and was brought to the emergency department (ED). Originally she was thought to be intoxicated, but her toxicology screens were negative and she was found to be severely hypothyroid [TSH 134 µIU/mL (134 mIU/L) and free T_4 <0.4 mg/mL (<5.15 pmol/L)] During that hospitalization she was diagnosed with myxedema coma and given a single IV dose of 200 mg hydrocortisone. Oral levothyroxine (LT_4) was started at a dose of 50 mcg/day. She was discharged 2 days later. She was diagnosed with Grave's disease 18 months ago while she was pregnant, and after being controlled on propylthiouracil and then methimazole, she underwent thyroidectomy. She was started in LT_4 after her thyroidectomy, but she had stopped taking it because she was too busy and she wasn't sure she really needed it anyway. She admits that she feels down and overwhelmed with having to take care of her child and work full time, and she wonders if she should just run away and end it all.

Past Medical History (PMH)

Grave's disease s/p thyroidectomy (12 months ago)

Post-thyroidectomy hypothyroidism

Depression "after my boyfriend left me and my baby"

Menorrhagia (12 months)

G1 P1 Ab 0

Family History

Father died of lung cancer at age 65. Mother died in car accident at age 60.

Social History

Patient works full time as a pharmacy technician at a busy chain pharmacy. She is single ("but I think I have a new boyfriend"). Her mother helps with child care.

Tobacco/Alcohol/Substance Use

Alcohol: denies use

Smoking: cigarette 1 pack/day since age 17

Admits to occasional marijuana use: "When I feel really down; I have a card so it's legal."

Allergy/Intolerance/Adverse Event history

NKDA

Medication History (Current)

Propranolol 20 mg po bid

Levothyroxine 50 mcg po q day

Calcium carbonate 500 mg q AM

Vitamin with iron q AM

Colace 100 mg po prn

Review of Systems

+ for fatigue, weakness "fuzzy" thinking, anxiety, constipation

Physical Exam

▶ **General**

Fatigued-appearing, somewhat overweight woman in no apparent distress (NAD).

▶ **Vital Signs**

BP 114/86 mm Hg, P 56, RR 12, T 36.4°C

Weight 149 lb. (68 kg)

Height 66 in. (167.6 cm)

Denies pain

▶ **Skin**

Dry-appearing skin and scalp; no rashes or lesions

▶ **HEENT**

PERRLA, EOMI; TMs appear normal.

▶ **Neck and Lymph Nodes**

Neck is supple and normal range of motion. Thyroid gland not palpable, well-healed thyroidectomy scar noted

▶ **Chest**

Clear, unlabored respirations, no shortness of breath (SOB) or wheezing

▶ **Cardiovascular**

Bradycardia but regular rhythm, normal S_1 and S_2, no murmurs

▶ **Abdomen**

Soft, nontender, bowel sounds active and normal, no organomegaly

▶ **Neurology**

Cranial nerves II-XII intact, sl delayed DTRs

▶ **Extremities**

Distal pulses 2+ bilaterally, no edema

▶ **Genitourinary**

Examination deferred

▶ **Rectal**

Examination deferred

Laboratory and Other Diagnostic Tests

	Conventional Units	SI Units
Na	134 mEq/L	134 mmol/L
K	4.4 mEq/L	4.4 mmol/L
Cl	96 mEq/L	96 mmol/L
CO_2	25 mEq/L	25 mmol/L
BUN	22 mg/dL	7.85 mmol/L
SCr	0.7 mg/dL	61.88 μmol/L
ClCr	123 mL/min	1.18 mL/s/m²
Glu	74 mg/dL	4.11 mmol/L
Ca	9.3 mg/dL	2.32 mmol/L
Mg	1.8 mg/dL	0.74 mmol/L
Phosphate	4.9 mg/dL	1.58 mmol/L
Hgb	12.5 g/dL	125 g/L; 7.75 mmol/L
Hct	40.1%	0.401
WBC	$5.4 \times 10^3/\mu L$	$5.4 \times 10^9/L$
MCV	81.2 μm³	81.2 fL
Albumin	4.2 g/dL	42 g/L
TSH	38.7 μIU/mL	38.7 mIU/L
Free T4	0.4 ng/dL	5.15 pmol/L
Total cholesterol	250 mg/dL	6.46 mmol/L
LDL cholesterol	198 mg/dL	3.80 mmol/L
HDL cholesterol	34 mg/dL	0.88 mmol/L
Urine HCG	negative	

Assessment

Thirty-two-year-old woman with overt hypothyroidism s/p thyroidectomy and nonadherence with LT_4. Pt may have s/s of depression.

Student Work-Up

Missing Information/Inadequate Data

Evaluate:	Patient database
	Drug therapy problems
	Care plan (by problem)

TARGETED QUESTIONS

1. What signs and symptoms of hypothyroidism does the patient have?
   Hint: See p. 682 in PPP

2. What is the cause of hypothyroidism in this patient?
   Hint: See p. 682 and Table 44-2 in PPP

3. What medications can cause hypothyroidism?
   Hint: See p. 682 and Table 44-2 in PPP

4. What are the triggers of myxedema coma?
   Hint: See p. 683 in PPP

5. What risks and adverse effects of therapy would you discuss with the patient?
   Hint: See p. 685 in PPP

6. Should the patient receive specific lipid-lowering pharmacotherapy?
   Hint: See p. 683 in PPP

FOLLOW-UP

Twelve months later, the patient feels much better and her thyroid tests are within normal limits. She is now married,

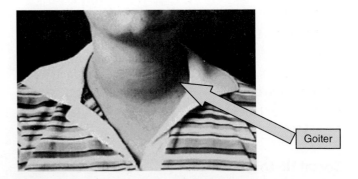

FIGURE 51-1. Goiter. (Adapted, with permission, from Gardner DG, Shoback D. Greenspan's Clffinical & Basic Endocrinology, 8th ed. New York, McGraw-Hill, 2007, Fig. 8-27A.)

and she and her husband want to have a child. If she becomes pregnant, what changes in her LT_4 therapy might be necessary?

Hint: See pp. 686 in PPP

🌐 GLOBAL PERSPECTIVE

Goiter, an enlargement of the thyroid gland, is caused by a variety of conditions, and can be associated with normal, excessive, or deficient thyroid function (Fig. 51-1). In developed countries, enlargement of the thyroid gland is most often associated with nodular goiter, autoimmune thyroiditis, and Grave's disease. However, in developing countries, iodine-deficient diet is commonly associated with goiter. Iodine deficiency and endemic goiter are especially common in women of childbearing age since pregnancy increases iodine requirements. Substances in the diet can also serve as goitrogens. Diets high in foods or herbal products containing cyanoglucosides (cassava, lima beans, maize, bamboo shoots, and sweet potatoes) release cyanide, which is then metabolized to thiocyanate, an agent that inhibits iodine transport. Foods or herbal products high in thioglucosides (cruciferous vegetables) can have a thionamide-like effect on the thyroid gland. Endemic goiter is easily treated with iodine supplementation (often in the form of iodized salt) and avoidance of dietary goitrogens.

CASE SUMMARY

- Thirty-two-year-old woman with overt hypothyroidism and dyslipidemia s/p Grave's disease and thyroidectomy.

- The patient appears to have adherence problems, which has resulted in inadequate thyroid replacement therapy.

- She has some signs and symptoms of depression that should be assessed.

For more information on the care plan and facilitator's guide please visit http://www.mhpharmacotherapy.com

52 Cushing's Syndrome

Devra K. Dang

PATIENT PRESENTATION

Chief Complaint

"Doctor, what are these stripes on my stomach?"

History of Present Illness

AB is a 52-year-old male who presents to his primary care physician's (PCP) office with complaints of several "stripes" on his abdomen that he has noticed appearing over the last month. He also noticed that he has gained ·7 lbs [3.2 kg] in the last 1-2 months, especially in the abdomen, and has attributed this to an inability to perform his usual exercise routine due to a worsening of asthma. He also complains of increasing fatigue and muscle weakness in his legs over the last several weeks, which also contributed to the lack of exercise. His wife accompanies him to the appointment and says that she noticed that he appeared to have gained weight in his face and that recently it looks "flushed."

Past Medical History

Hypertension (HTN) (7 years)

Asthma (since childhood); 3 exacerbations this year thus far—all requiring prednisone treatment, most recent exacerbation last month requiring emergency department visit

Allergic rhinitis (diagnosed 3 months ago after moving to a new house)

Family History

Mother is alive at age 82 with type 2 diabetes mellitus (T2DM) and osteoporosis; father is alive at age 80 with HTN. He has one sister, who is healthy.

Social/Work History

Married and lives with wife. Has a healthy 19-year-old son and 20-year-old daughter in college. Owns a restaurant.

Tobacco/Alcohol/Substance Use

Smokes half pack per day; occasional alcohol (1 glass with wine with dinner approximately 3 times/week); (–) illicit drug use

Allergies/Intolerances/Adverse Drug Events

No known drug/food allergies/intolerances/ADEs

Medications (Current)

Diltiazem ER 180 mg po bid; medication added this year after discontinuation of hydrochlorothiazide

Fluticasone/salmeterol DPI 500/250 mcg 1 inh bid; dose increased from 250/50 mcg approximately 3 months ago

Albuterol MDI 2 puffs q 4 h prn

Fluticasone 50 mcg spray 1 spray EN bid

Review of Systems

(+) Fatigue with muscle weakness in thighs; reports weight gain in his abdomen and wife reports weight gain in his face; (+) several reddish, purple striae on abdomen

Physical Examination

▶ *General*

Middle-aged Caucasian man in no apparent distress

▶ *Vital Signs*

BP 154/86 mm Hg, P 80, RR 16, T 37°C

Weight 200 lb. (90.9 kg)

Height 72 in. (183 cm)

Pain 0/10

▶ *Skin*

Thin, dry-appearing skin with several small bruises on legs; (–) rashes; reddish, purple striae visible on abdomen

▶ *HEENT*

Round face with facial plethora; PERRLA, EOMI; (–) sinus tenderness; TMs appear normal

▶ *Neck and Lymph Nodes*

(–) Lymphadenopathy; (–) carotid bruits, JVD, or thyromegaly

▶ *Chest*

Clear to auscultation bilaterally

▶ *Cardiovascular*

RRR, normal S_1, S_2; (–) S_3 or S_4

▶ *Abdomen*

Soft; not tender; obese with reddish, purple striae; (–) organomegaly

▶ *Neurology*

Grossly intact; DTRs normal

▶ *Genitourinary*

Examination deferred

▶ *Rectal*

Examination deferred

▶ *Musculoskeletal/Extremities*

Decreased muscle strength in upper and lower extremities bilaterally

LABORATORY TESTS

Collected at 3 p.m., Nonfasting

	Conventional Units	SI Units
Na	139 mEq/L	139 mmol/L
K	3.6 mEq/L	3.6 mmol/L
Cl	102 mEq/L	102 mmol/L
CO_2	24 mEq/L	24 mmol/L
BUN	17 mg/dL	6.1 mmol/L
SCr	0.8 mg/dL	71 μmol/L
Glu	170 mg/dL	9.35 mmol/L
Ca	9.6 mg/dL	2.4 mmol/L
Mg	1.9 mEq/L	0.95 mmol/L
Phosphate	3.7 mg/dL	1.2 mmol/L
Total cholesterol	200 mg/dL	5.17 mmol/L
LDL cholesterol (calculated)	122 mg/dL	3.15 mmol/L
HDL cholesterol	40 mg/dL	1.03 mmol/L
Triglycerides	190 mg/dL	2.15 mmol/L
Hgb	17 g/dL	170 g/L; 10.54 mmol/L
Hct	42%	0.42
MCV	86 μm³	86 fL
WBC	6.6×10^3/mm³	6.6×10^9/L
Platelets	280×10^3/mm³	280×10^9/L
Albumin	4 g/dL	40 g/L
Total bilirubin	0.5 mg/dL	8.6 μmol/L
Direct bilirubin	0.1 mg/dL	1.7 μmol/L
AST	32 IU/L	0.53 μkat/L
ALT	26 IU/L	0.43 μkat/L
Alkaline phosphatase	112 IU/L	1.87 μkat/L

Assessment

Fifty-two-year-old man with clinical presentation consistent with Cushing's syndrome.

Student Work-Up

Missing Information/Inadequate Data

Evaluate: Patient database

Drug therapy problems

Care plan (by problem)

TARGETED QUESTIONS

1. What signs and symptoms of Cushing's syndrome does the patient exhibit?

   Hint: See p. 703 in PPP

2. What is the likely etiology of Cushing's syndrome in this patient?

   Hint: See Table 45-4 on p. 702 in PPP

3. How should Cushing's syndrome in this patient be evaluated and treated?

   Hint: See pp. 704-707 in PPP

4. What patient education points should be provided regarding the Cushing's syndrome?

   Hint: See p. 708. Need to evaluate if he takes any nonprescription medications or herbals. Some of these may have corticosteroid activity (e.g., topical anti-itch medications) or may be adulterated with corticosteroids. in PPP

5. What are the most important things that the patient can do to improve his asthma control and avoid future exacerbations?

   Hint: See p. 247 in PPP

FOLLOW-UP

AB was referred to an endocrinologist for diagnostic testing. Which of the first-line screening tests for Cushing's syndrome may not be appropriate for AB given his medical history?

Hint: See p. 704 in PPP

☸ GLOBAL PERSPECTIVE

Cushing's syndrome is most commonly caused by chronic administration of exogenous glucocorticoids. Endogenous Cushing's syndrome is an uncommon disorder. According to European population-based studies, the incidence of endogenous Cushing's syndrome is 2-3 cases per 1 million inhabitants per year.[1] A study conducted in Spain reports that Cushing disease due to a pituitary adenoma is the most frequent cause of endogenous Cushing's syndrome, which is 5-6 times more frequent than adrenal Cushing's syndrome, with an incidence of 1.2 to 2.4 cases per 1 million inhabitants per year.[2] Treatment options for various types of endogenous Cushing's syndrome include surgery and pharmacotherapeutic options, which are discussed in the PPP Chapter 45.

CASE SUMMARY

- The patient's current clinical presentation and history point toward a diagnosis of corticosteroid-induced Cushing's syndrome. Topical corticosteroid therapy is rarely associated with Cushing's syndrome compared to systemic therapy, but case reports do exist especially when a drug interaction could increase the blood concentration of the corticosteroid.

- Discontinuation of the intranasal corticosteroid should be initiated and the allergic rhinitis treated with both an alternative drug class and trigger avoidance/minimization. Discontinuation of the inhaled corticosteroid is likely not possible given this patient's asthma history but there are several ways to minimize systemic exposure.

- To avoid a recurrence of this episode of drug-induced Cushing's syndrome, control of his asthma and allergic rhinitis is imperative. Careful attention should also be made whenever new medications are added, to avoid drug interactions that can increase systemic exposure of the inhaled corticosteroid for the management of his asthma.

- The patient should be educated about the possibility of adrenal insufficiency and symptoms of an acute adrenal crisis if testing is positive for secondary adrenal insufficiency.

REFERENCES

1. Nieman LK, Biller BM, Findling JW, et al. The diagnosis of Cushing's syndrome: An Endocrine Society Clinical Practice Guideline. J Clin Endocrinol Metab 2008;93:1526-1540.
2. Lindholm J, Juul S, Jorgensen AO, et al. Incidence and late prognosis of Cushing's Syndrome: a population-based study. J Clin Endocrinol Metab 2001;86:117-123.

For more information on the care plan and facilitator's guide please visit http://www.mhpharmacotherapy.com

53 Pregnancy

Kayce M. Shealy

PATIENT PRESENTATION

Chief Complaint
"I need relief from morning sickness."

History of Present Illness
Stacey Smith is a 32-year-old woman who presents to her primary care physician (PCP) for help with nausea related to pregnancy. She is approximately 11 weeks pregnant, and has been experiencing nausea with some vomiting for the past 6 weeks or so. This is her second pregnancy, and she experienced similar symptoms with her first child. She has experienced no other symptoms.

Past Medical History
Seasonal allergies
Hypothyroidism

Family History
Mother is alive at age 58 with migraines and hypertension (HTN). Father is alive at age 63 with hypothyroidism. She has one brother (age 36) who is healthy. She has one daughter who is healthy. There have been no multiple pregnancies in the family.

Social History
Born in the United States. Married and lives with her husband and 3-year-old daughter. Works full-time as a teacher. Usually does not eat breakfast. (+) Exercise (30-45 min 4 days/week). No pets.

Tobacco/Alcohol/Substance Use
(–) tobacco, alcohol, or illicit drug use

Allergies/Intolerances/Adverse Drug Events
No known drug allergies

Medications (Current)
Prenatal vitamin with DHA daily
Levothyroxine 50 mcg po once daily

Review of Systems
Nausea with some vomiting and fatigue; occasional headache

Physical Examination

▸ *General*

Normal weight African-American woman in no acute distress

▸ *Vital Signs*

BP 118/65 mm Hg, P 78 bpm, RR 12, T 36.2°C

Weight 137.2 lb. (62.4 kg)

Height 67 in. (170 cm)

Denies pain

▸ *Skin*

Normal

▸ *HEENT*

PERRLA, EOMI; TMs normal

▸ *Neck and Lymph Nodes*

Supple; enlarged thyroid

▸ *Chest*

Clear to auscultation

▸ *Breasts*

Slight tenderness; no nodule, discharge, or skin deformation

▸ *Cardiovascular*

RRR, normal S_1, S_2; (–) S_3 or S_4

▸ *Abdomen*

Not tender/not distended; (–) organomegaly

▸ *Neurology*

Grossly intact; DTRs normal

▸ *Genitourinary*

(–) discharge or lesions; cervix closed; bimanual examination normal; no urinary symptoms

▸ *Rectal*

Examination deferred

Laboratory Tests

TSH: 2.4 mIU/L (0.1 to 2.5 mIU/L)

Urinalysis: (+++) bacteria, (+) nitrite, (++) leukocyte esterase, trace blood

Assessment

Thirty-two-year-old woman, 11 weeks pregnant, wanting therapy for nausea/vomiting due to pregnancy.

Student Work-up

Missing Information/Inadequate Data

Evaluate: Patient database

Drug therapy problems

Care plan (by problem)

TARGETED QUESTIONS

1. What resources are available that provide data on medication use in pregnancy?

   Hint: See Table 47-4 in PPP

2. What nonpharmacologic and pharmacologic options would you discuss with the patient to help with nausea and vomiting?

   Hint: See Table 47-7 and p. 735 in PPP

3. What plan should you propose to address the urinalysis results?

   Hint: See Table 47-7 and p. 736 in PPP

4. How often should her TSH concentration be monitored and why?

   Hint: See Table 47-5 and pp. 741-742 in PPP

5. What treatment can be recommended for headache relief?

   Hint: See Table 47-7 and p. 735 in PPP

FOLLOW-UP

Nine weeks later, the patient returns for follow-up. She is taking her multivitamin and no longer needs the therapy recommended for nausea and vomiting. A follow-up urinalysis is normal, but her blood pressure is elevated. Her OB/GYN has recommended she be treated for gestational hypertension.

What do you suggest for management of nonsevere hypertension?

Hint: See Table 47-7 and p. 742 in PPP

⊙ GLOBAL PERSPECTIVE

Medication use in pregnancy should only be recommended when the benefit outweighs potential and perceived risk of treatment or lack thereof. Untreated medical conditions such as hypothyroidism and hypertension can lead to significant fetal and maternal morbidity and mortality. In addition, asymptomatic bacteriuria and urinary tract infections can lead to pregnancy complications. These conditions must be addressed and treated appropriately.

CASE SUMMARY

- Lifestyle modifications and drug therapy may be recommended for nausea and vomiting of pregnancy (NVP) in this patient. Lifestyle and diet modifications should be tried first, then medications can be recommended. The combination of pyridoxine and doxylamine are considered first line for use in NVP.

- Asymptomatic bacteriuria can lead to significant complications during pregnancy, and, therefore, should be treated.

- Routine monitoring of thyroid function is recommended as pregnancy can decrease the free fraction of thyroid hormone. Adjustments to medication dosing should be made appropriately.

- Acetaminophen is the preferred analgesic in pregnancy. Nonsteroidal anti-inflammatory agents, such as ibuprofen, should not be used during the third trimester.

- Gestational hypertension increases the risk of maternal and fetal morbidity and mortality, and should be treated. Methyldopa, labetalol, and nifedipine are considered first-line options for nonsevere hypertension.

For more information on the care plan and facilitator's guide please visit http://www.mhpharmacotherapy.com

54 Contraception

Shareen Y. El-Ibiary

PATIENT PRESENTATION

Chief Complaint

"I just had a baby, and I need a good hormonal birth control method. I am not ready to have another child anytime soon."

History of Present Illness

Jennifer Lawson is a 35-year-old woman who presents to her OB/GYN for a postpartum 4-week follow-up appointment status post caesarean section. She states she is extremely tired nursing her infant and sometimes feels dizzy. She feels very moody and seems to cry more easily so she started taking St. John's Wort because the medication her primary care physician (PCP) has not worked yet. She states that she is worried she might have another child too soon and barely can handle this one. She wants to make sure she does not get pregnant anytime soon. She just saw her PCP 8 days ago for the management of hypertension (HTN) and postpartum depression.

Past Medical History

HTN diagnosed immediately postpartum

Postpartum Depression newly diagnosed (6-month treatment course)

Family History

Father is alive at age 69 with HTN. Mother is alive at age 67 with osteoporosis and HTN. She has one sister who is healthy.

Social History

Married, one child, but plans to have another child in 2 years. Caucasian, English speaking, United States born.

Tobacco/Alcohol/Substance Use

Denies alcohol and tobacco use.

Allergies/Intolerances/Adverse Drug Events

NKDA

Medications (Current)

Labetalol 600 mg po bid

Sertraline 50 mg po daily

St. John's Wort 300 mg po tid

Prenatal vitamins

Review of Systems

Reports dizziness upon standing and sometimes just while sitting after laying down for a period of time.

Physical Examination

▶ **General**

Obese, well-appearing, Caucasian woman in no acute distress

▶ **Vital Signs**

BP 102/64 mm Hg, P 67, RR 12, T 36.2°C

Weight 198.4 lb. (90 kg)

Height 62 in. (157.5 cm)

▶ **Skin**

Supple, normal appearance

▶ **HEENT**

PERRLA, EOMI; (–) sinus tenderness; TMs appear normal

▶ **Neck and Lymph Nodes**

Thyroid gland smooth, slightly enlarged symmetrically; (–) thyroid nodules; (–) lymphadenopathy; (–) carotid bruits

▶ **Chest**

Clear to auscultation

▶ **Breasts**

Examination deferred

▶ **Cardiovascular**

RRR, normal S_1, S_2; (–) S_3 or S_4

▶ **Abdomen**

Not tender/not distended; (–) organomegaly; low transverse incision healing

▶ **Neurology**

Grossly intact; DTRs normal

▶ **Genitourinary**

Examination deferred

▶ **Rectal**

Examination deferred

Laboratory Tests

Fasting, Obtained this Morning

	Convectional Units	SI Units
Na	139 mEq/L	139 mmol/L
K	4.3 mEq/L	4.3 mmol/L
Cl	101 mEq/L	101 mmol/L
CO_2	25 mEq/L	25 mmol/L
BUN	10 mg/dL	3.6 mmol/L
SCr	0.62 mg/dL	47 μmol/L
Creatinine Clearance	>120 mL/min/ 1.73 m²	>2 mL/s/m²
Glu	95 mg/dL	5.27 mmol/L
Ca	9.1 mg/dL	2.28 mmol/L
Hgb	12.6 g/dL	126 g/L; 7.812 mmol/L
Hct	437.8%	0.378
WBC	8 × 10³/mm³	8 × 10⁹/L
AST	15 IU/L	0.25 μkat/L
ALT	22 IU/L	0.367 μkat/L
Alkaline phosphatase	42 IU/L	0.700 μkat/L

Assessment

Thirty-five-year-old postpartum, status post cesarean section, breastfeeding woman with postpartum depression, HTN, obesity, complaining of dizziness, and requesting a hormonal contraceptive

Student Work-Up

Missing Information/Inadequate Data

Evaluate: Patient database

Drug therapy problems

Care plan (by problem)

TARGETED QUESTIONS

1. What hormonal contraceptives should be avoided in this patient and why?

   Hint: See Table 48-3 in PPP

2. What risk factors does this patient have that are contraindications for use of combined hormonal contraceptives 4 weeks postpartum?

   Hint: See Table 48-3 in PPP

3. What medications or herbal products interact with combined hormonal contraceptives based on this patient's medication regimen?

   Hint: See p. 755 and Table 48-5 in PPP

4. What risks and adverse effects of hormonal contraceptives would you discuss with this patient?

   Hint: See p. 759 and Table 48-4 in PPP

5. How do this patient's needs influence the choice of hormonal contraceptive agents?

   Hint: Important to consider this patient's desire to have children in the near future and her age of 35 years. Consider the return to fertility of different contraceptive agents in this patient. The patient is also obese and contraceptive agents that heavily contribute to weight gain should also be avoided. See pp. 748-749 and pp. 751-752 in PP

FOLLOW-UP

Four weeks later, the patient returns for a 8-week follow-up appointment. Her dizziness has resolved after lowering her labetalol to 300 mg po bid. She has been taking her sertraline 50 mg po daily and continues to breastfeed. She states her mood has improved, and she no longer feels weepy or as sad. She has been taking her progestin-only pills every morning right after brushing her teeth, but missed a dose when she went out of town for a night.

What are some reasons her dizziness went away after lowering the labetalol dose? What are some reasons that her mood has improved 5 weeks after starting sertraline 50 mg po daily? What counseling would you provide the patient with regard to missing a progestin-only pill?

🌐 GLOBAL PERSPECTIVE

Hormonal contraception is mainly used for pregnancy prevention, but has other uses as well, such as treating acne, hirsutism, dysmenorrhea, menorrhagia, polycystic ovary syndrome, iron-deficiency anemia, premenstrual dysphoric disorder, and premenstrual syndrome. In the developing world, however, hormonal contraceptives are mainly desired for pregnancy prevention. Information provided by the Guttmacher Institute (http://www.guttmacher.org/pubs/AIU-2012-estimates.pdf Accessed May 18, 2015) states that in Eastern Africa an unmet need for contraception increased from 20% to 27% from 2008 to 2012 and from 50% to 56% in Southeast Asia. The information also cites that more than half (57%) of all reproductive age women (867 million women) in developing countries are in need of contraception. Approximately 42% (645 million) of women are using some form of modern contraception to prevent pregnancy, but about 15% (222 million) have unmet contraceptive needs. Contraception in developing countries may be particularly important in preventing abortions of unplanned babies, decreasing the spread of diseases such as HIV from partner to partner and mother to infant, preventing pregnancies in areas where risks of nonconsensual intercourse is high, and preventing pregnancies in women who have multiple children and cannot afford to have another. Increasing education and improving access related to contraception whether barrier, hormonal, or surgical in developing countries and in the United States may help to decrease unplanned pregnancies and prevent the associated consequences.

CASE SUMMARY

- The patient's contraceptive needs include an option compatible with breastfeeding and during the postpartum period. Ideally, this method could be a hormonal contraceptive that includes the following characteristics:

effective with her current weight, does not increase her weight significantly, does not increase her risk of stroke and CV risk because of her HTN status (though HTN is controlled), does not increase her risk of DVT while postpartum due to her risk factors of obesity and recent C-section, and has a quick return to fertility.

- A progestin-only pill or IUD would be appropriate in this patient with monitoring of mood symptoms in case the progestin worsens depression symptoms.

For more information on the care plan and facilitator's guide please visit http://www.mhpharmacotherapy.com

55 Anovulatory Bleeding

Jacqueline M. Lucey

PATIENT PRESENTATION

Chief Complaint

"I can't get pregnant."

History of Present Illness

Jamie Greene is a 29-year-old Caucasian female who presents to the clinic reporting irregular menstrual cycles and an inability to become pregnant for the past eight months. Her last menstrual cycle was two months ago and menarche occurred at age 13. Her menstrual cycle lasts 1-3 days and occur every 24-59 days. She denies painful or heavy menses.

Past Medical History

Exercise-Induced Asthma/bronchospasm (EIB) (13 years)
Seasonal allergic rhinitis (2 years)

Family History

Father is alive at age 56 with coronary heart disease (CHD), H/O myocardial infarction (MI) at age 49, dyslipidemia, and hypertension (HTN). Mother is alive at age 57 with osteopenia, HTN, dyslipidemia, and diabetes. She has one older brother (age 31) and one older sister (age 35) who are both alive and well.

Social/Work History

The patient is a married, heterosexual, sexually active female. She has been sexually active since age 17. She has had vaginal intercourse with multiple partners (3 men) in the past. She has been in a monogamous relationship for the past 5 years. She works full time at an ad agency.

Tobacco/Alcohol/Substance Use

Social drinker (2-4 glasses of wine per week); (–) tobacco use; (–) illicit drug use.

Allergies/Intolerances/Adverse Drug Events

NKDA

Medication History

▶ Current Medications

Albuterol HFA 2 puffs 15-30 minutes prior to exercise

Cetirizine 10 mg po once daily

Fluticasone proprionate 1 spray in each nostril bid

Ibuprofen 200 mg two tablets po prn headache (1-2 days per month)

▶ Past Medications

Yasmin® (Drospirenone/Ethinyl Estradiol)—discontinued 10 months ago

Review of Systems

EIB controlled with albuterol prior to exercise; occasional headache (HA) relieved with NSAID medication; seasonal allergies relieved with antihistamine; (–) GI upset, heartburn, or constipation, (–) abdominal pain; (–) change in urinary frequency; (–) dysuria; (–) vaginal discharge; (–) menorrhagia, (–) dysmenorrhea; LMP 53 days ago; age at menarche 13 years.

Physical Examination

▶ General

Obese-appearing, young, Caucasian woman in no apparent distress

▶ Vital Signs

BP 138/86 mm Hg, P 76, RR 12, T 37.0°C

Weight 190 lb. (86.4 kg)

Heigh 64 in. (162.6 cm)

Pain 0/10

▶ Skin

Normal-appearing nails; acne scars on forehead and cheeks; (–) rashes or lesions

▶ HEENT

PERRLA, EOMI; TMs appear normal; (+) hirsutism

▶ **Neck and Lymph Nodes**

No nodules

▶ **Chest**

Clear to auscultation bilaterally; (–) chest pain

▶ **Breasts**

Nontender; (–) masses

▶ **Cardiovascular**

RRR, normal S_1, S_2; (–) S_3 or S_4

▶ **Abdomen**

Soft, tender, nondistended; (–) hepatosplenomegaly

▶ **Neurology**

Grossly intact; DTRs normal

▶ **Extremities**

(–) edema; (+) pulses

▶ **Genitourinary**

Normal external appearance of labia; (–) lesions on cervix; (–) cervical motion tenderness; (–) vaginal discharge

▶ **Rectal**

Examination deferred

Laboratory and Other Diagnostic Tests
Today

- Urine pregnancy test: Negative
- Urine gonorrhea/chlamydia screening: Pending

Fasting, Obtained Today

	Conventional Units	SI Units
Na	138 mEq/L	138 mmol/L
K	4.3 mEq/L	4.3 mmol/L
Cl	104 mEq/L	104 mmol/L
CO_2	25 mEq/L	25 mmol/L
BUN	12 mg/dL	4.3 mmol/L
SCr	0.8 mg/dL	71 µmol/L
Glu	120 mg/dL	6.7 mmol/L
Hgb	13.2 g/dL	132 g/L; 8.18 mmol/L
Hct	37.2%	0.372
WBC	$6.9 \times 10^3/mm^3$	$6.9 \times 10^9/L$
Platelet	$255 \times 10^3/mm^3$	$255 \times 10^9/L$

Fasting, Obtained 1 year ago

	Conventional Units	SI Units
Na	140 mEq/L	140 mmol/L
K	4.5 mEq/L	4.5 mmol/L
Cl	102 mEq/L	102 mmol/L
CO_2	24 mEq/L	24 mmol/L
BUN	11 mg/dL	3.9 mmol/L
SCr	0.8 mg/dL	71 µmol/L
Glu	98 mg/dL	5.4 mmol/L
AST	23 IU/L	0.38 µkat/L
ALT	17 IU/L	0.28 µkat/L
Alk Phos	73 IU/L	L (1.22 µkat/L)
Hgb	12.9 g/dL	129 g/L; 8.00 mmol/L
Hct	36.5%	0.365
WBC	$5.5 \times 10^3/mm^3$	$5.5 \times 10^9/L$
Platelet	$220 \times 10^3/mm^3$	$220 \times 10^9/L$

Diagnostic Tests, Today

Pap smear: (–) cervical changes

Pelvic ultrasound: (–) masses or lesions, (+) ovarian cysts

Assessment

Twenty-nine-year-old obese woman with signs and symptoms consistent with polycystic ovarian syndrome (PCOS).

Student Work-Up

Missing Information/Inadequate Data

Evaluate: Patient database

Drug therapy problems

Care plan (by problem)

Complete a Pharmacotherapy Care Plan

Other missing information:

- Dietary habits
- Exercise routine
- Past full-term or miscarried pregnancies
- Fasting lipid panel
- Free or total testosterone

TARGETED QUESTIONS

1. What signs and symptoms of PCOS does the patient have?

   Hint: See p. 766 in PPP

2. Why are estrogen modulators the treatment of choice for patients with PCOS who desire pregnancy?

   Hint: See pp. 768-769 in PPP

3. What nonpharmacologic therapies have been shown to be beneficial in the treatment of PCOS?

   Hint: See pp. 767-768 in PPP

4. What risks and adverse effects of therapy would you discuss with the patient?

   Hint: See Table 49-1 in PPP

5. What chronic long-term complications of PCOS should the patient be screened for?

   Hint: See Table 49-3 in PPP

FOLLOW-UP

Three months later, the patient returns for follow-up. She reports her last menstrual cycle was 27 days ago. A urine pregnancy test is positive and is confirmed with a blood draw. Additional pertinent laboratory values include FBG 138 mg/dL (7.66 mmol/L); SCr 0.9 mg/dL (68.67 µmol/L), HgbA1c 6.7% (0.067). BP in the office today is 132/82 mm Hg. How would you manage this patient's anovulatory bleeding and cardiovascular risk factors at this time?

Therapy for withdrawal bleeding and induction of ovulation should be discontinued at this time to as the patient is now pregnant. Blood pressure is still below the goal of 140/90 mm Hg and treatment should not be initiated at this time. Low-moderate intensity aerobic exercise should be continued to prevent elevations in blood pressure during pregnancy as this would pose an additional risk to both the mother and fetus. This patient should be diagnosed with diabetes due to hemoglobin A1c ≥ 6.5% and fasting plasma glucose ≥ 126 mg/dL (7.00 mmol/L). Although the patient is pregnant, she should be diagnosed with diabetes as opposed to gestational diabetes as she is only 4 weeks pregnant and had an impaired fasting glucose at last visit. If elevated glucose levels are first diagnosed during weeks 24-28 of pregnancy, gestational diabetes would be the correct diagnosis. Metformin or insulin therapy should be initiated to control blood glucose concentrations as elevated levels are associated with neonatal risks.[1]

1. American Diabetes Association. Standards of Medical Care in Diabetes—2015. Diabetes Care 2015;38(Suppl. 1): S1-S2 | DOI:10.2337/dc15-S001.

🌐 GLOBAL PERSPECTIVE

Cardiovascular disease (CVD) varies among different ethnic backgrounds. It is known that African-American and Hispanic adults are at an increased risk of diabetes, hypertension, and dyslipidemia as well as associated long-term cardiovascular complications. More recently, polycystic ovary syndrome has been shown to increase the risk of cardiovascular disease risk factors, as these women tend to have higher rates of obesity, hypertension, and impaired fasting glucose or diabetes.[1,2] Since this finding, ethnic variations in the link between PCOS and cardiovascular disease have begun to be evaluated. While cardiovascular morbidity and mortality outcomes will take years to determine, risk factors associated with CVD in women with PCOS have been reported. In one study, black adolescent and adult women with PCOS had higher rates of metabolic syndrome, specifically, elevated glucose levels and lower levels of high-density lipoprotein compared to white adolescent and adult women with PCOS. The relative risk of metabolic syndrome was 2.65 (95% CI 1.29-5.4) in black adolescents and 1.44 (95% CI 1.21-2.6) in black adults compared to white adolescents and adults.[3] Hispanic women have also been shown to have higher rates of cardiovascular risk factors compared to non-Hispanic white women. These risk factors included increased abdominal obesity, dyslipidemia, and insulin resistance.[4] Knowledge of ethnic differences may be of benefit in the assessment and treatment of in women with PCOS, particularly when identifying early signs and symptoms of cardiovascular disease risk factors. Further studies are warranted to evaluate the link between PCOS and cardiovascular disease morbidity and mortality.

REFERENCES

1. Fauser BC, Tarlatzis BC, Rebar RW, et al. Consensus on women's health aspects of polycystic ovary syndrome (PCOS): the Amsterdam ESHRE/ASRM-Sponsored 3rd PCOS Consensus Workshop Group. Fertil Steril. 2012;97:28-38.

2. Dokras A. Cardiovascular disease risk in women with PCOS. Steroids. 2013;78:773-776.

3. Hillman JK, Johnson LNC, Limaye M, et al. Black women with polycystic ovary syndrome (PCOS) have increased risk for metabolic syndrome and cardiovascular disease compared with white women with PCOS. Fertil Steril. 2014 Feb;101(2):530-5. doi:10.1016/j.fertnstert.2013.10.055.

4. Sam S, Scoccia B, Yalamanchi S, Mazzone T. Metabolic dysfunction in obese Hispanic women with polycystic ovary syndrome. Hum Reprod. 2015 Jun;30(6):1358-64. doi:10.1093/humrep/dev073.

CASE SUMMARY

- The patient's current clinical picture is consistent with anovulatory bleeding secondary to PCOS. Therapy with oral medroxyprogesterone acetate to induce withdrawal bleeding and an estrogen modulator to induce ovulation should be initiated.

- Given the patient's family history and personal risk factors for cardiovascular disease, the patient should be screened for hypertension, diabetes, and dyslipidemia.

- Fertility should occur in one to five cycles. If fertility does not occur, additional work-up and referral may be necessary.

KEY REFERENCES/READINGS

1. Legro RS, Barnhart HX, Schlaff WD, et al. Clomiphene, metformin, or both for infertility in the polycystic ovary syndrome. N Engl J Med 2007;356:551-566.
2. Tang T, Lord JM, Norman RJ, Yasmin E, Balen AH. Insulin-sensitising drugs (metformin, rosiglitazone, pioglitazone, D-chiro-inositol) for women with polycystic ovary syndrome, oligo amenorrhoea and subfertility. Cochrane Database Syst Rev 2012;5:CD003053-CD003053.
3. Tredway D, Schertz JC, Bock D, Hemsey G, Diamond MP. Anastrozole vs. clomiphene citrate in infertile women with ovulatory dysfunction: a phase II, randomized, dose-finding study. Fertil Steril 2011;95:1720-1724

For more information on the care plan and facilitator's guide please visit http://www.mhpharmacotherapy.com

56 Menopause

Tracy M. Hagemann

PATIENT PRESENTATION

Chief Complaint

"I can't stand these symptoms anymore! I can't sleep, I'm having bad hot flashes, and my family says that I'm so cranky they are considering a long vacation without me."

History of Present Illness

NG is a 45-year-old Caucasian woman who presents to her primary care physician complaining of hot flashes, sleep disturbances, and irritability that have been increasing in severity over the last 3 months. She admits to interruptions in her day several times per week due to profuse sweating and mood swings. She is awakened with an average of 1-2 hot flashes nightly. In addition, she has had a recent onset of vaginal dryness that is causing dyspareunia that is not relieved by lubricants, and has reported that she has had two urinary tract infections during the last 2 months. Her menstrual periods have been decreasing in frequency over the past year.

Past Medical History

Hypothyroidism (8 years)

Ductal Carcinoma In Situ, ER positive—treated with radiation, lumpectomy 6 years ago; completed 5 years of tamoxifen treatment last year

Past Surgical History

Right breast lumpectomy (5 years ago)

Cesarean section (14 years ago)

Appendectomy (14 years ago)

Family History

Father is 70 and has coronary heart disease (CHD) and bipolar disorder. Mother is 68, has hypertension (HTN), is a survivor of thyroid cancer, and had a thyroidectomy 10 years ago. NG has one sister, age 42, in good health.

Social History

NG is a married mother of two children, ages 18 and 14. She has been married for 22 years. She works as an office manager for a cardiologist practice.

Tobacco/Alcohol/Substance Use

2-3 alcoholic drinks/week; (–) tobacco or illicit drug use

Allergies/Intolerances/Adverse Drug Events

None

Medications (Current)

Levothyroxine 100 mcg po daily

Calcium with vitamin D 600 mg/400 IU po bid

Multivitamin one tablet po q 24 h

Ibuprofen 200 mg po prn joint pain after exercising

Review of Systems

Several incidences of painful intercourse; (+) dyspareunia; also episodes of increased body temperature and irritability; (+) vasomotor symptoms; (+) night sweats; (–) chest pain; (–) palpitations; (–) tachycardia

Physical Examination

▶ **General**

Forty-five-year-old Caucasian woman in no acute distress

▶ **Vital Signs**

BP 112/70 mm Hg, P 70, RR 16, pulse O_2 98% (0.98), T 97.4°F (36.3°C)

Weight 132 lb. (60 kg)

Height 66 in. (167.6 cm)

Pain score 0/10

▶ **Skin**

Denies history of skin cancer. No rashes or new or unusual skin lesions

▶ **HEENT**

PERRLA, EOMI; intact without nystagmus, conjunctivas clear, sclera anicteric, canals clear, oropharynx clear without exudate

▶ **Neck and Lymph Nodes**

No masses or crepitance, symmetric, thyroid without nodularity, midline trachea

▶ **Breasts**

No discrete nodules, scar on right breast

▶ **Cardiovascular**

Regular rate and rhythm, no murmurs, no jugular venous distention

▶ **Lungs**

Clear to auscultation

▶ **Abdomen**

No tenderness, organomegaly, or masses; appendectomy and cesarean scars

▶ **Neurology**

No history of seizures, migraines, falls, or vertigo

▶ **Genitourinary**

No urinary problems, negative for renal stones

▶ **External Genitalia**

No unusual findings

▶ **Vagina**

Minimally atrophic mucosa

▶ **Psychiatric**

Mood swings, irritability

Laboratory Tests

Fasting, Obtained this Morning

	Conventional Units	SI Units
Na	136 mEq/L	136 mmol/L
K	4.9 mEq/L	4.9 mmol/L
Cl	107 mEq/L	107 mmol/L
CO_2	23 mEq/L	23 mmol/L
BUN	7 mg/dL	2.5 mmol/L
SCr	0.7 mg/dL	62 μmol/L
Glu	72 mg/dL	3.9 mmol/L
Ca	8 mg/dL	2 mmol/L
Mg	1.6 mEq/L	0.80 mmol/L
Phosphate	3.7 mg/dL	1.20 mmol/L
Hgb	12.8 g/dL	128 g/L; 7.93 mmol/L
Hct	38.5%	0.385
WBC	$6 \times 10^3/mm^3$	$6 \times 10^9/L$
MCV	$87 \ \mu m^3$	87 fL
Albumin	3.9 g/dL	39 g/L
TSH	3.2 μIU/mL	3.2 mIU/L
Free T_4	0.96 ng/dL	12.4 pmol/L
Total cholesterol	180 mg/dL	4.65 mmol/L
LDL cholesterol	75 mg/dL	1.94 mmol/L
HDL cholesterol	85 mg/dL	2.19 mmol/L
TG	80 mg/dL	0.90 mmol/L

Student Work-Up

Missing Information/Inadequate Data

Evaluate:
Patient database
Drug therapy problems
Care plan (by problem)

TARGETED QUESTIONS

1. What signs and symptoms of menopause does NG have?
   Hint: See p. 776 in PPP

2. What factors in NG's medical history must we consider when deciding upon medication therapy?
   Hint: See Figure 50-1 in PPP

3. What nonpharmacologic therapy would be recommended in NG's case?
   Hint: See p. 777 in PPP

4. What are the pharmacotherapy options for NG's menopausal signs/symptoms?
   Hint: See pp. 782-783 in PPP

5. What risks and adverse effects of therapy would you discuss with NG?
   Hint: See pp. 781-782 in PPP

FOLLOW-UP

When NG returns for her follow-up appointment 6 weeks later, she reports that she stopped taking the paroxetine 2 weeks ago because she was having severe headaches, unrelieved by over-the-counter analgesics. She does not want to restart the paroxetine. Her vasomotor symptoms are unchanged from her last visit, however, she is noticing a little relief of her vaginal dryness and sexual intercourse is less painful since starting the vaginal low-dose estrogen. What do you recommend to treat her vasomotor symptoms?

Hint: See p. 782 in PPP

🌐 GLOBAL PERSPECTIVE

Menopause happens to every woman once she reaches the end of her reproductive ability and is a physiological change. However, when comparing how menopause manifests itself through signs and symptoms across cultures, the results vary greatly. Signs and symptoms of menopause differ in quality and quantity. Use of medication or alternative therapies can vary considerably as well.

CASE SUMMARY

- NG's clinical condition is consistent with menopause and pharmacotherapy should be initiated, but consideration of her history of estrogen-positive breast cancer will limit some of the pharmacotherapy options for her.

- Use of topical low-dose estrogen and an SSRI are acceptable first-line therapy given her history of breast cancer. Systemic use of hormone replacement therapy (HRT) should be avoided.

- Close follow-up (4-6 weeks) may be desired initially to ensure success of medication therapy, and then 6-month follow-up would be acceptable.

REFERENCES

1. North American Menopause Society. Estrogen and progesterone use in postmenopausal women: 2010 position statement of The North American Menopause Society. Menopause 2010 Mar;17(2):242-55.

2. Holmberg L, Iversen OE, Rudenstam CM, Hammar M, Kumpulainen E, et al. Increased risk of recurrence after hormone replacement therapy in breast cancer survivors. J Natl Cancer Inst 2008;100(7):475-82.

3. Krause MS, Nakajima ST. Hormonal and nonhormonal treatment of vasomotor symptoms. Obstet Gynecol Clin North Am 2015;42(1):163-79.

For more information on the care plan and facilitator's guide please visit http://www.mhpharmacotherapy.com

57 Erectile Dysfunction

Mary Lee   Roohollah Sharifi

PATIENT PRESENTATION

Chief Complaint

Patient complains of impotence for the past year. His sexual partner is unsatisfied and has encouraged him to seek medical help, just like on those television commercials. The patient says that he has a desire for sex, but that his desire is less now than when he was younger. At today's clinic visit (March 16, 2015) patient is requesting medication to improve his performance.

History of Present Illness

Robert Smith is a 65-year-old white male with erectile dysfunction. He is in a stable relationship with a significant other, and they have lived together for many years. He describes her as a physically attractive, 47-year-old female who works full time as an accountant. The patient also reports no change in his personal life in the past year: he is in a stable full-time job as a store manager, enjoys his work and colleagues, and has no family-related concerns.

Prior to this clinic visit, the patient describes himself as very healthy, with just a few aches and pains associated with aging. Typically, he only sees a doctor for an annual physical exam and only takes medications as needed for various episodic problems.

Past Medical History

Heartburn, since 2012. Heartburn is precipitated by spicy foods. Although he tries to avoid spicy foods, sometimes the urge is uncontrollable and he "pays for it." Omeprazole controls heartburn. On average, he takes omeprazole 20 mg once a week.

Knee pain. This resulted from a ski injury sustained about 35 years ago. Periodically, if he walks too much, he has knee pain. This responds to naproxen 250 mg po prn.

Hemorrhoids. Has self-managed this with Preparation H for many years. He has not had rectal bleeding. Hemorrhoids are just uncomfortable and painful.

High blood pressure, documented at last clinic visit 2 months ago. Patient reports that he has not/is not receiving any medication for this. He was instructed to lose weight, exercise, and reduce his salt intake by not adding salt to his food once it was served to him.

Family History

Father is alive, and has hypertension and hypercholesterolemia. Mother is alive, and has hypertension. Has two younger sisters, both alive and well.

Social History

Patient is in stable relationship with long-time female partner.

Tobacco/Alcohol/Substance Use

Noncontributory. Reports only a glass of wine for special occasions.

Medications (Current)

Omeprazole 20 mg po prn

Naproxen 250 mg po prn

Preparation H ointment 1 applicatorful to rectum at bedtime

Review of Systems

This patient complains only of erectile dysfunction for the past year. Has no other complaints.

Physical Examination

▶ *General*

Well-developed, well-nourished white male

▶ *Vital Signs*

BP 165/95 mm Hg (higher than last year). BP was repeated × 2 and was consistently 165/95 mm Hg, P 72, RR 16, T 37°C

Weight 190 lb. (86.4 kg)

Height 68 in. (172.7 cm)

No pain

▶ **Skin**

(–) Rashes or lesions

▶ **HEENT**

PERRLA, EOMI

▶ **Neck and Lymph Nodes**

Thyroid gland is smooth and symmetrical; (–) thyroid nodules; (–) lymphadenopathy; (–) carotid bruits

▶ **Chest**

Clear to auscultation and percussion

▶ **Cardiovascular**

RRR, no murmurs, (–) S_3, (+) S_4

▶ **Abdomen**

Soft, not tender to palpation; no masses or organomegaly

▶ **Neurology**

Grossly intact, deep tendon reflexes normal

▶ **Extremities**

No edema; good range of motion; (4+) left and right pedal pulses

▶ **Genitourinary**

Digital rectal exam: prostate mildly enlarged, symmetric, no nodules or induration

Penis: normal

Testes: both normal sized

Scrotum: normal

Perineum: normal

▶ **Rectal**

External hemorrhoids only

Normal sphincter tone

Laboratory and Other Diagnostic Tests

	03/16/2015	03/16/2015
	Conventional Units	SI Units
Na	140 mEq/L	140 mmol/L
K	4.0 mEq/L	4 mmol/L
Cl	106 mEq/L	106 mmol/L
CO_2/HCO_3	24 mEq/L	24 mmol/L
BUN	14 mg/dL	5.00 mmol/L urea
Serum creatinine	0.9 mg/dL	79.56 µmol/L
Glucose (fasting)	82 mg/dL	4.55 mmol/L
Total Ca	9.1 mg/dL	2.28 mmol/L
Mg	2.2 mEq/L	1.1 mmol/L
PO_4	2.9 mg/dL	0.94 mmol/L
Hemoglobin	14 g/dL	140 g/L
Hematocrit	44%	0.44
WBC	$6.2 \times 10^3/mm^3$	6.2×10^9/L
Platelet	$350 \times 10^3/mm^3$	350×10^9/L
Albumin	4.5 d/dL	45 g/L
Bilirubin (total)	1.0 mg/dL	17.10 µmol/L
Bilirubin (direct)	0.2 mg/dL	3.42 µmol/L
AST	45 IU/L	0.75 µkat/L
ALT	45 IU/L	0.75 µkat/L
Alk phos	100 IU/L	1.67 µkat/L
Testosterone	250 ng/dL	8.68 nmol/L

03/16/2015 International Index of Erectile Function score 10.

Assessment

Patient reports erectile dysfunction for the past year and decreased sexual desire. Based on the IIEF (international index of erectile function) score, erectile dysfunction is of moderate severity. He has received no treatment to date. Erectile dysfunction is probably organic in nature, and may be caused by/exacerbated by untreated hypertension, omeprazole, and hypogonadism.

Hypertension could be contributing to the patient's erectile dysfunction. Will reinforce weight reduction, exercise, low-sodium intake. Will treat hypertension with valsartan 80-320 mg po daily or enalapril 5-40 mg po daily, if medication is needed. Once blood pressure is under control, will check to see if sexual function improves.

For gastroesophageal reflux, will discontinue omeprazole, which could be contributing to the patient's erectile dysfunction. Will instruct patient to minimize trigger foods, lose weight, and elevate head of the bed. If necessary, to control pain, will recommend antacid/alginic acid (Gaviscon) 2 tablets or 15 mL po after meals and at bedtime. Will check to see if sexual function improves after omeprazole is stopped.

If serum testosterone is low, will confirm initial low serum testosterone level by repeating the lab test. If the patient has confirmed hypogonadism, will start testosterone supplementation, which often restores both libido and erectile function. Will start phosphodiesterase type 5 inhibitor only if these measures fail to improve sexual function.

For hemorrhoids, will check to see if patient has symptoms that require Preparation H ointment, which includes phenylephrine 0.25%, a vasoconstrictor, that could be systemically absorbed and contribute to hypertension. If the patient has minimal/mild symptoms, will encourage the patient to maintain a high fiber diet, drink fluids during the day, avoid constipation, avoid lifting heavy objects, avoid straining, and maintain good perianal hygiene. If patient has itching and pain, he could try sitz baths several times a day. Anorectal medication should be reserved if these measures fail.

Student Work-Up

Missing Information/Inadequate Data

Evaluate: Patient database

Drug therapy problems

Care plan (by problem)

Additional information:

- Has a serum testosterone level been obtained in the past year.

- Has the patient used any over the counter or herbal products for erectile dysfunction? If yes, what has he tried?

- Is this patient providing a complete medical and medication history? If we are not sure, we should request a copy of his medical records. We need to make sure that this patient does not have any medical disorders or is not taking any medications that are contraindications to treatment for erectile dysfunction.

TARGETED QUESTIONS

1. List five major pharmacological classes of medications that can cause erectile dysfunction.

   Hint: See Table 51-2 in PPP

2. Is this patient a candidate for a vacuum erection device? What are the advantages and disadvantages of using a vacuum erection device in this patient?

   Hint: See p. 791 in PPP

3. Identify key differences among the phosphodiesterase type 5 inhibitors used for erectile dysfunction.

   Hint: See pp. 791-792 and Table 51-4 in PPP

4. Summarize key counseling points when educating a patient about a phosphodiesterase type 5 inhibitor so that optimal results can be achieved.

   Hint: See pp. 791-792 in PPP

5. Assume that this patient is started on intramuscular testosterone cypionate injections every month. Is this medication indicated in this patient? Explain your answer.

   Hint: See p. 794 in PPP

FOLLOW-UP

Assume that the patient's erectile dysfunction does not improve after an adequate treatment trial of testosterone supplements and a therapeutic dosing regimen of phosphodiesterase type 5 inhibitor. What other treatment options could be considered in this patient?

Hint: See pp. 791-792 and 794 in PPP

⊙ GLOBAL PERSPECTIVE

Although medications that are FDA-labelled for management of erectile dysfunction are to be used as monotherapy, use of combinations of medications or adding a medication to a vacuum erection device have been reported to be effective in the published literature particularly when a single agent loses effectiveness. Such combinations include testosterone supplementation plus a phosphodiesterase type 5 inhibitor; or a vacuum erection device plus a phosphodiesterase inhibitor or alprostadil.

CASE SUMMARY

- Prior to starting a phosphodiesterase type 5 inhibitor for erectile dysfunction, a patient's medical history and medication list should be evaluated to identify any conditions or medications that could contribute to the patient's sexual dysfunction. If present, the condition(s) or medication(s) should be addressed first.

- Symptomatic hypogonadism of aging is characterized by decreased libido and erectile dysfunction and low serum testosterone levels. Testosterone supplementation is indicated to increase sexual drive; erectile function often improves as sexual drive improves.

- Phosphodiesterase type 5 inhibitors are medications of first choice and vacuum erection devices are a modality of first choice for management of erectile dysfunction.

For more information on the care plan and facilitator's guide please visit http://www.mhpharmacotherapy.com

58 Benign Prostatic Hyperplasia

Mary Lee   Roohollah Sharifi

PATIENT PRESENTATION

Chief Complaint

"I can't get a good night's sleep. I have to go to the washroom 3-4 times each night. What's worse is that during the day, I am having accidents because I can't get to the toilet fast enough. When I have to urinate, I can't hold it until I get to the rest room. On February 1, 2015 when I was in the Urology Clinic, you had prescribed medication for my problem, but I have not been able to get the prescription filled. My insurance doesn't cover it and it is too expensive for me to afford. I am here now on March 1, 2015 to get a different prescription for my urinary problem."

History of Present Illness

Sam Jones is a 68-year-old white male with lower urinary tract symptoms (LUTS), who first presented to the Urology Clinic on February 1, 2015. At that time, the patient's American Urological Association (AUA) symptom score was 16, peak urinary flow rate was 8 mL/second, post void residual urine volume was 10 mL. A digital rectal exam was performed. The prostate was enlarged, approximately 30 g, soft and symmetrical, with no nodularity or induration. Blood tests were ordered for PSA, BUN, and serum creatinine. At that time, a clinical diagnosis of benign prostatic hyperplasia was made and alfuzosin 10 mg po daily was prescribed. Patient was unable to start medication because alfuzosin is not covered on his insurance plan and it was too expensive. At the time, the patient decided to wait for his next follow-up Urology Clinic visit in one month to discuss the medication problem with the urologist. In the meantime, on 2/9/2015, he returned for some blood testing which had been ordered by his family medicine doctor and the urologist. Patient is now requesting a different prescription for his urinary problem.

Past Medical History

Essential hypertension (since 2009)

Hyperlipidemia (since 2013)

Overweight

Family History

Father died of a stroke and mother died of "old age." His older brother was recently diagnosed and started medical treatment for benign prostatic hyperplasia and is responding well.

Social History

Patient is happily married, and has no children

Tobacco/Alcohol/Substance Use

Has been sober for 30 years, after joining Alcoholics Anonymous

Does not smoke or use recreational drugs

Allergies/Intolerances/Adverse Drug Events

Amoxicillin causes hives and a swollen tongue. This reaction occurred more than 58 years ago when the patient was 10 years old.

Medications (Current)

Alfuzosin 10 mg po daily (Although prescribed on February 1, 2015, patient never got the prescription filled)

Chlorthalidone 25 mg po daily (since 2013)

Lovastatin 20 mg po daily (since September 30, 2014)

Multivitamin 1 capsule po daily

ASA 81 mg po daily

Review of Systems

This patient complains of only bothersome nocturia and urinary incontinence during the day. He has no other complaints.

Physical Examination

▶ **General**

Well-developed, overweight male.

▶ **Vital Signs**

BP 152/90 mm Hg, P 89, RR 16, T 37°C

Weight 215 lb. (97.7 kg)

Height 70 in. (177.8 cm)

No pain

▶ **Skin**

(–) Rashes or lesions

▶ **HEENT**

PERRLA, EOMI

▶ **Neck and Lymph Nodes**

Thyroid gland is smooth and symmetrical; (–) thyroid nodules; (–) lymphadenopathy; (–) carotid bruits

▶ **Chest**

Clear to auscultation and percussion.

▶ **Cardiovascular**

RRR, no murmurs, (–) S_3, (–) S_4

▶ **Abdomen**

Soft, not tender to palpation; no masses or organomegaly.

▶ **Neurology**

Grossly intake; deep tendon reflexes normal

▶ **Extremities**

No edema; good range of motion; (4+) left and right pedal pulses

▶ **Genitourinary**

Digital rectal examination was not repeated at this visit since it was performed only 4 weeks ago. Normal external genitalia. No costovertebral ankle tenderness.

▶ **Rectal**

Exam deferred since it was performed only 4 weeks ago

Laboratory and Other Diagnostic Tests

	2/9/2015	2/9/2015
	Conventional Units	SI Units
Na	140 mEq/L	140 mmol/L
K	3.5 mEq/L	3.5 mmol/L
Cl	102 mEq/L	102 mmol/L
CO_2/HCO_3	29 mEq/L	29 mmol/L
BUN	14 mg/dL	5.00 mmol/L
Serum creatinine	1.2 mg/dL	91.56 μmol/L
Glucose	95 mg/dL	5.27 mmol/L
Cholesterol	225 mg/dL	5.82 mmol/L
Triglycerides	104 mg/dL	1.18 mmol/L
HDL	32 mg/dL	0.83 mmol/L
LDL	170 mg/dL	4.40 mmol/L
PSA	1.8 ng/mL	1.8 μg/L

2/1/2015: American Urological Association Symptom Score 16, peak urinary flow rate 8 mL/second, post void residual urine volume 10 mL

3/9/2015: American Urological Association Symptom Score 16, peak urinary flow rate 9 mL/second, post void residual urine volume 0 mL

Assessment

Patient was diagnosed 4 weeks ago with probable benign prostatic hypertrophy with moderate LUTS. Alfuzosin 10 mg po qd was prescribed to manage symptoms, however, the prescription was not filled because it was not covered on this patient's insurance plan and it was too expensive. Need to start the patient on an alternative α-adrenergic antagonist. Will initiate terazosin immediate release formulation. It is available as a generic formulation and will also lower blood pressure, which would be beneficial for this patient.

Patient's hypertension is not well-controlled on chlorthalidone. Patient tolerates it well. Serum potassium is normal. Addition of α-adrenergic antagonist for BPH to current antihypertensive regimen may lower blood pressure, which would be beneficial for this patient.

Patient's most recent lipid panel shows inadequate control of hyperlipidemia on current dose of lovastatin. Patient admits to poor compliance with low cholesterol diet and is overweight. Will refer to a dietician for retraining on low cholesterol, low calorie diet and importance of daily exercise regimen. Will refer patient back to Family Medicine to increase dose of lovastatin (effective range, 20-80 mg/day).

Student Work-Up

Missing Information/Inadequate Data

Evaluate:
- Patient database
- Drug therapy problems
- Care plan (by problem)

Additional information:

TRUS assessment of prostate volume/size (for a more accurate assessment of prostate size); estimated creatinine clearance; history of recurrent urinary tract infection, hematuria, or other complications of benign prostatic hyperplasia; assessment of patient's compliance with medications for hypercholesterolemia and hypertension; steps patient has taken to lose weight, increase physical activity, and initiate a low salt/low cholesterol diet.

TARGETED QUESTIONS

1. Review the urologic tests performed on 2/1/2015. What do the results imply about the severity of this patient's BPH?

   Hint: See Table 52-1 and Table 52-2 in PPP

2. Doxazosin is available as an extended release formulation for BPH. What are the clinical advantages of the extended release formulation over the immediate release formulation?

   Hint: See p. 804 in PPP

3. Alfuzosin was originally prescribed in this patient. What are the potential advantages of this particular alpha adrenergic antagonist when compared to other agents in the same pharmacologic class?

   Hint: See p. 804 in PPP

4. Finasteride or dutasteride was not recommended for this patient. Why not?

   Hint: See pp. 805-806 in PPP

5. Is this patient a candidate for prostate surgery?

   Hint: See Figure 52-1 in PPP

FOLLOW-UP

The patient was stabilized on terazosin 10 mg po daily. After 6 weeks, his AUA symptom score is 11. His nocturia is improved and he wakes up only 0-1 times each night. However, he still has some urgency and incontinence that interfere with his daily activities.

Is there any medication that might be helpful for management of irritative symptoms?

   Hint: See pp. 806-807 in PPP

☉ GLOBAL PERSPECTIVE

The use of phytotherapy for symptomatic management of benign prostatic hypertrophy is highly variable in countries outside of the United States. However, in the United States, the American Urological Association has taken the position that there is inadequate evidence from prospective, controlled clinical trials that justifies the use of phytotherapy for treatment of benign prostatic hypertrophy.

CASE SUMMARY

- For symptomatic management of benign prostatic hypertrophy, α-adrenergic antagonists are first-line treatment. Several characteristics differentiate α-adrenergic antagonists, including: functional and pharmacologic uroselectivity, immediate or extended release dosage formulation, single versus multi-source availability, and adverse effect profile.

- 5-α-reductase inhibitors are preferentially prescribed in patients who are at risk of progression of benign prostatic hypertrophy, which include those patients with a prostate of 40 g or larger, or a serum PSA of 1.6 ng/mL or higher.

- An anticholinergic agent can be added to an α-adrenergic antagonist for improved management of irritative voiding symptoms, for example, urgency.

- Tadalafil 5 mg po qd can be used for LUTS. Because of its cost, it is best to use this in patients who have both benign prostatic hypertrophy and erectile dysfunction.

- Mirabegron enhances urine storage in the bladder and is an alternative to an anticholinergic agent, particularly in those patients who do not tolerate anticholinergic adverse effects.

KEY REFERENCES

1. American Urological Association Guideline-Management of benign prostatic hyperplasia 2010 (reviewed and validity confirmed 2014). www.auanet.org/education/clinical-practice-guidelines.cfm (last accessed 3/24/2015).

For more information on the care plan and facilitator's guide please visit http://www.mhpharmacotherapy.com

59 Urinary Incontinence: Overactive Bladder

Andrea S. Franks

PATIENT PRESENTATION

Chief Complaint

"My overactive bladder problems have gotten worse over the last few weeks. I can barely make it to the restroom in time."

History of Present Illness

Gloria Jones is a 66-year-old female who comes to clinic for a hospital discharge follow-up appointment. She was recently hospitalized with heart failure, and was started on a new regimen including a diuretic (furosemide 40 mg twice daily). She has previously not used medications for incontinence, and was able to manage her overactive bladder with behavioral management like frequent, scheduled trips to the restroom and pelvic floor muscle rehabilitation. She states she is taking her furosemide 40 mg twice daily most days, but sometimes skips the afternoon dose if she is out running errands because she is afraid she won't make it to the rest room on time. She would like to take a medicine her friend recommended, Detrol LA.

Past Medical History

Overactive bladder (diagnosed 2 years ago)

Hypertension (for 15 years)

Heart failure, reduced ejection fraction (HFREF) (diagnosed 2 years ago)

Depression (diagnosed 1 year ago)

Dry eye syndrome (diagnosed at age 45)

Family History

Mother died of heart problems in her 70s

Father died of stroke in his 80s

Social History

Married, lives with husband; 2 adult children who live independently

Tobacco/Ethanol/Substance Use

Denies tobacco or alcohol; drinks 3 cups of caffeinated coffee each morning, and 1 cup midafternoon

Allergies/Intolerances/Adverse Drug Events

No known drug allergies. Antihistamines aggravate dry eye syndrome.

Medications (Current)

Lisinopril 40 mg po q 24 h

Metoprolol succinate 100 mg po q 24 h

Furosemide 40 mg po twice daily

Potassium Chloride 20 mEq po q 24 h

Sertraline 50 mg po q hs

Calcium carbonate 500 mg po twice daily with meals

Acetaminophen 500 mg/diphenhydramine 25 mg po hs prn aches and pains/insomnia

Review of Systems

The patient has urge urinary incontinence and reports 1-2 accidents per week. She complains of urinary urgency and sometimes cannot make it to the bathroom in time. She urinates as frequently as every 1 to 2 hours during the day and awakens twice nightly with a strong urge to void. You administer the Overactive Bladder Symptom Score (OABSS) and she scores 6 overall. She was recently hospitalized with a heart failure exacerbation that presented with weight gain, dyspnea, and lower extremity edema. With the new addition of furosemide, she has no complaints related to her heart failure.

Physical Examination

▶ *General*

Overweight Caucasian female in no acute distress.

▶ *Vital Signs*

BP 130/80 mm Hg, P 70, RR 18, T 36.3°C

Weight 174 lb. (79 kg)

Height 64 in. (157 cm)

▶ *Skin*

Healthy-appearing skin, no rashes or lesions

▸ **HEENT**

Normal exam

▸ **Neck and Lymph Nodes**

No lymphadenopathy or masses

▸ **Chest**

Clear to auscultation

▸ **Breasts**

No masses

▸ **Cardiovascular**

RRR; no murmurs appreciated

▸ **Abdomen**

Nontender, nondistended; positive bowel sounds

▸ **Neurology**

Grossly intact, motor strength 5/5 symmetrical, normal reflexes

▸ **Genitourinary**

Normal exam

▸ **Rectal**

Examination deferred

Laboratory Tests

	Conventional Units	SI Units
Na	140 mEq/L	140 mmol/L
K	4.0 mEq/L	4.0 mmol/L
CL	100 mEq/L	100 mmol/L
Bicarbonate	24 mEq/L	24 mmol/L
BUN	12 mEq/L	4.3 mmol/L
Serum creatinine	1.2 mEq/L	106 μmol/L
Glucose	104 mEq/L	5.8 mmol/L
Urinalysis		
pH	5.2	
WBC	0/lpf	
RBC	0/lpf	
Leucocyte esterase	(−)	
Nitrites	(−)	

Assessment

Sixty-six-year-old female with signs and symptoms consistent with urge urinary incontinence/overactive bladder and other comorbidities.

TARGETED QUESTIONS

1. What signs and symptoms of urge urinary incontinence (UUI) does the patient have?

   Hint: See pp. 812-813 in PPP

2. What class of agents is treatment of choice for patients with urge urinary incontinence and why?

   Hint: See pp. 816-818 in PPP

3. What medication could be aggravating this patient's overactive bladder?

   Hint: See Table 53-1 in PPP

4. What potential adverse effects or drug interactions would you be concerned with in this specific patient if initiating tolterodine?

   Hint: See pp. 816-818 and Table 53-4 in PPP

5. What additional changes could be made to this patient's pharmacotherapy that could improve her overactive bladder symptoms?

   Hint: See Table 53-1 in PPP

FOLLOW-UP

One month later, the patient returns for a refill of tolterodine long-acting. She reports moderate improvement in her overactive bladder symptoms, with this documented in a bladder diary. However, she complains of dry eyes. What actions, if any, would you take?

   Hint: See p. 816 in PPP

⊙ GLOBAL PERSPECTIVE

While different cultures approach urinary incontinence differently, it is a universal problem with a significant socioeconomic impact. In developing countries where girls are forced to marry and bear children very young, they often experience incontinence following childbirth. Unfortunately, absorbent products are generally not available in these areas. The sense of shame, embarrassment, and reluctance to seek treatment for urinary incontinence is common across many cultures and countries.

CASE SUMMARY

- The patient has symptoms of urge urinary incontinence that appear to interfere with her quality of life.
- Managing her diuresis and fluid balance for heart failure must be balanced with treating her symptoms of urge urinary incontinence.

- Her insomnia could be related to her nocturia, and the nonprescription medication she takes for insomnia might have a cumulative effect with the drug class of choice for treating urge urinary incontinence/overactive bladder.

For more information on the care plan and facilitator's guide please visit http://www.mhpharmacotherapy.com

60 Drug Allergy

Lauren S. Schlesselman

Daniel J. Ventricelli

PATIENT PRESENTATION

Chief Complaint

"I was working in the animal research lab when I was bitten by one of the lab rats. I was in a hurry so I was not wearing gloves. When I tried to pick up the rat, he turned and bit my hand."

History of Present Illness

Abby Picket is a 26-year-old woman who presents to the emergency department with a rat bite to her left hand. While working on a behavioral research project involving rats, the patient attempted to pick up one of the rats. The rat turned around and bit the patient who was not wearing protective gloves. The patient describes attempting to shake the rat from her hand. When the rat let go of her hand, it escaped through a small hole in the wall. The rat's whereabouts remain unknown. Damage to the hand confirms rat-inflicted damage to the skin and muscles on the palm of her left hand.

On arrival at the hospital, pressure is applied to the wound to stop bleeding. When bleeding was controlled, cleaning of the wound began with soap and water, followed by application of 3 stitches to close the wound. The wound was then covered with antibiotic ointment and a clean dressing. During this time, a single dose of amoxicillin/clavulanate 875/125 mg was orally administered. Within 30 minutes of the dose, the patient began complaining of shortness of breath (SOB), abdominal pain, itchiness, nausea, and rapid heart rate. Nurse noted audible wheezing and pruritis on trunk and arms.

Past Medical History

No significant medical history

Family History

Father is alive with no significant medical history at age 64. Mother is alive with no significant medical history at age 62. She has two young sisters who are healthy.

Social History

Research student pursuing degree in psychology. Single, lives with her dog; has no children. Works full time at the college campus research lab.

Tobacco/Alcohol/Substance Use

(+) Social drinker; (–) tobacco or illicit drug use

Allergies/Intolerances/Adverse Drug Events

Cephalosporin (anaphylaxis)

Codeine (nausea)

Ibuprofen (GI upset and abdominal pain)

Meperidine (hallucinations)

Medications (Current)

No outpatient medications

Physical Examination

▶ **General**

Young, Caucasian woman in acute distress

▶ **Vital Signs**

BP 90/45 mm Hg, P 98, RR 16, T 37.2°C

Weight 134.2 lb. (61 kg)

Height 68 in. (172.7 cm)

Pain 4 (scale 0–10)

▶ **Skin**

Clammy skin

Bite and tearing of the skin on palm of left hand is 1 inch (2.5 cm) long with underlying tissue and muscle damage; minor bleeding at site; (+) urticaria on trunk and arms

▶ **HEENT**

PERRLA, EOMI; (–) trace periorbital edema; (–) sinus tenderness

▶ **Neck and Lymph Nodes**

(–) Lymphadenopathy; (–) carotid bruits

▶ **Chest**

Audible wheezing

▶ **Breasts**

Examination deferred

▶ **Cardiovascular**

Normal rhythm; tachycardia; normal S_1, S_2; (–) S_3 or S_4

▶ **Abdomen**

Not tender/not distended; (–) organomegaly

▶ **Neurology**

Grossly intact; deep tendon reflexes normal

▸ *Genitourinary*

Examination deferred

▸ *Rectal*

Examination deferred

Laboratory Tests

Nonfasting

	Conventional Units	SI Units
Na	141 mEq/L	141 mmol/L
K	4.1 mEq/L	4.1 mmol/L
Cl	99 mEq/L	99 mmol/L
CO_2	24 mEq/L	24 mmol/L
BUN	20 mg/dL	7.14 mmol/L
SCr	0.8 mg/dL	71 μmol/L
Glu	140 mg/dL	7.77 mmol/L

Assessment

Twenty-six-year-old woman with signs and symptoms consistent with anaphylaxis following antibiotic administration; also with signs consistent for animal bite.

Student Work-Up

Missing Information/Inadequate Data

Evaluate: Patient database

   Drug therapy problems

   Care plan (by problem)

TARGETED QUESTIONS

1. What signs and symptoms of anaphylaxis does the patient have?

   Hint: See p. 831 in PPP

2. What are the treatments of choice for patients with anaphylaxis?

   Hint: See Table 54-3 in PPP

3. What classes of medications are frequently associated with anaphylaxis?

   Hint: See Table 54-2 in PPP

4. What are the odds of cross-reactivity with β-lactams?

   Hint: See p. 831 in PPP

5. For the nonantibiotic medications listed on her allergy/intolerance/adverse reaction list, does she have a true allergy to any of them that would prevent her from taking these medications in the future?

   Hint: See p. 831 in PPP

FOLLOW-UP

Upon follow-up, you learn that the patient has not completed her full course of doxycycline treatment due to nausea and vomiting associated with the antibiotic. While deciding another alternative therapy options, the doctor has asked you to provide the treatment team with information pertaining to the desensitization protocol for penicillin agents and the risk associated with this treatment option.

   Hint: See p. 835 and Table 54-6 in PPP

⊙ GLOBAL PERSPECTIVE

As the study of medical genetics continues to evolve and expand, our understanding of genotype association with medication hypersensitivity will also evolve. Studies have already found that HLA B*1502, found predominantly in patients of Southeast Asian ancestry, is associated with increased risk of carbamazepine hypersensitivity, while HLA B*5801, found in Southeast Asian, Japanese, and European ancestry, is associated with allopurinol hypersensitivity. Different interleukin-4 variants associated with different ethnic groups, in particular Chinese, Italians, and Caucasians, are associated with increased hypersensitivity to beta-lactams. In the near future, expanding recommendations on testing prior to treatment with certain agents is anticipated in certain ethnic populations as rapid methods of detection are identified.

CASE SUMMARY

- Her current clinical picture is consistent with a rat bite and antibiotic therapy should be initiated to prevent infection.

- Cross-allergenicity has been reported between penicillins and cephalosporins.

- The patient's reactions to amoxicillin/clavulanate include; SOB, abdominal pain, itchiness, nausea, rapid heart rate, wheezing, and urticaria on her trunk and arms, which are signs and symptoms consistent with anaphylaxis.

- The treatment of anaphylaxis includes discontinuation of the causative agent, immediate intervention with epinephrine, and subsequent intervention with normal saline infusion and epinephrine infusion if she is not responding to immediate intervention procedures and volume resuscitation.

- An oral course of doxycycline 100 mg twice per day for 14 days is an appropriate treatment alternatives for this patient due to her allergy to cephalosporins and penicillins.

- Desensitization is a potentially life-threatening procedure and requires continuous monitoring in a hospital setting. It is required for penicillin-allergic patients when penicillin is clearly the only treatment option.

For more information on the care plan and facilitator's guide please visit http://www.mhpharmacotherapy.com

61 Solid Organ Transplantation

Kimberly A. Trobaugh   Rita R. Alloway

PATIENT PRESENTATION

Chief Complaint

"I think I'm okay. I'm just here for my routine clinic visit."

History of Present Illness

Anthony ("Tony") Aconi is a 64-year-old Caucasian male with a past medical history significant for end-stage renal disease (ESRD) secondary to hypertension (HTN) who underwent a living unrelated donor (LURD) kidney transplant 3 months ago (4 antigen mismatch). This was his first transplant, and he did not have any other sensitizing events prior to transplant. Pretransplant testing revealed a current and peak cytotoxic panel reactive antibody (PRA) of 0% and a United Network for Organ Sharing (UNOS) calculated PRA (cPRA) of 0%. Prior to transplant, he was on peritoneal dialysis for 4 months. At time of transplant, patient received rabbit antithymocyte globulin (rATG) as induction therapy along with a rapid steroid taper. Current maintenance immunosuppression includes tacrolimus and mycophenolate mofetil. Patient was also on nystatin for 1 month posttransplant for fungal prophylaxis and is currently on valganciclovir and trimethoprim/sulfamethoxazole for cytomegalovirus (CMV) and *Pneumocystis* pneumonia (PCP) prophylaxis, respectively, with planned duration of 6 months per institutional policy (see pretransplant serologies below). Since Mr. Aconi's renal function immediately posttransplant was creatinine clearance (CrCl) less than 60 mL/min (1.0 mL/s), his valganciclovir dose was renally adjusted. However, his serum creatinine (SCr) has been slowly trending downward to around 1.3 to 1.4 mg/dL (114.9 to 123.8 μmol/L). Although the clinic team has discussed increasing his valganciclovir dose since he is experiencing improved renal function, the patient has been maintained on the reduced dose. Patient has been coming to clinic for a routine visit and labs every 2 weeks and is in clinic today for regular follow-up. His labs 2 weeks ago showed an increase in his SCr to 1.57 mg/dL (138.8 μmol/L), with repeat labs obtained today. Patient reports a subjective decrease in urine output today but states that he "had the 'stomach bug' that's been going around" earlier in the week with significant diarrhea for about 48 hours. He has been having trouble getting himself rehydrated since that time.

Past Medical History

ESRD secondary to HTN

S/P LURD kidney transplant 3 months ago (induction rATG × 4 doses)

HTN (22 years)

Past Surgical History

S/P LURD kidney transplant (3 months ago)

Inguinal hernia repair (6 years ago)

Family History

Mother: deceased (breast cancer, age 68)

Father: deceased (stroke, age 82)

Sibling: 1 brother (age 58) with HTN and hyperlipidemia

Social/Work History

Marital status: Married (42 years)

Children: 2 sons (ages 33 and 38)

Part owner of restaurant (runs with his brother)

Tobacco/Alcohol/Substance Use

Tobacco use: former smoker ("social smoker" × 32 years); never used smokeless tobacco

Alcohol use: 1 can of beer, once per week

Drug use: never used

Allergies

No known drug allergies

Current Medication List

Prograf (tacrolimus) 5 mg po bid

Cellcept (mycophenolate mofetil, MMF) 1000 mg po bid

Valcyte (valganciclovir) 450 mg po daily (renally dose adjusted)

Trimethoprim/sulfamethoxazole (TMP/SMX) 1 single-strength (SS) tablet (400-80 mg) po daily

Amlodipine 5 mg po daily

Metoprolol tartrate 50 mg po bid

Pantoprazole 40 mg po daily, before breakfast

Review of Systems

Recently with diarrhea (about 6-7 episodes per day) × 48 hours (last episode day before yesterday). Also with abdominal pain/cramping at that time. Negative for nausea/vomiting. Positive for subjective decrease in urine output. Negative for increased urgency or frequency of urination; difficulty or painful urinating; and hematuria. All other systems reviewed and are negative.

Physical Exam

► General

Obese white male who is well-groomed and appears his stated age; in NAD

► Vital Signs

BP 138/86 mm Hg (sitting), dropped to 122/74 upon standing; HR 58; RR 18; T 36.4°C (97.5°F)

Weight 243 lb. (110.2 kg)

Height 69 in. (175.3 cm)

Pain 0/10

► HEENT

PERRLA; EOMI

► Chest

Lungs clear to auscultation bilaterally

► Cardiovascular

RRR; (+) S_1, S_2; (–) murmurs; (–) edema

► Abdomen

Soft, nontender, nondistended; (+) bowel sounds; no organomegaly

► Neurology

A&O × 3; CN II-XII intact; no focal deficits

Laboratory and Other Diagnostic Tests

Laboratory Findings (Fasting)

	Conventional Units	SI Units
Na	138 mEq/L	138 mmol/L
K	3.9 mEq/L	3.9 mmol/L
Cl	101 mEq/L	101 mmol/L
CO_2	23 mEq/L	23 mmol/L
BUN	38 mg/dL	13.6 mmol/L
SCr	1.69 mg/dL	149.4 μmol/L
eGFR (MDRD)	44 mL/min/1.73 m²	
Glu	105 mg/dL	5.8 mmol/L
Ca	9.6 mg/dL	2.4 mmol/L
Mg	2.1 mg/dL	0.86 mmol/L
Phos	3.8 mg/dL	1.23 mmol/L

Albumin	3.8 g/dL	38 g/L
WBC	$2 \times 10^3/\mu L$	$2 \times 10^9/L$
ANC	1400/μL	$1.4 \times 10^9/L$
Hgb	12.4 g/dL	124 g/L
Hct	37%	0.37
Plt	$175 \times 10^3/\mu L$	$175 \times 10^9/L$
Tacrolimus	16.4 ng/mL	16.4 mcg/L

Quant CMV DNA PCR	328,877 cells/mL	329×10^6 copies/L
Quant BKV DNA PCR	0 cells/mL	0 copies/L
Quant EBV DNA PCR	0 cells/mL	0 copies/L

Pre-transplant serologies:
Recipient

- CMV negative
- EBV positive

Donor

- CMV positive
- EBV positive

Assessment

Mr. Aconi is a 64-year-old Caucasian male who is 3 months S/P LURD kidney transplant and presents with increasing SCr and other abnormal laboratory findings consistent with CMV viremia.

Student Work-Up

Missing Information/Inadequate Data

Evaluate:
Patient database
Drug therapy problems
Care plan (by problem)

Additional information:

Additional assessment of renal function/causes of renal dysfunction, for example, urine output, urinalysis, fractional excretion of sodium (FENa), renal ultrasound to assess for obstruction, volume status to assess for dehydration.

TARGETED QUESTIONS

1. What are the patient's risk factors for development of CMV disease?

   Hint: See p. 854 in PPP

2. What therapeutic options are available for the treatment of CMV disease? How do these therapies differ from those used for CMV prophylaxis?

   Hint: See p. 854 and Table 55-6 in PPP

3. What clinical and/or laboratory parameters should be monitored to determine treatment efficacy? How long should treatment be continued in this patient?

   Hint: See p. 854 in PPP

4. What is the "next step" in management of the patient's CMV disease once he has successfully completed treatment as evidenced by resolution of clinical symptoms and virologic clearance?

   Hint: See p. 854 in PPP

FOLLOW-UP

Mr. Aconi was started on treatment-dose valganciclovir, with dose adjusted based on renal function.

1. What if the patient had come into clinic with complaints of abdominal pain and persistent diarrhea (about 6-7 episodes per day) for the past week. Assuming all laboratory findings remain unchanged, how would this change your management of the patient?

2. What if the patient's viral load (as per CMV PCR testing) remains essentially unchanged after 2 weeks of treatment with IV ganciclovir at an appropriate dose. How would this change your management of the patient?

3. What if the patient later experiences a rejection episode to be treated with a course of rATG. The team asks for your recommendation for CMV prevention. What would your recommendation be to the team?

⊙ GLOBAL PERSPECTIVE

CMV infection is a common complication of solid organ transplantation. The virus is found throughout all geographic locations and socioeconomic groups, and it is estimated that up to 80% of all adults in the United States (greater than 90% worldwide) are infected with CMV, which most often lies dormant in the body throughout life. In patients whose immune system is weakened (including transplant recipients who take immune-suppressing medications) the CMV virus can be reactivated and cause illness. The use of CMV-seropositive donor organs is a particular risk for reactivation of infection in the immunosuppressed recipient posttransplant, with highest risk of infection being in seronegative transplant recipients (R-). The use of potent immunosuppressive agents posttransplant for treating rejection further increases the risk of developing CMV disease, with T-cell depleting antibody therapies being principally associated with an increased risk of viral infections. Symptoms of infection may range from those of a common viral syndrome to severe disease with tissue involvement and damage to the transplanted organ. Several antivirals have proven effective in preventing and treating CMV, with valganciclovir and IV ganciclovir considered the agents of choice in most organ transplant recipients.

CASE SUMMARY

- Organ transplant recipients are at increased risk of infectious diseases, which are a chief cause of early morbidity and mortality. Posttransplant infections generally occur in a standard pattern; therefore, prevention is a key management strategy.

- Patient presents with increasing SCr and other abnormal laboratory findings consistent with CMV viremia. Prompt initiation of appropriate antiviral therapy and reduction in maintenance immunosuppression with appropriate laboratory monitoring is crucial to achieve virologic clearance.

For more information on the care plan and facilitator's guide please visit http://www.mhpharmacotherapy.com

62 Osteoporosis

Allison Ann Presnell   Beth Bryles Phillips

PATIENT PRESENTATION

Chief Complaint

"I am here for my annual wellness visit."

History of Present Illness

KD is a 74-year old Caucasian female who presents to the family medicine clinic for a routine physical and annual wellness visit. She has been an active patient since 1992, and is in relatively good health. However, recently she has been tired and sluggish during the day, stating her energy level isn't what it used to be. She fell in her home 6 months prior and broke her left wrist, requiring surgery for a plate and screws hardware insertion. The fall happened during a Braves baseball game when she got up for a glass of iced tea and tripped over her beagle, Lilly. She has had several dual-energy X-ray absorptiometry (DXA) scans for bone mineral density, and the most recent measurement has shown a worsening of bone health. She has never received prescription treatment for osteoporosis. When asked about her diet, she reports consuming 4-5 dairy foods per day (milk in cereal, yogurt, and at least 2 servings of cheese) and 3-4 cups of coffee per day, which has been consistent for most of her adult life. She also seems to have trouble with balance lately, but can't attribute it to a definite cause. She experiences episodes of dizziness when she gets up in the morning or has been sitting in her living room chair for long periods of time. She does report having a dry mouth. She states she started using Tylenol PM 2 capsules every night approximately 7-8 months ago because she was having trouble sleeping. She also has had problems with heartburn "on and off" over the years, but believes omeprazole controls her symptoms well.

Past Medical History

Osteoporosis status post (s/p) wrist fracture requiring surgical hardware insertion (6 months prior)

Gastroesophageal reflux disease (GERD)

Barrett's esophagus, s/p pneumatic (balloon) dilation for achalasia

Hypertension

Dyslipidemia

Family History

Mother deceased at age 85 due to Alzheimer's type dementia, hip fracture at age 84. Father deceased at age 32 (military plane crash). She has one brother, 72, with osteoarthritis.

Social History

The patient is a recent widow and lives alone. She has 3 children and 5 grandchildren. She is a retired school teacher.

Tobacco/Alcohol/Substance Use

Social drinker—approximately 1 drink per week; former tobacco user with 44-pack year smoking history, (–) illicit drug use

Allergies/Intolerances/Adverse Drug Events

Neomycin (rash), sulfa (rash)

Medications (Current)

Omeprazole 20 mg daily

Atorvastatin 20 mg QHS

Atenolol 25 mg daily

Lisinopril 10 mg daily

Calcium carbonate 600 mg twice daily

Acetaminophen/diphenhydramine 500/25 mg (Tylenol PM®) 2 capsules q HS prn

Review of Systems

(+) for heartburn treated with omeprazole, and dry mouth; Denies back or hip pain, (+) kyphosis

Physical Exam

▶ **General**

Thin, elderly woman who looks to be her stated age, mild kyphosis present

▶ **Vital Signs**

Sitting BP 108/74 mmHg, P 58 bpm

Standing BP 87/65 mmHg, P 60 bpm

RR 16, T 36.2°C

Height 63 in. (160 cm)

Weight 117 lb. (53 kg)

BMI 20.7 kg/m²

Denies pain

▶ **Skin**

Normal turgor and color; warm

► **HEENT**

PERRLA, EOMI; disks flat; fundi with no hemorrhages or exudates, (+) Barrett's esophagus

► **Neck and Lymph Nodes**

No lymphadenopathy, thyromegaly, or carotid bruits

► **Chest**

Clear to auscultation bilaterally

► **Breasts**

No tenderness, masses on palpation

► **Cardiovascular**

RRR; normal S_1 and S_2; no S_3 or S_4; no m/r/g

► **Abdomen**

Not tender/Not distended; (–) organomegaly

► **Neurology**

A & O × 3; CN II–XII intact; DTR 2+

► **Extremities**

Cool, normal color, dorsalis pedis pulse weak

► **Genitourinary**

Exam deferred

► **Rectal**

Exam deferred

Laboratory Tests

Fasting, Obtained 2 days Ago

	Conventional Units	SI Units
Na	135 mEq/L	135 mmol/L
K	4.2 mEq/L	4.2 mmol/L
Cl	100 mEq/L	100 mmol/L
CO_2	29 mEq/L	29 mmol/L
BUN	14 mg/dL	5.0 mmol/L
SCr	0.8 mg/dL	70.1 μmol/L
Glu	99 mg/dL	5.5 mmol/L
Ca	9.3 mg/dL	2.3 mmol/L
TSH	2.5 μU/mL	2.5 mU/L
25(OH)D	21 ng/mL	52.4 nmol/L
Hgb	15.5 g/dL	9.61 mmol/L
Hct	48%	0.48
WBC	7.4×10^3/mm³	7.4×10^9/L
MCV	76 μm³	76 fL

Total cholesterol	179 mg/dL	9.9 mmol/L
LDL cholesterol	102 mg/dL	5.7 mmol/L
HDL cholesterol	48 mg/dL	2.7 mmol/L
Triglyceride	148 mg/dl	mmol/L

Other

Bone Mineral Density

5 years ago

Total Hip	T score –1.1
Femoral Neck	T score –1.2
Lumbar Spine	T score –1.4

Today

Total Hip	T score –2.2
Femoral Neck	T score –2.2
Lumbar spine	T score –2.36

Assessment

Seventy-four-year-old female with signs of osteoporosis; bone densitometry consistent with osteopenia.

Student Work-Up

Missing Information/Inadequate Data

Evaluate:	Patient database
	Drug therapy problems
	Care plan (by problem)

TARGETED QUESTIONS

1. What signs and symptoms of osteoporosis does the patient have?

   Hint: See p. 864 in PPP

2. What risk factors does this patient have for osteoporosis?

   Hint: See pp. 863-864 in PPP

3. What nonpharmacologic recommendations are important for her treatment plan?

   Hint: See pp. 866-867 in PPP

4. What is your assessment of her calcium and vitamin D, including requirements and dietary intake? What recommendations should be made regarding supplementation or treatment?

   Hint: See p. 867 in PPP

5. Is this patient a candidate for drug therapy? What additional calculations are needed to determine if treatment is warranted?

   Hint: See pp. 867-872 and 875 in PPP

FOLLOW-UP

What if her vitamin D measured 8 weeks later is 38 ng/dl? What recommendations should be made for this patient?

🌐 GLOBAL PERSPECTIVE

Osteoporosis causes a bone fracture every 3 seconds around the world, totaling 9 million fractures every year. This skeletal disorder, caused by a bone remodeling imbalance, results in fractures accounting for 0.83% of global burden of noncommunicable diseases. Osteoporosis affects more than 75 million people in the United States, Europe, and Japan.[1,2,3] Globally, osteoporosis affects men and women of all races, but the highest risk of osteoporotic fractures is present in white and Asian postmenopausal women.[4] It is estimated that 1-in-3 women and 1-in-5 men over age 50 will experience an osteoporotic fracture in their lifetime.[5,6,7] The European Foundation for Osteoporosis and Bone Disease (EFFO) as well as the National Osteoporosis Foundation (NOF) in the United States define osteoporosis as a bone mineral density (BMD) greater than or equal to 2.5 standard deviations below the BMD of a young healthy individual of the same sex (known as a *T*-score). Diagnosis is often validated by a *T*-score measured by a dual-energy X-ray absorptiometry (DXA), but availability and cost vary from country to country.[8] Additionally, fracture risk varies greatly among nations, amounting to a 10-fold variance in hip fracture risk among European countries. Scandinavia owns the highest hip fracture risk in the world.[9] The lowest absolute hip fracture risk is found in developing countries, which may be attributed to lower overall life expectancy.[10] It is projected that by 2050, the incidence of hip fractures will double in North America, increase fivefold in Asia, and increase sevenfold in Latin America.[11]

CASE SUMMARY

- This patient has never received treatment to reduce the risk of osteoporotic fractures. Her risk factors should be evaluated to determine if the benefits of drug therapy outweigh the risks. Her history of Barrett's esophagus with previous dilation for achalasia affects choice of drug therapy.

- Adequate calcium and vitamin D supplementation is needed to optimize osteoporosis treatment. This patient is receiving large amounts of elemental calcium through her diet. Additional supplementation should be evaluated, with special consideration for concurrent proton pump inhibitor use. Vitamin D is essential for calcium absorption. Her vitamin D is low and treatment should be considered.

- Medications that cause anticholinergic and sedation side effects should be avoided due to increased risk of falls. Additionally, orthostatic hypotension and vitamin D insufficiency contribute to fall risk. Based on status of orthostatic hypotension and bradycardia, patient may also benefit from a change in antihypertensive drug therapy.

REFERENCES

1. Johnell O and Kanis JA. An estimate of the worldwide prevalence and disability associated with osteoporotic fractures. Osteoporos Int 2006;17:1726.
2. Kanis JA. WHO Technical Report, University of Sheffield, UK. 2007;66.
3. Kanis JA, Oden A, Johnell O, Jonsson B, De Laet C, Dawson A. The burden of osteoporotic fractures: a method for setting intervention thresholds. Osteoporos Int 2000;12:417–427.
4. Diseases and Conditions: Osteoporosis. (2014, December 13). Retrieved May 29, 2015, from http://www.mayoclinic.org/diseases-conditions/osteoporosis/basics/definition/con-20019924.
5. Melton LJ 3rd, Atkinson EJ, O'Connor MK, et al. Bone density and fracture risk in men. J Bone Miner Res 1998;13:1915.
6. Melton LJ 3rd, Chrischilles EA, Cooper C, et al. Perspective. How many women have osteoporosis? J Bone Miner Res 1992;7:1005.
7. Kanis JA, Johnell O, Oden A, et al. Long-term risk of osteoporotic fracture in Malmo. Osteoporos Int 2000;11:669.
8. Kanis jA, Torgerson D, Cooper C. Comparison of the European and USA practice guidelines for Osteoporosis. Trends Endocrinol Metab. 2000 Jan-Feb;11(1):28-32.
9. Kanis JA, Johnell O, De Laet C, et al. International variations in hip fracture probabilities: implications for risk assessment. J Bone Miner Res 2002;17:1237.
10. WHO Scientific Group on the Assessment of Osteoporosis at Primary Health Care Level. Summary Meeting Report. Geneva: World Health Organization; 2007.
11. Gullberg B, Johnell O and Kanis JA. World-wide projections for hip fracture. Osteoporos Int 1997;7:407.

For more information on the care plan and facilitator's guide please visit http://www.mhpharmacotherapy.com

63 Rheumatoid Arthritis

Susan P. Bruce

PATIENT PRESENTATION

Chief Complaint

"My hands are so sore. I can hardly use them in the morning."

History of Present Illness

Winnie Stewart is a 68-year-old postmenopausal woman presenting to the rheumatologist for evaluation and treatment of rheumatoid arthritis (RA). Winnie was diagnosed with RA approximately 10 years ago. Approximately 6 months ago, the rheumatologist initiated methotrexate/etanercept combination therapy. At today's visit, she reports significant difficulty with dressing (especially buttons, zippers, and tying her shoes) and meal preparation. She has experienced progressive morning stiffness, now lasting for 2-3 hours daily. This is frustrating for her because her hobbies require steady and controlled use of her hands.

Past Medical History

Dyslipidemia (15 years)

Chronic obstructive pulmonary disease (diagnosed 6 months ago)

Osteoporosis (3 years)

Menopause (at age 56)

Family History

Father had CAD (coronary artery disease) and died of MI (myocardial infarction) at age 62. Mother had RA and died from complications of heart failure at age 65. Her only sister has dyslipidemia and hypertension. One son and two daughters are alive and well.

Social/Work History

Winnie, a retired schoolteacher, spends her time volunteering at the local food bank and participating in her favorite hobbies, which include hand quilting and needlepoint. She has health insurance/prescription coverage available through her retirement benefits.

Tobacco/Alcohol/Substance Use

(+) Tobacco—1 ppd × 40 years; quit 5 years ago (+) alcohol use (1 glass of wine with dinner) (−) illicit drug use

Allergies/Intolerances/Adverse Event History

Penicillin—rash

Medication History

She has trialed penicillamine, gold salts, sulfasalazine, NSAIDs, high dose prednisone, methotrexate monotherapy, and methotrexate/infliximab combination therapy without success.

Current Medications

Methotrexate 15 mg po weekly

Etanercept 50 mg sc weekly

Atorvastatin 80 mg po daily

Alendronate 35 mg po once weekly

Albuterol 2 puffs every 4-6 hours as needed

Folic acid 1 mg po daily

Review of Systems

Generalized malaise and fatigue unchanged since last evaluation; (−) fevers, night sweats, adenopathy, dry eyes, oral ulcers, or skin rashes; morning cough productive of clear sputum, resolves 15 to 30 minutes after arising; (−) hemoptysis, chest pain, shortness of breath, exertional chest discomfort, abdominal pain, or diarrhea; initial difficulty falling asleep at night due to joint discomfort, but then sleeps soundly once asleep

Physical Examination

▸ **General**

Thin, middle-aged, white woman in obvious discomfort

▸ **Vital Signs**

BP 152/88 mm Hg, P 80, RR 19, T 36.8°C

Weight 120 lb (54.5 kg)

Height 62 in. (157.5 cm)

Pain rated as 5/10

▸ **Skin**

(−) Rashes, lesions or evidence of vasculitis

▶ **HEENT**

(–) Conjunctival or sclera injection; (–) oral or nasal ulcers; mucus membranes moist

▶ **Neck and Lymph Nodes**

(–) Adenopathy, thyromegaly, or masses

▶ **Cardiovascular**

RRR; S_4 gallop present; (–) S_3 gallop or rubs

▶ **Abdomen**

Scaphoid and nontender; (–) masses, hepatomegaly, or splenomegaly

▶ **Neurology**

Grossly intact; deep tendon reflexes normal

▶ **Extremities**

Small olecranon nodules bilaterally; 1+ synovitis and tenderness of the bilateral dorsal wrists; 2+ synovitis of the right metacarpophalangeal (MCP) joints and 1+ synovitis of the left MCP joints; 1+ synovitis and tenderness of the bilateral proximal interphalangeal joints (PIP) joints; 2+ synovitis and tenderness of the right metatarsophalangeal (MTP) joints and 1+ synovitis of the left MTP joints; (–) joint effusions.

▶ **Genitourinary**

Examination deferred

▶ **Rectal**

Normal sphincter tone; (–) masses; stool brown and (–) guaiac

Laboratory and Other Diagnostic Tests

Fasting, Obtained 1 week Ago

	Convectional Units	SI Units
Na	138 mEq/L	138 mmol/L
K	3.9 mEq/L	3.9 mmol/L
Cl	102 mEq/L	102 mmol/L
CO_2	23 mEq/L	23 mmol/L
BUN	16 mg/dL	5.7 mmol/L
SCr	1.1 mg/dL	97 µmol/L
Glu	102 mg/dL	5.66 mmol/L
Ca	9.1 mg/dL	4.55 mmol/L
Mg	1.8 mEq/L	0.9 mmol/L
Phosphate	3.2 mg/dL	1.03 mmol/L
Hgb	10.2 g/dL	6.32 mmol/L
Hct	31%	0.31
MCV	81 µm³	81 fL
Albumin	4 g/dL	40 g/L
AST	30 IU/L	0.50 µkat/L
ALT	36 IU/L	0.60 µkat/L

Assessment

Sixty-eight-year-old woman with signs, symptoms, and laboratory tests consistent with RA of moderate-disease activity and poor prognostic factors.

Student Work-Up

Missing Information/Inadequate Data

Evaluate:	Patient database
	Drug therapy problems
	Care plan (by problem)

TARGETED QUESTIONS

1. On the basis of established disease activity, which medications are appropriate for the treatment of RA in this patient?

   Hint: See Figure 57-1 in PPP

2. Which comorbid conditions related to RA or its treatment must also be addressed for this patient?

   Hint: See p. 876 in PPP

3. What is the most appropriate treatment for each comorbid condition?

   Hint: See pp. 876-877 in PPP

4. What pharmacologic and nonpharmacologic measures should your patient education plan include?

   Hint: See pp. 881-882 in PPP

5. What tests can be utilized to determine if the medications(s) are effective?

   Hint: See p. 886 in PPP

⊙ GLOBAL PERSPECTIVE

With the increased use of biologic disease-modifying antirheumatic drugs (DMARDs), it is increasingly important to consider global implications of such treatment. For example, patients receiving biologic DMARDs, especially TNF inhibitors, are at an increased risk of tuberculosis as a result of previous or current exposure. Continuous clinical vigilance must be maintained to evaluate every patient to consider current risk and risk management. In addition, patients traveling to areas with increased risk of tuberculosis exposure must be aware of their risk and encouraged to communicate it back to their healthcare providers. Other risks include hepatitis B, hepatitis C, and herpes zoster. In summary, it is critical that all health care providers involved with the care of a patient with RA are aware of immunization history, medication use, adverse effect risk, and follow up parameters.

CASE SUMMARY

- Winnie is experiencing RA with moderate disease activity.
- She requires an adjustment in therapy in order to alleviate disease symptoms.
- Her comorbid conditions must also be evaluated and subsequent treatment adjusted.

- Overall, patients with RA require a comprehensive medication evaluation to insure appropriate treatment regimens for RA and comorbid conditions.

For more information on the care plan and facilitator's guide please visit http://www.mhpharmacotherapy.com

64 Osteoarthritis

Eric Dietrich Charlie Michaudet
Steven M. Smith

PATIENT PRESENTATION

Chief Complaint

"My right knee hurts every day now."

History of Present Illness

Adele Johnson is a 68-year-old African-American woman presenting to her primary care physician complaining of right knee pain that had been intermittent for the past 2 years but has become more constant over the past 3 months. She is a former collegiate track-and-field athlete and she has been active all her life. She does not recall any trauma or specific injury to her right knee. She describes her pain as dull in nature, usually worsening as the day goes on but improving with rest. She does not report any stiffness or swelling but feels some instability, as if her knee is giving out sometimes. She is seeking medical care regarding her knee pain for the first time. She was taking Tylenol extra strength 500 mg once or twice a week previously but is now taking 500 mg twice daily for the past 4 weeks. She states she has been able to get through the day with this regimen, but she still has pain during the day. She has gained 8 pounds in 6 months and would like to be able to exercise. However, the pain limits her from being able to run and take long walks on a regular basis. One of her friends recently received a "shot in her knee" and has had great relief of her pain, so she would like to discuss that option. Lastly, she wants to know your opinion regarding glucosamine-chondroitin as she has heard it prevents joint breakdown and is safer than painkillers.

Past Medical History

Hypertension (23 years)
Stage III chronic kidney disease
NSAID-induced peptic ulcer disease (45 years ago)
Hyperlipidemia
Overweight

Family History

Father with type 2 diabetes and hypertension
Mother with hypertension

Social/Work History

She is currently a public relation employee of a university Athletic Association. Married with two children, aged 20 and 23.

Tobacco/Alcohol/Substance Use

Social drinker; no smoking; No illicit drug use

Allergy/Intolerance/Adverse Event History

Shellfish (unknown reaction)

Medications (Current)

Amlodipine 10 mg po once daily
Lisinopril 20 mg po once daily
Acetaminophen 500 mg po twice daily
Multivitamin po once daily
Simvastatin 40 mg po once daily

Review of Systems

General: no fever or chills. Weight gain.

CV: no chest pain, palpitations, leg swelling.

MSK: right knee pain and instability. No swelling or stiffness. No other joint involvement.

Neuro: no weakness or numbness.

Skin: negative.

Physical Examination

▶ *General*

Pleasant African-American woman, well nourished, in no acute distress.

▶ *Vital Signs*

BP 128/72 mm Hg, P 62/min, RR 14/min, T 36.6°C (97.9°F)
Weight 187 lb. (84.8 kg)
Height 68 in. (172.7 cm)
BMI 29.3 kg/m²

▶ *Skin*

No lesions or rash

▶ *HEENT*

PERRL, EOMI; TMs normal appearing

▶ *Respiratory*

Unlabored, clear to auscultation

▶ *Cardiovascular*

RRR, normal S_1, S_2; no S_3 or S_4; normal peripheral pulses

▶ *Abdomen*

Soft, nontender, not distended; no organomegaly; good bowel sounds

▶ *Neurology*

Grossly intact, no numbness or weakness. Gait is normal. Normal tone and coordination.

▶ *Musculoskeletal*

Right knee with no deformity, swelling or discoloration. Mild tenderness to palpation; medial joint line but no pain over quadriceps muscle, patella, patella tendon, pes anserine, medial collateral ligament, lateral collateral ligament. Range of motion is abnormal with full extension but flexion to 100 degrees. Strength is grossly 5/5 with normal sensation and pulses. Anterior and posterior cruciate ligaments assessment is normal as well as medial and lateral collateral ligament assessment. Other joints look normal and are not painful.

Laboratory Tests
Fasting

	Conventional Units	SI Units
Na	143 mEq/L	143 mmol/L
K	4.1 mEq/L	4.1 mmol/L
Cl	103 mEq/L	103 mmol/L
CO_2	24 mEq/L	24 mmol/L
BUN	12 mg/dL	4.3 mmol/L
SCr	1.6 mg/dL	141 μmol/L
eGFR (CKD-EPI)	44 mL/min	0.42 mL/s/m^2
Glu	98 mg/dL	5.44 mmol/L
Urinary microalbumin: creatinine ratio	47 mg/g	5.32
Total cholesterol	205 mg/dL	5.30 mmol/L
LDL cholesterol (calculated)	115 mg/dL	2.97 mmol/L
HDL cholesterol	37 mg/dL	0.96 mmol/L
Triglycerides	162 mg/dL	1.83 mmol/L

Imaging

Right knee x-ray showing medial compartment joint space narrowing with ostcophytcs.

Assessment

Sixty-eight-year-old, overweight, African-American woman with symptoms, physical findings and x-ray consistent with osteoarthritis of the right knee.

Student Work-Up

Missing Information/Inadequate Data

Evaluate:
- Patient database
- Drug therapy problems
- Care plan (by problem)

TARGETED QUESTIONS

1. What evidence from the history and physical exam are consistent with a diagnosis of osteoarthritis in this patient?

   Hint: See pp. 890-891 in PPP

2. What dose and duration of acetaminophen constitutes an adequate trial before moving on to additional treatment options?

   Hint: See pp. 891 and 894 in PPP

3. Would you consider this patient a candidate for NSAID therapy with a selective COX-2 inhibitor? What factors would help differentiate choosing between a nonselective NSAID and a COX-2 inhibitor?

   Hint: See pp. 894-895 in PPP

4. How effective is glucosamine/chondroitin in the treatment of OA? Would you recommend glucosamine/chondroitin for this patient?

   Hint: See p. 896 in PPP

5. How would you counsel the patient on the benefits and risks of intra-articular corticosteroids and hyaluronic acid?

   Hint: See p. 896 in PPP

FOLLOW-UP

Mrs. Johnson does well following implementation of your therapeutic plan. However, she still experiences occasional knee pain, especially during times of exercise or when she stands on her feet for prolonged periods of time.

What non-pharmacological options are available to help reduce pain and improve her functioning?

Hint: See p. 891 in PPP

⊙ GLOBAL PERSPECTIVE

Osteoarthritis is the most common rheumatic disease worldwide; however, the prevalence of OA varies widely across geographic regions. Prevalence rates in Europe approximate those in North America and generally do not exceed 10%. In contrast, the prevalence in developing regions can range from 3% to 20%. These differences are probably more closely associated with differences in populations than geographic location because the development of OA is not predicated solely on environmental factors. For example, when compared with North American Caucasians, Asians exhibit higher rates of symptomatic knee OA, but lower rates of hip and hand OA. This finding may be attributable to the higher proportion of rural farmers and hard laborers in many Asian regions than in North America. Thus, the prevalence of OA in any region reflects population differences in age, lifestyle, genetics, and occupational history.

CASE SUMMARY

- The overall clinical picture is consistent with OA of the right knee.
- Nonpharmacologic therapies should reduce further joint damage and improve joint stability.

For more information on the care plan and facilitator's guide please visit http://www.mhpharmacotherapy.com

65 Gout and Hyperuricemia

William Joshua Guffey

PATIENT PRESENTATION

Chief Complaint
"My left hand is swollen and hurts after starting this new gout medicine."

History of Present Illness
Robert Harrison is an 82-year-old Caucasian male who presents to his primary care physician (PCP) complaining of an acute gout attack. The patient has a 20-year history of gout with 2-3 acute attacks per year. He was recently started on febuxostat 2 weeks ago for chronic hyperuricemia. He was on allopurinol several years ago but thinks that they may have stopped it due to a rash. He became concerned when his hand started swelling with redness and warmth present after starting a medicine that he was told would decrease his risk for a gout attack. Swelling noted in the joints of the left hand and wrist. He has tried to alleviate his current pain with ice packs and hydrocodone/acetaminophen which provided minimal relief.

Past Medical History
Gout

Chronic atrial fibrillation

Hypertension

Osteoarthritis

Benign prostatic hyperplasia (BPH)

History of prostate cancer

Family History
Father had diabetes mellitus type 2 and died from a myocardial infarction at age 66; mother died from stomach cancer at age 73.

Social History
Widowed and lives at home; has one child and visits at least once weekly; retired as a school teacher 15 years ago.

Tobacco/Alcohol/Substance Use
Denies alcohol consumption × 25 years; lifetime nonsmoker; denies any illicit drug use

Allergies/Intolerances/Adverse Drug Events
No known drug allergy

Medications (Current)
Amlodipine 5 mg po daily for hypertension

Lisinopril/hydrochlorothiazide (HCTZ) 20/12.5 mg po daily for hypertension

Febuxostat 40 mg po daily for gout

Tamsulosin 0.4 mg po daily for BPH

Finasteride 5 mg po daily for BPH

Hydrocodone/acetaminophen 5/325 mg po q 4-6 hours as needed for pain

Pantoprazole 40 mg po daily as needed for stomach

Warfarin 5 mg po q PM or as directed by clinic

Docusate/senna 50/8.6 mg po qhs as needed for bowel movements

Promethazine 25 mg po 3 times daily as needed for nausea

Review of Systems
Chronic pain from osteoarthritis usually controlled with hydrocodone/acetaminophen; denies any recent chest pain, shortness of breath, abdominal pain, unusual bruising or bleeding, or changes in bladder or bowel habits.

Physical Examination

▶ **General**

Obese, elderly, Caucasian male in acute distress

▶ **Vital Signs**

BP 153/89 mm Hg, P 83, RR 18, T 37.1°C, SpO$_2$ 98% (0.98)

Weight 222 lb. (100.9 kg)

Height 66 in. (167.6 cm)

Reports pain score of 7/10

▶ **Skin**

Warm and dry to touch; (+) erythema and swelling of 1-3 metacarpophalangeal joints of the left hand and left wrist.

▶ **HEENT**

PERRLA, EOMI; (–) sinus tenderness; TMs appear normal

▶ **Neck and Lymph Nodes**

Supple, nontender; no carotid bruit; no jugular venous distention

▶ **Chest**

Clear to auscultation

▶ **Cardiovascular**

RRR, normal S_1, S_2; (–) S_3 or S_4; good pulses equal in all extremities

▶ **Abdomen**

Obese; soft, nontender/nondistended; (–) organomegaly

▶ **Neurology**

Alert and oriented × 3; cranial nerves II to XII grossly intact; deep tendon reflexes normal

Laboratory Tests

Lab	Conventional Units	SI Units
Na	135 mEq/L	135 mmol/L
K	4.1 mEq/L	4.1 mmol/L
Cl	104 mEq/L	104 mmol/L
CO_2	23 mEq/L	23 mmol/L
BUN	23 mg/dL	8.21 mmol/L
SCr	1.98 mg/dL	175 µmol/L
eCrCl	32 mL/min/1.73 m²	0.31 mL/s/m²
Glucose	102 mg/dL	5.66 mmol/L
Total Ca	8.7 mg/dL	2.175 mmol/L
Mg	1.9 mEq/L	0.95 mmol/L
PO_4	3.2 mg/dL	1.03 mmol/L
Hgb	12.6 g/dL	7.81 mmol/L
Hct	37%	0.37 (fraction)
MCV	97 µm³	97 fL
WBC	$5.9 \times 10^3/\mu L$	$5.9 \times 10^9/L$
Neutrophils	66%	0.66 (fraction)
Eosinophils	3%	0.03 (fraction)
Basophils	1%	0.01 (fraction)
Lymphocytes	20%	0.20 (fraction)
Monocytes	10%	0.10 (fraction)
Bands	0%	0 (fraction)
Platelet	$120 \times 10^3/\mu L$	$120 \times 10^9/L$
Prothrombin Time	36.8	
INR	3.1	
Uric Acid	2.9 mg/dL	172.4 µmol/L

Assessment

Eighty-two-year-old man with signs, symptoms, and laboratory tests consistent with gout

Student Work-Up

Missing Information/Inadequate Data

Evaluate: Patient database

Drug therapy problems

Care plan (by problem)

TARGETED QUESTIONS

1. What signs and symptoms of gout does the patient have?

   Hint: See p. 902 in PPP

2. What risk factors for the development of gout are present in the patient?

   Hint: See pp. 901-902 in PPP

3. What would be the best treatment regimen for acute gout attack in this patient?

   Hint: See Table 59-1 and Figure 59-2 in PPP

4. What risks and adverse effects of therapy would you discuss with the patient?

   Hint: See pp. 903-904 and 909 in PPP

5. What lifestyle modification patient education points should be discussed with the patient regarding the prevention of future gout attacks?

   Hint: See pp. 905-906 and 908 in PPP

FOLLOW-UP

6. How would you treat this patient differently without the presence of comorbid conditions?

   Hint: See Figure 59-2 in PPP

7. What risks and adverse effects of therapy would you discuss with the patient using this treatment?

   Hint: See pp. 903-909 in PPP

8. What approach would you use for determining a treatment regimen for an acute gout attack in a young, pregnant female?

⊕ GLOBAL PERSPECTIVE

Gout is the most common form of inflammatory arthritis in the United States and Western Europe. It is a condition caused by an abnormality of uric acid metabolism, resulting in hyperuricemia. The findings from the Rochester Epidemiology Project have estimated the annual incidence of gout in the United States as 62 cases per 100,000 people. Over the past decade, the prevalence of gout in the United States has significantly increased due to several factors, including changes in diet, increased use of medications associated with the development of gout, increased rates of hypertension, dyslipidemias, metabolic syndrome, diabetes, and renal impairment, and an increase in the overall population life expectancy. Until recent years, there have been few new developments in therapeutic options for the management of gout. Despite the availability of these new options, these therapies are reserved only for those unresponsive to traditional treatments and can be costly to those who receive them. To help decrease the incidence of gout and hyperuricemia, it is important for health care professionals to educate patients at risk for developing gout on the signs and symptoms of gout, potential drug interactions, and therapeutic lifestyle changes, including weight reduction and avoidance of foods high in purine content.

CASE SUMMARY

- Clinical picture is consistent with an acute gout attack secondary to a lack of anti-inflammatory agent during initiation of a urate lowering therapy. An appropriate pain and anti-inflammatory management therapy should be initiated.

- Although the risk of gout increases with elevated serum uric acid concentrations, levels may actually be normal during an acute attack and should not be an indicator of exclusion or severity of a gout attack.

- Colchicine would be a reasonable initial therapy for this patient with a dose of 1.2 mg po immediately followed by 0.6 mg po 1 hour later (1.8 mg/day) and then 0.6 mg po 1-2 times daily for 6 months while initiating urate lowering therapy. The patient should be educated on appropriate use and potential gastrointestinal side effects.

- Pharmacotherapy options may be limited in presence of other comorbid disease states and lifestyle modifications, including weight reduction and avoidance of substances with high purine content, should also be implemented.

For more information on the care plan and facilitator's guide please visit http://www.mhpharmacotherapy.com

66 Glaucoma

Jon P. Wietholter

PATIENT PRESENTATION

Chief Complaint

"I swear my vision is getting worse. It seems like everything is closing in around me and I'm not able to see as well as I used to."

History of Present Illness

Aidan Joseph is a 67-year-old Caucasian male presenting to your clinic for a follow-up appointment regarding the management of his type 2 diabetes mellitus (T2DM). While interviewing Mr. Joseph, his main complaint centers on his worsening vision. He tells you he was diagnosed with glaucoma about 3 years ago, and since then his vision has seemed to slowly deteriorate. When asked about this vision loss, he claims to be primarily losing his peripheral vision and that it's been much more noticeable over "the last 1-2 weeks." He also mentions that he was admitted to the hospital "about a week ago" for a chronic obstructive pulmonary disease (COPD) exacerbation. Due to these worsening complaints you call the physician you work with at the clinic to do a more thorough physical examination of Mr. Joseph.

Past Medical History (PMH)

COPD (diagnosed 5 years ago)

POAG (diagnosed 3 years ago)

Hypertension (HTN) (diagnosed 25 years ago)

Type 2 diabetes mellitus (diagnosed 10 years ago)

Family History

Father is alive (age 97) with only medical problem being HTN. Mother passed away from a myocardial infarction (MI) at age 76. She also had a history of glaucoma and T2DM. He has no siblings.

Social/Work History

Retired from a factory job at age 62. Married for 46 years and currently lives with his wife. Has three children, aged 45, 43, and 39.

Tobacco/Alcohol/Substance Use

Currently smoking 1.5 ppd cigarettes. Had smoked 2 ppd for 47 years but cut back to 1.5 ppd when he was diagnosed with COPD. (–) Illicit drug use. (–) Alcohol consumption

Allergy/Intolerance/Adverse Event History

Allergic to amoxicillin (anaphylaxis)

Medications (Current)

Albuterol inhaler two puffs every 4 hours as needed

Tiotropium 18 mcg inhaled daily

Prednisone 20 mg orally daily for 3 days, then 10 mg orally daily for 4 days (total of 14 days of corticosteroid treatment for COPD exacerbation)

Brimonidine 0.15%, 1 drop in each eye daily

Nifedipine XL 30 mg orally daily

Carvedilol 6.25 mg orally twice daily

Metformin 500 mg orally twice daily

Glipizide 5 mg orally twice daily

Review of Systems

Physical Exam

▶ **General**

Patient is in no acute distress. He is able to talk in complete sentences with no noticeable shortness of breath. Overall, he seems to be relatively comfortable.

▶ **Vital Signs**

BP 152/79 mm Hg, HR 95, RR 18, T 36.5°C, O_2 sat: 92% on room air

Weight 260 lb. (118 kg)

Height 72 in. (183 cm)

Pain score 0/10

▶ **Skin**

No acute rashes or lesions

▶ **HEENT**

EOMI; open anterior chamber angles noted; optic disc cupping noted in both eyes; IOP 30 mm Hg (4.0 kPa) in right eye on examination; IOP 32 mm Hg (4.2 kPa) in left eye on examination; TMs appear normal; (–) sinus tenderness; (–) eye pain or redness

▶ **Neck and Lymph Nodes**

No thyroid nodules or lymphadenopathy present

▶ **Chest**

Mild wheezing on auscultation; (–) rhonchi; mildly decreased breath sounds diffusely; (–) accessory muscle usage

▶ **Cardiovascular**

Regular rate and rhythm; heart sounds noted to be somewhat distant

▶ **Abdomen**

Nontender; (–) organomegaly

▶ **Neurology**

Grossly intact; deep tendon reflexes normal

▶ **Extremities**

No signs of cyanosis; (–) peripheral edema; good pulses in all four extremities; no signs of peripheral neuropathy

▶ **Genitourinary**

Deferred

▶ **Rectal**

Deferred

Laboratory and Other Diagnostic Tests

None during this clinic visit outside of the IOP's documented in HEENT portion of physical exam.

Assessment

This is a 67-year-old male with signs, symptoms, and physical examination consistent with uncontrolled worsening primary open-angle glaucoma.

Student Work-Up

Missing Information/Inadequate data

Evaluate: Patient database

Drug therapy problems

Care plan (by problem)

Additional Information:

- What is this patient's central corneal thickness?
- What insurance does this patient have? Can he afford a more expensive option for glaucoma treatment?
- Is this patient using any OTC and/or herbal medications?
- Has this patient ever had any adverse effects with common preservatives contained in eye drops (e.g., benzalkonium chloride)?
- Do we have any previous IOP measurements?

- Do we have any previous pulmonary function test (PFT) results?
- Do we have any previous blood pressure readings?
- Do we have any previous blood glucose or Hgb A_1c levels?
- How is his inhaler technique?
- How is his instillation technique when using his eye drops?
- Is this patient compliant with his medications?
- Do we have any further information regarding his hospitalization from a week ago?

TARGETED QUESTIONS

1. What is(are) the goal(s) of therapy in the management of this patient's glaucoma?

   Hint: See p. 925 in PPP

2. What are the most appropriate pharmacotherapeutic options at this time and what adverse effects should be monitored for with each possible treatment option?

   Hint: See pp. 925 and 927 in PPP. Additionally, review Table 61-5 in PPP

3. Does this patient have any concomitant diseases or current medications that may affect his glaucoma or your medication recommendation(s) for the management of his glaucoma?

   Hint: Review each class of medications considered for the management of this patient's glaucoma to avoid/minimize any unwanted adverse effects (See "Pharmacologic Therapy" on pp. 929-931 in PPP). Consider the concomitant disease states this patient has been diagnosed with. Additionally, review which medications and/or classes of medications could potentially worsen and/or exacerbate Mr. Joseph's glaucoma (See "Special Considerations: Drug Induced Glaucomas" on p. 931 in PPP)

4. If this patient had instead presented with closed anterior angles on ophthalmic examination and significant ocular pain, what recommendation(s) would you have made?

   Hint: See on pp. 927 and 929 in PPP

5. How should you counsel this patient regarding appropriate ophthalmic medication administration technique?

   Hint: See "Application of Ophthalmic Solutions or Suspension" on p. 932 in PPP

FOLLOW-UP

Two weeks later, the patient returns to your clinic for a follow-up appointment. He claims that he feels like his vision hasn't worsened at all over the last 2 weeks, but that he gets a bad taste in the back of his throat when administering "his new eye drop." Additionally, he feels like his "eye color is changing" and is extremely concerned about this.

What should you tell the patient regarding his complaints and what counselling point(s) should you make during this visit?

Hint: Review common adverse effects from the "Pharmacologic Therapy" section on pp. 929-931 in PPP. Additionally, review "Application of Ophthalmic Solutions or Suspension" on p. 932 in PPP and "Pharmacologic Therapy" on pp. 929-931 in PPP for any potential counselling point(s) that may help Mr. Joseph.

☯ GLOBAL PERSPECTIVE

Glaucoma is a disease state that affects people of all races and nationalities. Although many different countries and cultures use medications and procedures similar to those used in the United States, many practitioners around the world turn to acupuncture or herbal remedies to aid in the treatment of glaucoma. Traditional Chinese medicine suggests that glaucoma is primarily due to "fire" carrying excess fluids to the eye. Although this may seem complicated, the practice of traditional Chinese medicine has been around for centuries and can be used to appropriately place acupuncture needles, typically at points to sedate the liver and stomach channels, or to select the appropriate herbal remedies (e.g., Xie Gan Jie Yu Tang and Wu Ling San) and/or eye drops (e.g., puerarin and alkaloids from erycibe) for the clinical scenario.

CASE SUMMARY

- This patient presentation is consistent with worsening primary open-angle glaucoma (POAG) that may have been aggravated by systemic corticosteroids prescribed for a COPD exacerbation.

- Multiple treatment options exist for management of this patient's POAG including increasing the frequency of brimonidine to 2-3 times per day or via replacement of brimonidine with an ocular hypotensive lipid. The final decision should take past medical history, cost, dosing frequency, adverse effect profiles, overall efficacy, and patient preferences into account to provide the most appropriate recommendation.

- Initial follow-up monitoring should take place in 2-4 weeks and adjustment of therapy should be based on efficacy (initial goal is at least a 25% reduction in IOP) and tolerability of the recommended therapy.

For more information on the care plan and facilitator's guide please visit http://www.mhpharmacotherapy.com

67 Allergic Rhinitis

David A. Apgar

PATIENT PRESENTATION

Chief Complaint
"What can you recommend for my red, itchy eyes?"

History of Present Illness (HPI)

Scarlet Skalera is a 62-year-old woman who presents to your community pharmacy setting with a complaint of red, itchy eyes. Both eyes are affected.

She has had these symptoms in various degrees of severity for many years. However, during the last 6-8 weeks, when plants have started to bloom and the weather has been windy, her symptoms have been much worse than usual. She has read in the lay press about what experts call a "pollen vortex" this year. Based on that, she expects to have severe symptoms for quite some time. In addition, she has some eye and other "hay fever" symptoms all the time, regardless of the season and the weather.

Both eyes itch intensely, albeit intermittently, most of her waking hours. Sometimes the symptoms interfere with her sleep. There is also some stinging and burning quality, as well as some watering or tearing of the eyes.

Especially in the recent weeks, symptoms have been daily. They negatively affect her quality of life (she has particular trouble concentrating and reading). She thinks her productivity is decreased due to the symptoms because it is hard to stay on task without rubbing her eyes, blowing her nose and otherwise dealing with her symptoms. She avoids some social situations and interactions due to embarrassment about her symptoms.

While some symptoms occur even when she is inside her home, they are markedly worsened, especially in the last few weeks, when she is outside. Windy days are particularly troublesome. Another setting that worsens symptoms is when one of the household cats (there are two) sleep near her head on her side of the bed.

There are numerous additional symptoms. She has frequent, sometimes profuse, clear watery nasal discharge most days. She has abrupt onset of prolonged episodes of sneezing at least 3 times each week. She also has severe nasal congestion, usually after these sneezing episodes. The congestion is often associated with a headache around her eyes, and some decreased hearing. It can interfere with sleep when it occurs in the evening. She admits to itching of her nose and sometimes in the roof of her mouth.

Years ago she used diphenhydramine for allergy symptoms. It helped some (nose symptoms more than eye symptoms),

but it made her very sleepy, even for part of the next day. This limited her use to 2-3 times a week at most. More recently she has tried both oral loratadine and oral cetirizine. They cause minimal sleepiness, but they also do not help as much as the diphenhydramine. About 4 years ago she got a prescription from her primary care physician (PCP) for fluticasone propionate nasal spray. This seemed to help all (even her eye) symptoms after using it twice daily for about 10 days in a row. However, after that, she reduced the frequency to once daily (at bedtime) because she noticed that it caused an unpleasant taste, some sore throat, and sometimes tended to dry her nose enough to cause some bleeding. If she could fall asleep quickly, bedtime use was better tolerated than the first thing in the morning. However, the bad taste sometimes interfered with getting to sleep. Currently, she uses this agent only once or twice a week, at bedtime. She has also tried ketotifen eye drops, but had trouble using it 3 times a day as recommended.

She has been told by health care providers that she has "hay fever" and thinks that her worsened symptoms lately are due to the "pollen vortex" that has been in the news. She knows that her "indoor" symptoms are probably mostly due to the cats in the house. However, her husband agreed to adopt a dog, so she will tolerate his cats. They launder the bedclothes and vacuum the bedroom very frequently, because the animals sometimes sleep in the bed with them. There is no carpet and no material window coverings anywhere in their home.

Review of Systems

She denies her eyes being "stuck shut" in the morning. She also denies vision changes, eyeball pain, and extreme sensitivity to bright light. She denies purulent or bloody nasal discharge (except as mentioned above, sometimes in association with intranasal steroid use). She does not have ear pain or ear discharge. Besides the occasional sore throat in association with intranasal steroid use, she only has brief morning sore throat that she thinks is due to mouth breathing from nasal congestion. She only coughs occasionally, and it is due to the nasal discharge "dripping down" her throat. She denies wheezing and trouble breathing. She does not have chest pain. She has no significant loss of appetite, upset stomach, throwing up or diarrhea in association with hay fever symptoms. She has no urinary or "women's" symptoms. She does not have diffuse or frequent aches or pains. She denies trouble moving her arms, legs, head or shoulders. She does not experience weakness, numbness or tingling. She denies skin lesions and rash. She has not had fever or chills with her hay fever symptoms.

Past Medical History

Scarlet has some other chronic medical conditions including dyslipidemia and the post-menopausal state.

Past Surgical History

S/P appendectomy (as a child) and bilateral salpingo-oophorectomy (at age 56, for an ovarian mass).

Family History

Patient was adopted and nothing is known about her birth parents or her genetic makeup.

Social History

Scarlet is a retired school nurse, who is married, and lives with her husband in a home with one dog and two cats. She and her husband each have one son, each from a previous relationship. She spends her time babysitting the grandchildren, reading, gardening, and volunteering at a local memory-care facility. She denies all tobacco and illicit (street) drug use. She has one beer or one glass of wine 3-4 nights per week.

Allergies/Intolerances/Adverse Effects

She is known to be allergic to various pollens and to cats. However, she has never had specific allergen testing, so does not know what specific pollens and cannot rule out allergy to house dust mite, molds, or cockroaches. She has no medication allergies. She has had itching after a morphine injection (in association with the last surgery), but was told it is just a side effect. She has had what sounds like an episode of *C. difficile* associated diarrhea from an unknown antibiotic (given for an upper respiratory tract infection) about 10 years ago. See HPI for details about diphenhydramine and intranasal fluticasone propionate adverse reactions.

Current Medications

Lovastatin 20 mg q hs for dyslipidemia

Angeliq (drospirenone 0.5 mg and estradiol 1 mg) one tablet every day for hormone replacement therapy (HRT)

As above, fluticasone propionate nasal spray 1 spray into both nostrils 1-2 times each week and loratadine 10 mg or cetirizine 10 mg 1 tablet orally once a day, 3-4 times per week for AR symptoms

Acetaminophen 500 mg 1-2 tablets prn HA, aches/pains (less than 4 tablets/month)

Ginger tea prn for upset stomach (less than once/month)

She claims that all immunizations are up to date

Physical Examination

Done to the extent possible, in the back room of a community pharmacy with limited equipment.

▶ *General*

WDWN Caucasian adult woman who appears her stated age. Good historian. Sophisticated health literacy. No evidence of trauma or pain, and denies pain.

▶ *Vital Signs*

Afebrile to touch of forehead. Radial pulse regular at about 60/minute. Respiratory rate about 12/minute during interview. BP not taken.

▶ *Eyes*

Pt wearing glasses for driving and can read newsprint at arms length. With aid of flashlight, her pupils are equal and react to light. Light does not cause discomfort. Visual fields not evaluated. Her pupils react to accommodation. Eye movements are symmetrical. The corneae are clear bilaterally, without evidence of abrasion. There is no hyphema and no hypopyon. There is diffuse bilateral bulbar conjunctival injection, but no limbal flush. There is some lower bilateral palpebral conjunctival injection. There is minimal clear watery discharge at both medial canthi, but no evidence of purulence or crusting. Lids and lashes are normal without purulence or crusting.

▶ *Ears*

Hearing is grossly normal based on whispered conversation. No obvious discharge from either ear. No pain on pinna traction or tragus pressure. No periauricular adenopathy.

▶ *Nose*

Midline without trauma or deformity. With aid of flashlight, there is no evidence of septal deviation or perforation. The nasal mucosa is boggy and bluish in color. There is minimal opaque discharge, without evidence of trauma, bleeding or purulence.

▶ *Sinuses*

No pain or discomfort on palpation or percussion of frontal, ethmoid or maxillary sinuses.

▶ *Mouth*

Oral mucosa normal pink. Good oral/dental hygiene. Breath is not fetid.

▶ *Throat*

Tonsils somewhat enlarged, but pink without exudate. Uvula pink and midline. Posterior pharynx patent but with some redness, streaking and lymphoid hyperplasia. Soft palate somewhat red.

▶ *Neck*

Full range of motion without pain or restriction, supple, without adenopathy.

► *Lungs*

No evidence of respiratory distress during normal conversation. With aid of stethoscope, auscultation of posterior lung fields and upper anterior lung fields, through clothing, reveals no adventitious sounds (crackles, rhonchi or wheezes).

► *Other Components Of Exam*

Breast, cardiovascular, abdominal, neurologic, musculoskeletal, dermatologic, genitourinary/rectal, and endocrine all deferred as noncontributory or inappropriate to perform in the community setting.

Laboratory Values

At last visit to PCP and gynecologist for annual physical done about 3 months ago. Results are by patient's history (again, she is a retired nurse):

Complete blood count, urinalysis (without culture), basic metabolic profile (electrolytes, BUN, creatinine) were all "within normal limits" but she does not recall specific values.

PAP smear—reported as normal.

Screening mammogram—reported as category 1 (negative or no lesions).

Note well that the patent has never had any sort of specific allergen testing procedures.

Assessment

Allergic rhinitis/conjunctivitis, suboptimal control

Dyslipidemia, unknown control and cardiovascular risk

Post-menopausal on HRT

Student Work-Up

Missing Information/Inadequate Data

Evaluate:
    Patient database

    Drug therapy problems

    Care plan (by problem)

Additional information:

More detail about role of the patient's husband relative to avoidance of cat allergen.

More detail about severity and significance of adverse effects of intranasal fluticasone propionate.

Results of most recent lipid panel.

Determination of cardiovascular risk by either Framingham Risk Criteria (from NCEP 2001) or newer Pooled Cohort Equations (from ACC/AHA 2013 Dyslipidemia Guideline).

More information about duration of patient's HRT and attendant thromboembolic risks.

TARGETED QUESTIONS

1. How is this patient's complaint best characterized?

   Hint: See Table 63-2 and the last paragraph of the Introduction to Chapter 63 (p. 949) in PPP

2. a. What typical manifestations of her chief complaint diagnosis does she experience?

   Hint: See the Typical Symptoms section of the Clinical Presentation and Diagnosis of Allergic Rhinitis box (p. 951) in Chapter 63 of PPP

   b. What nontypical manifestation of her chief complaint diagnosis does she experience?

   Hint: See the Other Symptoms section of the Clinical Presentation and Diagnosis of Allergic Rhinitis box (p. 951) in Chapter 63 of PPP

3. What general therapeutic options are available to her?

   Hint: See Table 63-3 and Table 63-4 in PPP

4. Describe an initial pharmacologic plan for this patient, at this time. Offer alternatives where appropriate.

   Hint: See portions of Pharmacologic Therapy section of text (pp. 951-953) as well as appropriate portions of Table 63-9 in PPP

5. Discuss her specific limitations to optimizing the management of her chief complaint diagnosis. What can be offered to her to overcome these limitations?

   Hint: See portions of text that concern adherence, avoidance of allergens and patient education in the Summary of Treatment (pp. 958 and 961), Outcome Evaluation (p. 961), and Patient Care Process (p. 961) sections in Chapter 63 of PPP

FOLLOW-UP

How would your recommendations change (see Targeted Question 4, above) if the index patient was younger and 2 months pregnant, but all other elements of the case were the same?

Hint: See Special Populations, Pregnant Women section of text (p. 958)

↻ GLOBAL PERSPECTIVE

Allergic rhinitis is a common condition worldwide. It is being recognized more frequently in many developing countries, probably due to increasing urbanization and industrialization resulting in people being exposed to new and different potential pollutants and allergens. This has been termed "Westernization." The major differences in approach to the management of AR in countries other than the United States involve affordability of health care and medications in general, and availability of specific medication by individual country. This difference is less than a few years ago, with the recent introduction of a second intranasal corticosteroid product available over-the-counter. However, there are more options for immunotherapy in many developed countries outside the United States (administered by both subcutaneous and sublingual routes). And, there are differences in the availability of specific oral, intranasal, and intraocular antihistamine products throughout the world.

CASE SUMMARY

- The categorization of the patient's AR is easily determined from Table 63-2, and this helps determine the order of optimal management.

- The patient presents with what may sound like primary and isolated allergic conjunctivitis. However, by thoroughly evaluating the chief complaint, with a systematic process for the history of present illness, it becomes clear that the patient really has allergic rhinitis. A suggested system for HPI includes seven basic elements (location, onset, quality, quantity, setting, associated symptoms, modifying factors) and a final question that asks the patient what she thinks is causing the problem. Frequently, this question reveals important information, not already established. The patient has all four of the typical symptoms of AR plus a major component of allergic conjunctivitis (see Clinical Presentation and Diagnosis of Allergic Rhinitis). Nothing in the presentation suggests a more serious, sight-threatening ocular condition.

- The optimal approach to her category of AR is easily from Tables 63-3, 63-4, and 63-9.

- There are two limitations to optimization of this patient's management. These are inadequate avoidance of some (especially cat) allergen, and inadequate adherence to the most beneficial mode of pharmacologic therapy (instranasal corticosteroid) due to adverse effects. Conceptually, the student must realize that the health care provider's role is limited to educating the patient and their support system and encouraging implementation of appropriate avoidance and adherence strategies. Patients ultimately decide what they will and will not accept from among the various suggestions and recommendations. The health care provider cannot dictate action steps.

REFERENCES

1. Krouse JH. Allergic rhinitis: journeys and experiences (editorial). Otolaryngol Head Neck Surg 2015;152(2):193-194.
2. Seidman MD, Gurgel RK, Lin SY, et al. Clinical practice guideline: allergic rhinitis executive summary. Otolaryngol Head Neck Surg 2015;152(2):197-206.
3. Recommending over-the-counter options for allergic rhinitis. Pharmacist's Letter 2014;Self study course #140207.

For more information on the care plan and facilitator's guide please visit http://www.mhpharmacotherapy.com

68 Conjunctivitis

Michelle L. Hilaire   Jaime R. Hornecker

PATIENT PRESENTATION

Chief Complaint

"My eyes are so red and watery. It started 3 days ago in my right eye while I was traveling with my family on vacation out of state. The light really makes my eyes water right now. I feel like my left eye is starting to get affected too. I've got to get back to work since I was on vacation all last week."

History of Present Illness

Julia Watson is a 39-year-old woman who comes to see her physician because currently her right eye is red and watering. Three days ago, she noticed that her right eye was irritated and looked a little red, but assumed it was because she had been up late while traveling with family. She tried Visine, but did not notice much difference. Yesterday while waiting for her airplane, she noticed that she had to wipe away watery discharge from her right eye several times. This seemed to get worse as she was on the airplane. Today when she woke up, her left eye looked the same as the right. She thinks they look redder than yesterday and are watering more and now she is light-sensitive. She mentions that her niece was coughing and sniffling and having watery eyes when they were visiting.

Past Medical History

Seasonal Allergies

GERD (diagnosed 3 years ago)

Hypertension (HTN) (diagnosed 5 years ago)

Obesity

Family History

Mother has osteoporosis and HTN, and is alive at age 68. Father had pancreatic cancer and died at age 60. She has a sister, who has hyperlipidemia.

Social History

Married and lives with her husband of 15 years; has two children. Works as a medical assistant at a local doctor's office. Started walking with kids 1 mile 3 days a week for exercise.

Tobacco/Alcohol/Substance Use

Social drinker (four drinks per week)

(–) Tobacco or illicit drug use

Allergies/Intolerances/Adverse Drug Events

Penicillin (breaks out in hives)

Medications (Current)

Esomeprazole 20 mg po daily

Lisinopril 10 mg po daily

Calcium carbonate 1000 mg po q 12 h

Vitamin D 1000 international units po daily

Acetaminophen 325 mg po prn headache

Ibuprofen 200 mg po prn pain

Cetirizine 10 mg po daily during allergy season

Review of Systems

(+) Eye discharge and tearing in both eyes

(–) Double vision and blind spots

Occasional headaches relieved with pain reliever

Physical Examination

▶ *General*

Well-developed, well-nourished, Caucasian female in no acute distress. Speech is clear and affect is appropriate.

▶ *Vital Signs*

BP 156/82 mmHg, P 70, RR 14 (easy and nonlabored), T 36.8°C

Weight 218 lb. (99 kg)

Height 66 in. (167.6 cm)

Denies pain

▶ *Skin*

Dry-appearing skin and scalp

(–) Rashes or lesions

▶ *HEENT*

Vision 20/40 in each eye with glasses

Both eyes—conjunctiva red and slightly swollen

PERRLA

EOMI

Ear canals without erythema, swelling, discharge, or cerumen

► **Neck and Lymph Nodes**

Physical examination of neck is unremarkable; (–) thyroid nodules; (–) lymphadenopathy; (–) carotid bruits

► **Chest**

Clear to auscultation bilaterally with no wheezing, ronchi, or rales

► **Breasts**

Examination deferred

► **Cardiovascular**

RRR

Normal S_1, S_2 (–) S_3 or S_4

No murmurs, rubs, or gallops

► **Abdomen**

Nontender/nondistended

(–) Organomegaly

► **Neurology**

Cranial nerves II to XII intact (I not assessed at this visit)

Deep tendon reflexes normal

No complaints of weakness, numbness, or loss of coordination

► **Genitourinary**

Examination deferred

► **Rectal**

Examination deferred

Laboratory Tests

Fasting, Obtained 3 months Ago

	Conventional Units	SI Units
Na	140 mEq/L	140 mmol/L
K	4.1 mEq/L	4.1 mmol/L
Cl	107 mEq/L	107 mmol/L
CO_2	28 mEq/L	28 mmol/L
BUN	11 mg/dL	5.4 mmol/L
SCr	0.9 mg/dL	80 µmol/L
Ca	9.4 mg/dL	2.35 mmol/L
Mg	1.6 mEq/L	0.80 mmol/L
Phosphate	3.1 mg/dL	1 mmol/L
Hgb	12.0 g/dL	8.4 mmol/L
Hct	37.4%	0.374
WBC	$7.2 \times 10^3/mm^3$	$7.2 \times 10^9/L$
MCV	89 mm^3	89 fL
Albumin	3.9 g/dL	39 g/L

Hemoglobin A1c	6.2%	0.062
Glucose	91 mg/dL	5.05 mmol/L
Total cholesterol	105 mg/dL	2.72 mmol/L
Triglycerides	110 mg/dl	1.24 mmol/L
LDL cholesterol	120 mg/dL	3.10 mmol/L
HDL cholesterol	40 mg/dL	1.03 mmol/L

Assessment

Thirty-nine-year-old woman with signs and symptoms consistent with viral conjunctivitis (pink eye).

Student Work-Up

Missing Information/Inadequate Data

Evaluate: Patient database

Drug therapy problems

Care plan (by problem)

TARGETED QUESTIONS

1. What types of conjunctivitis exist?

   Hint: See pp. 936-940 in PPP

2. What is the primary cause of viral conjunctivitis?

   Hint: See p. 938 in PPP

3. What nonpharmacologic measures can be used to relieve symptoms?

   Hint: See p. 938 in PPP

4. What pharmacologic therapy should be used to treat viral conjunctivitis?

   Hint: See pp. 938-939 in PPP

5. When should the patient see significant improvement in the viral conjunctivitis?

   Hint: See p. 939 in PPP

FOLLOW-UP

Two weeks later, the patient returns for follow-up. Her symptoms have resolved, but she notes that her husband and oldest son are experiencing similar symptoms.

What actions, if any, would you take? What nonpharmacologic measures would you share with the patient?

   Hint: See p. 938 in PPP

🌐 GLOBAL PERSPECTIVE

Conjunctivitis is a worldwide ophthalmic disorder and viral conjunctivitis is one of the most common forms. This condition is very contagious and poses a significant health problem in schools and workplaces where touch contamination is poorly controlled. Poor living conditions can contribute to continuous cases of viral conjunctivitis as household items such as towels and pillows are shared. If the etiology of the conjunctivitis is not clear, the patient should be referred to an eye care practitioner.

CASE SUMMARY

- Her current clinical picture is consistent with viral conjunctivitis. Although it is self-limiting, the patient needs to observe nonpharmacologic measures to avoid

spreading conjunctivitis to others. This is essential due to her job in health care.
- Antibiotic medications should be avoided in viral infections.

For more information on the care plan and facilitator's guide please visit http://www.mhpharmacotherapy.com

69 Psoriasis

Meghan K. Sullivan

PATIENT PRESENTATION

Chief Complaint

"My hands and feet are stiff and sore."

History of Present Illness

Jacob Garvey is a 55-year-old male who presents to his primary care provider today for a 12-week follow-up appointment. JG is complaining of pain and stiffness in his hands and feet. JG states that he was been taking ibuprofen "around the clock" to help control his pain. JG states that he has been experiencing this pain for approximately 3 weeks, but did not seek help knowing that he had an appointment scheduled.

Past Medical History

Gout (35 years ago)

Psoriasis diagnosed (30 years ago)

Dysplastic nevi diagnosed (30 years ago)

Hypertension (HTN) (2 years)

Hypertriglyceridemia (2 years)

Depression (1 year)

Pre-Diabetes (12 weeks)

Family History

Mother is alive at the age of 82 with a history of dyslipidemia, hypertension, and breast cancer. Father is alive at age 83 with a history of hypertension, dyslipidemia, atrial fibrillation, and gout. He has three sisters, all of whom are healthy.

Social History

The patient is an owner and operator of a local plumbing company. He lives with his wife of 23 years and has two children, both of whom are away at college leaving him and his wife as empty nesters for the first time.

Tobacco/Alcohol/Substance Use

Drinks 1-2 beers per day; (−) tobacco or illicit drug use

Allergies/Intolerances/Adverse Drug Events

Sulfa antibiotics (rash as child)

Medications (Current)

Betamethasone dipropionate 0.1% cream: apply to affected area 2-4 times daily

Cyclosporine 100 mg: 1 capsule tid

Ibuprofen 200 mg: 2 tablets po q 4-6 h

Metoprolol 25 mg: 1 tablet bid

Omega-3/DHA 1 gram: 3 capsules q daily

Sertraline 25 mg: 1 tablet q daily

Unscented moisturizers: apply to affected area PRN

Valsartan and HCT 80/12.5 mg: 1 tablet q daily

Review of Systems

(+) Pain and stiffness, (+) multiple lesions around the hairline on scalp, nape of neck and elbows, (+) pruritis, (+) depression

Physical Examination

▸ *General*

The patient appears to be distressed about the pain and stiffness in his hands and feet.

▸ *Vital Signs*

BP 138/88 mm Hg, P 68, RR 18, T 37.2°C

Weight 265 lb. (120 kg)

Height 72 in. (173 cm)

Pain is 8/10 and complains of moderate pruritus

▸ *Skin*

Lesions on scalp, nape of neck and elbows

▸ *HEENT*

TMs normal; PERRLA

▸ *Neck and Lymph Nodes*

Within normal limits

▸ *Chest*

Within normal limits

▸ *Breasts*

Within normal limits

▶ *Cardiovascular*

Within normal limits

▶ *Abdomen*

Within normal limits

▶ *Neurology*

Reflexes normal

▶ *Genitourinary*

Examination deferred

▶ *Rectal*

Examination deferred

Laboratory Tests

Fasting blood glucose obtained during the appointment: 117 mg/dL (6.49 mmol/L)

Basic chemistry panel collected at last office visit: All values within normal limits except fasting blood glucose 111 mg/dL (6.16 mmol/L) on 05/28/2015

Assessment

Fifty-five-year-old male with multiple comorbidities presents with signs/symptoms consistent with onset of psoriatic arthritis (PsA) and psoriatic flare-up.

Student Work-Up

Missing Information/Inadequate Data

Evaluate: Patient database

Drug therapy problems

Care plan (by problem)

TARGETED QUESTIONS

1. What comorbidities are associated with psoriasis?

   Hint: See p. 965 in PPP

2. What are the general characteristics, signs and symptoms of plaque psoriasis?

   Hint: See p. 966 in PPP

3. What are the goals of therapy for psoriatic arthritis (PsA)?

   Hint: See pp. 966-967 in PPP

4. What factors may be contributing to the increased severity of JG's plaque psoriasis and the onset of psoriatic arthritis?

   Hint: See p. 966 in PPP

5. What factors must be taken into consideration in identifying the right therapy for a patient with psoriasis?

   Hint: See p. 967 in PPP

FOLLOW-UP

JG returns to the office 4 weeks later for a follow-up appointment. JG reports significant improvement in his pain and stiffness (4/10 on pain scale). His lesions have improved dramatically.

What actions will you take, if any, to enhance the therapeutic effect of the patient's current therapy?

What additional steps will you take to ensure that he enters remission and experiences minimal flare-ups for his psoriasis?

☼ GLOBAL PERSPECTIVE

Psoriasis is a common chronic inflammatory disease of the skin that is seen in people throughout the world. Incidence and prevalence of psoriasis continues to be studied on an ongoing basis. It is thought that psoriasis dates back to Biblical times as a similar disorder is made mention of in the Bible. Throughout the years, the diagnosis of psoriasis has changed as more has been understood about the disease. Several patterns have been identified in studies that have been conducted in patients suffering from psoriasis. However, these findings cannot always be deemed conclusive for the fact that many patients do not seek medication attention for the treatment of psoriasis. Observations include a greater incidence of psoriasis seen in patients living in regions further from the equator. Studies conducted in Australia show that people residing in southern Australia are more likely to experience psoriasis than those residing in northern Australia. The opposite is true for a study conducted in Norway, helping to prove the theory that those residing close to the equator are less likely to suffer from the disease. In terms of race, Caucasians have been found to have psoriasis more often than those of Asian or African descent. Lifestyle plays a large role in the incidence and prevalence of the disease as well. Individuals living in third-world countries are less likely to have psoriasis in comparison to developed countries where smoking, stress, and obesity are more prominent and have been shown to increase a person's risk for developing the disease.

CASE SUMMARY

- JG's current condition can be classified as the onset of psoriatic arthritis and a psoriasis flare-up in conjunction with multiple comorbidities.

- The psoriatic flare-up is most likely due to a drug-induced exacerbation of psoriasis as well as recent life events.

- Onset of psoriatic arthritis is unpredictable and does not have to correlate with the severity of psoriasis.

- Many factors must be taken into consideration when selecting appropriate therapy to ensure relief of sign/symptoms of both psoriasis and psoriatic arthritis, especially in conjunction with therapy for JG's comorbidities.

For more information on the care plan and facilitator's guide please visit http://www.mhpharmacotherapy.com

70 Acne

Jean E. Cunningham

PATIENT PRESENTATION

Chief Complaint

"I'm tired of my constant acne!"

History of Present Illness

NP is a 28-year-old female picking up a refill on her oral contraceptive (drospirenone/ethinyl estradiol). When counseling was offered, she shares her frustration that her acne is not improving and nothing she does seems to help. She is in her sister's wedding in 3 months and would really like to see improvement in her skin before the big day, and wants to know if there is anything else she should consider. On further questioning and examination, you find that the patient has severe acne on her cheeks, chin, neck, chest, and back, which seems to intensify around the start of her cycle. The patient has tried several different products without much success several times (recently about a year ago) and usually uses a name brand "Acne Solution." She has tried facials, but did not notice much improvement. She is considering trying an oil cleansing method that her friend who is really into essential oils has told her about (1 part castor oil and 3 parts olive oil) because she has heard it works miracles. She was on a strict gluten-free diet a few years ago for her own wedding and felt like that might have helped her skin some. She is overwhelmed with the amount of medications she takes to help with her skin and she is not noticing that much improvement.

Past Medical History

Acne (severe)

Family History

NP is married with no children. Both of her parents are alive and well (mother has arthritis; father has high blood pressure). She has two younger sisters with no known medical issues. She and her husband would like to start a family soon, especially once he finishes graduate school (in about 2 months).

Social History

NP leads an active lifestyle (exercises 3-4 times a week) and works as a structural engineer for a large company (spends a lot of time on the phone and at her desk) and sells jewelry in her free time.

Tobacco/Alcohol/Substance Use

NP does not smoke but does drink socially a few times a week. She denies substance use or abuse.

Allergies/Intolerances/Adverse Drug Events

Developed a rash when she took sulfamethoxazole/trimethoprim as a child

Medications (Current)

Drospirenone/ethinyl estradiol 1 po daily (has taken for 3 years)

Spironolactone 50 mg po daily (started last month)

Adapalene/Benzoyl peroxide gel apply daily (started about 2 months ago)

Minocycline 100 mg po daily (has taken before, started last month, has 1 refill remaining)

Tea tree oil applies prn

Multivitamin daily

"Acne Solutions" facial wash daily

Review of Systems

Painful swelling and redness located on cheeks, chin, upper back, and chest/neck area; (+) papues, pustules, open and closed comedones, moderately painful lesions; (+) scarring; (–) dry skin; (–) hyperpigmentation; (+) nodules.

Physical Examination

▶ *General*

Pleasant demeanor, motivated to try something that will work.

▶ *Vital Signs*

Weight 145 lb. (65 kg)

Height 69 in. (175 cm)

BP, HR, pulse: normal

▶ *Skin*

A combination of red, solid, elevated lesions and vesicles; (+) papules, pustules, nodules, and scaring located on cheeks, chin, upper back, and exposed chest/neck area; (+) open and closed comedones on upper back

► *HEENT*

Grinds her teeth at night; has retainer

Assessment

28-year-old female with signs, symptoms, and physical examination consistent with severe acne possibly hormonally related.

Student Work-Up

Missing Information/Inadequate Data

Evaluate: Patient database

                      Drug therapy problems

                      Care plan (by problem)

TARGETED QUESTIONS

1. What distinguishes NP's symptoms from moderate acne?
   Hint: See p. 979 of PPP

2. Would topical antibiotics be appropriate in this patient? Why or why not?
   Hint: See p. 981 of PPP

3. What is the optimal time-frame of lesion improvement for each of NP's acne medications?
   Hint: See pp. 979-980 of PPP

4. What medications should NP discontinue if she stops her oral contraceptive and begins "trying for a family"?
   Hint: See pp. 979-980 of PPP

5. Are any of NP's medications suboptimally dosed?
   Hint: See Table 65-2 in PPP

FOLLOW-UP

Three months later, NP is picking up a prescription for prenatal multivitamins and is considering other options for her acne now that she has discontinued her drospirenone/ethinyl estradiol, spironolactone, and adapalene/benzoyl peroxide (her minocycline was discontinued once she completed her last refill). She is now wondering what options she has to help with her skin while she is trying to get pregnant.

What treatment options are available for NP's severe acne now that she is trying to get pregnant?

Hint: See pp. 979-980 of PPP

⊘ GLOBAL PERSPECTIVE

Acne affects races and skin types differently and may present with different clinical manifestations depending on the affected patient. Although acne is considered the most common disease in the United States, it is also common in other countries, but in different forms. Cystic acne is commonly found in countries such as Spain, Italy, Iran, and other countries in the Mediterranean region. African-Americans or people of other ethnicities can also develop a certain type of acne commonly associated with the use of oil or ointment-based hair pomades. Although the primary cause of acne depends on pathogenic factors, additional factors, whether culturally related or not, such as the use of occluding cosmetic and hair products, certain medications, disease states, and items worn directly against skin that obstruct skin pores can worsen acne and should be identified, discussed, and avoided if possible.

CASE SUMMARY

- Her current clinical picture is consistent with severe papular pustular acne not responding to her current therapy, and alternative treatments should be initiated.

For more information on the care plan and facilitator's guide please visit http://www.mhpharmacotherapy.com

71 Atopic Dermatitis

Kim W. Benner

PATIENT PRESENTATION

Chief Complaint

"Madison has had a red rash on her elbows and knees and it is now starting on her face spreading up on her scalp. She scratches it all the time and it seems to be getting worse despite the use of lotion and an over-the-counter steroid cream."

History of Present Illness

Madison is a 12-month-old female who presents to her pediatrician with a 3-month history of a pruritic and erythematous rash on the inside of her elbows and knees, that has now spread to her face and scalp. The lesions on her elbows and knees contain some erythematous papules. Madison frequently scratches at all the lesions. The mother had been using lotion on Madison's skin but as the lesions worsened, she tried a nonprescription hydrocortisone cream. Madison's mother transitioned her from breast milk to formula approximately 3 months ago and has recently been introducing new foods into her diet; she tried cow's milk that seemed to worsen her skin. The addition of eggs was also was associated with increasing skin lesions and gastrointestinal upset.

Past Medical History

Mother reports Madison was a full-term delivery with no complications and went home with family on day of life #2. She reports episodes of colic and gastrointestinal distress prompting the mother to change formulas several times after 6 months of exclusive breast feeding. Even when Madison was younger, her mother reports noticing many bouts of "dry, red skin" to which she would apply baby lotion. The rashes would come and go but around 3 months ago, they progressively flared and spread to adjacent areas. The rashes have also appeared to worsen simultaneously with the addition of foods to her diet, such as cow's milk and eggs.

Family History

Maternal history of asthma, controlled with inhalers

Paternal history of allergic rhinitis; (+) smoking in home

Social/Work History

Noncontributory

Allergy/Intolerances/Adverse Event History

Potentially allergic to milk and eggs per mother's report

Medication History

Nonprescription hydrocortisone cream prn to skin lesions

Review of Systems

Cutaneous examination reveals symmetric, brightly erythematous, lesions on the antecubital fossae and extensor aspects of the knees. Similar, although milder, erythematous lesions are present on her face and scalp.

Physical Exam

▶ **General**

Active, alert toddler who appears playful and in no acute distress. Occasionally rubs at active lesions.

▶ **Vital Signs**

BP 85/60 mm Hg, HR 105, RR 25, T 36.4°C

Weight 21 lb. (9.5 kg)

Height 30 in. (76.2 cm)

▶ **Skin**

Generalized xerosis; (+) pruritic, erythematous papules and vesicles on antecubital and popliteal fossa of arms and legs. Pruritic lesions also present on face and scalp. Diaper markings are present on her torso.

▶ **HEENT**

PERRLA, EOMI, nares moist with mucus; Dennie-Morgan fold (atopic pleat) present

▶ **Neck and Lymph Nodes**

Not significant

▶ **Extremities**

Xerosis on hands and feet

▶ **Genitourinary**

Noncontributory; patient is in a diaper with some mild redness on the buttocks

Laboratory and Other Diagnostic Tests

	Conventional Units	SI Units
Na	136 mEq/L	136 mmol/L
K	4.0 mEq/L	4.0 mmol/L

Cl	103 mEq/L	103 mmol/L
CO_2	23 mEq/L	23 mmol/L
BUN	13 mg/dL	4.6 mmol/L
SCr	0.4 mg/dL	35.36 μmol/L
Glu	170 mg/dL	9.35 mmol/L
Creatinine clearance	91 mL/min/1.73 m²	0.88 mL/s/m²
Ca	9.1 mg/dL	4.55 mmol/L
Mg	1.8 mEq/L	0.9 mmol/L
Phosphate	3.2 mg/dL	1.0 mmol/L
Hgb	12 g/dL	120 g/L; 7.44 mmol/L
Hct	35%	0.35
Serum IgE	2.20 IU/mL (normal 20 to 100)	
Eosinophils	9%	0.09

Assessment

Twelve-month-old female with signs and symptoms consistent with atopic dermatitis (AD)

Student Work-Up

Missing Information/Inadequate Data

Evaluate: Patient database

Drug therapy problems

Care plan (by problem)

TARGETED QUESTIONS

1. What signs and symptoms of AD does the patient have?

2. What significant findings in Madison's history contribute to the development of her AD?

    Hint: Her history of food allergies and positive family history of asthma and allergic rhinitis all are consistent with atopy and thus development of atopic dermatitis.

3. What nonpharmacologic therapy can you recommend for Madison?

4. Is a topical corticosteroid the treatment of choice for her? If so, what potency of steroid should be utilized?

    Hint: See p. 987 and Table 65-4 in PPP

5. What are the second-line options available for the acute control of AD?

FOLLOW-UP

Four weeks later, Madison and her mother return to clinic and states that after using the prescribed initial therapy, the lesions are slightly improved. The mother notices that some of Madison's skin is now discolored. They are curious as to any alternative medicine options that exist for the treatment of AD.

What alternative therapy is available for these AD lesions?

☉ GLOBAL PERSPECTIVE

Atopic dermatitis (AD) is a common skin disorder that appears to be increasing in other countries. AD is often associated with triggers such as food allergies. The incidence of food allergies can differ around the world and is increasing in developing countries. It can be seen more in the urban environment and some studies have shown an increasing prevalence of allergen sensitization in children born in families living on farms. In addition, differing prevalence rates can be seen in other countries due to variations in diets. For example, rice allergies occur more often in Asia where rice is a major component of the Asian diet, whereas corn allergies may be more prevalent in the United States since corn derivatives are commonplace in the U.S. diet. The most common food allergies in many countries include milk, eggs, peanuts, tree nuts, fish, shellfish, soy, wheat and sesame. Seed allergies, especially sesame, have been reported to be increasing in some countries. The United States has the FDA to mandate appropriate labeling for possible allergens in the food supply; third-world countries may not have safeguards in place for consumers to heed caution of possible allergic triggers. Often exposure to extreme hot or cold temperatures can be a cause of an exacerbation, so inhabitants of such environments worldwide may suffer exacerbations more (or less) often.

CASE SUMMARY

- Madison's current skin lesions (and history) are consistent with atopic dermatitis. She has been using lotion as needed and a low dose steroid cream with no improvement. Therefore, the next step would be a higher potency topical steroid.

- Second line therapy for AD could include topical tacrolimus/pimecrolimus or phototherapy.

- Nonpharmacologic therapy is essential in AD and includes liberal use of emollients, avoidance of triggers, short lukewarm baths, use of nonirritating soaps and fabrics, and keeping fingernails short.

REFERENCE

1. American Academy of Dermatology. Guidelines of care for the management of atopic dermatitis. J Am Acad Dermatol 2014;71:116-132.

For more information on the care plan and facilitator's guide please visit http://www.mhpharmacothcrapy.com

72 Iron-Deficiency Anemia

Dawne Cylwik

PATIENT PRESENTATION

Chief Complaint

"I have been feeling really down lately, and I just have not had energy to do anything."

History of Present Illness

Sarah Simmens is a 19-year-old female who presents to her University's outpatient psychiatry clinic with complaints of fatigue and depression that have worsened over the past several months. She has not had the energy to go to her freshman classes and instead is taking long naps in the middle of the day. Despite eating only a single vegetarian meal daily, she is adherent to her insulin regimen.

Past Medical History

Type I diabetes mellitus (T1DM) (diagnosed at age 6)

Major Depressive Disorder (diagnosed at age 17)

History of suicide attempt via medication overdose (age 17)

Family History

Father is 52 and has T1DM and GERD. Mother is 51 and has a history of ovarian cancer, in remission, and hypothyroidism. She has 1 sibling in college with no significant medical conditions.

Social History

She works part time in a biochemistry research laboratory. Her family lives about 2 hours away in another city.

Tobacco/Alcohol/Substance Use

She drinks alcohol socially on weekends with friends. She denies tobacco and substance use.

Allergies/Intolerances/Adverse Event History

Olanzapine (rash)

Medications (Current)

Fluoxetine 10 mg po every morning

Lantus 13 units at bedtime

Novolog dosed using correction factor of 60 and insulin to carbohydrate ratio of 1:20

Review of Systems

(+) Anhedonia, difficulty concentrating, poor appetite, fatigue, frequent headaches, shortness of breath; (–) SI/HI, polydipsia, polyuria, recent infection, SOB, hematuria, hematochezia, melena or epitaxis. Menstrual cycles occur every 28 days (7 pads/day), with LMP 6 days ago.

Physical Examination

> #### General

Thin, pale, white female who appears stated age looking mildly disheveled.

> #### Vital Signs

BP 114/70 mm Hg, P 110, RR 22, T 37°C

Weight 130 lb. (59 kg)

Height 69 in.

> #### Skin

Brittle nails; dry and cracked skin; small bruises on abdomen

> #### HEENT

PERRLA; EOM intact; moist mucus membranes of oral cavity; no retinopathy; pale conjunctiva

> #### Neck and Lymph Nodes

No lymphadenopathy or thyromegaly

> #### Chest

Clear to auscultation bilaterally

> #### Breasts

Examination deferred

> #### Cardiovascular

RRR; normal S_1 and S_2; (–) S_3 and S_4

> #### Abdomen

Soft; nontender, nondistended; (+) bowel sounds; no rebound/guarding; no masses

▶ **Neurology**

A&O × 3; blunted affect; normal deep tendon reflexes; PHQ9 score 15, denied SI/HI

▶ **Extremities**

Abnormal monofilament with decreased sensation bilaterally in heels; no edema; (+) pedal pulses; no rashes

▶ **Genitourinary**

Examination deferred

▶ **Rectal**

(−) Stool guaiac

Laboratory Tests

Fasting, Obtained Next Day After Appointment

	Conventional Units	SI Units
Na	139 mEq/L	139 mmol/L
K	3.9 mEq/L	3.9 mmol/L
Cl	98 mEq/L	98 mmol/L
CO_2	24 mEq/L	24 mmol/L
BUN	15 mg/dL	5.35 mmol/L
SCr	0.9 mg/dL	80 μmol/L
Glu	115 mg/dL	6.38 mmol/L
Ca	8.7 mg/dL	2.17 mmol/L
AST	15 IU/L	0.25 μkat/L
ALT	24 IU/L	0.4 μkat/L
Albumin	2.8 g/dL	28 g/L
Hgb	8.1 g/dL	81 g/L; 5.02 mmol/L
Hct	27%	0.27
WBC	$7 \times 10^3/mm^3$	$7 \times 10^9/L$
RBC	$4.42 \times 10^6/\mu L$	$4.42 \times 10^{12}/L$
MCV	$61 \mu m^3$	61 fL
MCHC	30.1 g/dL	301 g/L
RDW	19.7%	0.197
Iron	11 mcg/dL	1.97 μmol/L
TIBC	477 mcg/dL	85.4 μmol/L
TSAT	2%	0.02
Ferritin	6 ng/mL	6 mcg/L
TSH	2.41 μU/mL	2.41 mU/L
HgA1C	6.7%	0.067

Peripheral blood smear
Microcytic, hypochromic RBCs

Assessment

Nineteen-year-old female with signs, symptoms and laboratory results consistent with iron-deficiency anemia.

Student Work-Up

Missing Information/Inadequate Data

Evaluate: Patient database
             Drug therapy problems
             Care plan (by problem)

TARGETED QUESTIONS

1. What signs and symptoms of iron-deficiency anemia does this patient have? What laboratory values support this diagnosis?

   Hint: See p. 995 and Table 66-2 in PPP

2. What are potential causes of iron-deficiency anemia?

   Hint: See pp. 993-994 in PPP

3. What therapy options are available to treat iron-deficiency anemia in this patient?

   Hint: See pp. 996-997 and Table 66-4 in PPP

4. Is this patient a candidate for iron infusion therapy? Discuss why or why not.

   Hint: See p. 998 in PPP

5. What risks and adverse effects of oral iron therapy would you discuss with the patient? How can this patient prevent recurrence?

   Hint: See p. 1001 and Table 66-3 in PPP

FOLLOW-UP

The patient returns to your clinic in 1 month. She reports being unable to tolerate the oral ferrous sulfate and decided to stop taking it after only using the supplements for one week. Her provider decides to initiate intravenous iron dextran.

What monitoring is required with use of intravenous iron dextran? What additional counseling should the patient receive regarding adverse effects associated with use of this medication?

Hint: See p. 998 in PPP

🌐 **GLOBAL PERSPECTIVE**

Iron-deficiency anemia is the leading cause of anemia worldwide and is estimated to affect more than 2 billion people, with prevalence highest in Central and West Africa and South Asia. The causes of iron-deficiency anemia vary by location. In developing countries, the anemia typically results from insufficient dietary intake secondary to famine, poverty and malnutrition. Blood loss secondary to intestinal worm colonization by organisms causing schistosomiasis and hookworm infections are also common causes. By contrast, causes in higher-income countries are attributed to dietary choices and/or pathologic conditions.

Although iron-deficiency anemia is frequently asymptomatic, it is not benign. In children, the disease can cause decreased cognitive performance and lead to delays in development of physical and cognitive functioning. In pregnancy, iron-deficiency anemia is associated with decreased birth weight, and increased risk of preterm labor and mortality of newborn and mother. It can also precipitate heart failure and cause restless leg syndrome.

Overall, patients with iron-deficiency anemia should receive therapy with iron supplementation to improve quality of life and allow economic productivity. Emerging evidence with in vitro studies suggests that caution should be advised in countries where malaria is endemic, as iron-deficiency is potentially protective against malarial infections. More studies are needed to elucidate this correlation and to improve how iron-deficiency anemia is treated in these areas.

CASE SUMMARY

- The patient's clinical picture is consistent with iron-deficiency anemia resulting from a combination of inadequate dietary intake of iron and blood loss during menstruation.

- The patient should receive oral iron replacement therapy with 200 mg elemental iron daily in divided doses.

KEY REFERENCES

Camaschella C. Iron-deficiency anemia. N Engl J Med 2015;372:1832-43.

For more information on the care plan and facilitator's guide please visit http://www.mhpharmacotherapy.com

73 Vitamin B₁₂ Deficiency Anemia

Janice L. Stumpf

PATIENT PRESENTATION

Chief Complaint

"My Crohn's has flared. I'm so tired and haven't been able to go to work all week."

History of Present Illness

Carmen Brown is a 29-year-old white female who presents to her physician with complaints of abdominal cramping and diarrhea over the past week associated with a 3 lb weight loss. She notes a lack of energy for several months, affecting her ability to work and play with her kids. She once rode her bike 3 miles to work each morning, but has stopped because of fatigue.

Past Medical History

Crohn's disease (10 years – ileal lesions)

Gravida 2, para 2

Family History

Mother with Crohn's disease, otherwise healthy. Father with hypertension. No siblings.

Social History

Vegetarian since Crohn's diagnosis at age 19 years—no meat, poultry, or dairy; eats fish and eggs. Married with 2 children, ages 14 months and 3 years. Nursing assistant at long-term care facility.

Tobacco/Alcohol/Substance Use

Occasional alcohol (one to two glasses wine monthly); no tobacco; no illicit drugs

Allergies/Intolerances/Adverse Drug Events

Penicillin—rash

Medications (Current)

Mesalamine (Pentasa®) extended release capsules 1 g po 4 times daily

Ibuprofen 400 mg po prn menstrual cramps

Review of Systems

Fatigue for several months; abdominal cramping and non-bloody diarrheal stools shortly after eating; recent weight loss; weakness during exercise; sore, tender tongue, making eating difficult; menstrual cramps relieved with ibuprofen; dry skin; fingernails break easily

Physical Examination

▶ *General*

Petite, thin, white female who appears pale and somewhat uncomfortable

▶ *Vital Signs*

BP 118/72 mm Hg, P 88, RR 18, T 37.2°C

Weight 103 lb. (46.8 kg)

Height 63 in. (160.0 cm)

Moderate crampy abdominal pain after eating only

▶ *Skin*

Pale, dry skin noted

▶ *HEENT*

PERRLA; glossitis: tongue smooth and red

▶ *Neck and Lymph Nodes*

Thyroid normal size; no lymphadenopathy noted

▶ *Chest*

Clear to auscultation

▶ *Breasts*

Normal breast examination

▶ *Cardiovascular*

RRR; normal S_1, S_2; (–) S_3 or S_4

▶ *Abdomen*

Right lower quadrant tenderness; no distention; no rebound tenderness

▶ *Neurology*

Grossly intact; normal deep tendon reflexes and sensory examination; some muscle weakness noted

► *Extremities*

Cold extremities; fingernails short and brittle

Laboratory and Diagnostic Tests

	Conventional Units	SI Units
Na	142 mEq/L	142 mmol/L
K	3.6 mEq/L	3.6 mmol/L
Cl	100 mEq/L	100 mmol/L
CO_2	22 mEq/L	22 mmol/L
BUN	12.8 mg/dL	4.6 mmol/L
SCr	0.6 mg/dL	53 μmol/L
Glu (nonfasting)	160 mg/dL	8.9 mmol/L
Ca	9.0 mg/dL	2.25 mmol/L
Phosphate	3.4 mg/dL	1.10 mmol/L
Albumin	3.5 g/dL	35 g/L
WBC	$6 \times 10^3/mm^3$	$6 \times 10^9/L$
Hgb	10.8 g/dL (108 g/L)	108 g/L; 6.70 mmol/L
Hct	31.4%	0.314
RBC	$3.04 \times 10^6/\mu L$	$3.04 \times 10^{12}/L$
MCV	$102.2 \ \mu m^3$	102.2 fL
MCH	31.8 pg/cell	
MCHC	34.4 g/dL	344 g/L
RDW	14.5%	0.145
Plasma folate	10.6 ng/mL	24 nmol/L
Vitamin B_{12}	128 pg/mL	94.5 pmol/L
Hemoccult	negative	

Assessment

Thin, pale 29-year-old female who presents with symptoms of Crohn's disease flare (diarrhea, abdominal cramping) as well as complaints of fatigue, muscle weakness, and tongue tenderness, likely related to anemia.

Student Work-Up

Missing Information/Inadequate Data

Evaluate: Patient database

Drug therapy problems

Care plan (by problem)

TARGETED QUESTIONS

1. With what signs and symptoms of anemia does the patient present?

   Hint: See p. 995 and Table 66-2 in PPP

2. What is the likely etiology of the patient's anemia?

   Hint: See p. 995 and Table 66-3 in PPP

3. How should the patient's anemia be treated?

   Hint: See p. 999 and Table 66-3 in PPP

4. What parameters should be monitored after treatment is initiated?

   Hint: See p. 1001 in PPP

FOLLOW-UP

The patient returns to the clinic 6 months later, happily reporting that she is now 18 weeks pregnant. She continues on a regimen of cyanocobalamin 1000 mcg intramuscularly once monthly. Her Hgb and Hct levels are within the normal range and she has no symptoms of anemia; however, her serum cyanocobalamin concentration is again low.

What may account for the low serum cyanocobalamin concentration?

Hint: The patient's pregnancy may be increasing her vitamin B_{12} requirements, leading to early signs of deficiency. In addition, high doses of folic acid can correct the macrocytic anemia associated with vitamin B_{12} deficiency, so she should be questioned regarding the use of folate supplements. However, in light of her adherence to parenteral cyanocobalamin maintenance therapy and lack of clinical symptoms and laboratory measures consistent with anemia, it is unlikely that the patient is again deficient in vitamin B_{12}. Instead, low serum vitamin B_{12} concentrations unrelated to anemia have been described during pregnancy. In vitamin B_{12}–deficient states, serum methylmalonic acid and homocysteine concentrations will be increased. Results of these determinations may therefore allow differentiation between pregnancy-related decreases in serum cyanocobalamin concentrations and true deficiency

🌐 GLOBAL PERSPECTIVE

Macrocytic anemia caused by micronutrient deficiencies occurs worldwide in those suffering from malnutrition. Vitamin B_{12} is available from a variety of animal sources, including meat, fish, poultry, eggs, and dairy products; however, populations without ready access to these foods and who instead rely on plant sources for the majority of their calorie intake may develop deficiencies. Malabsorption of vitamin B_{12} is more often the cause of deficiency in advanced nations, in which dietary ingestion is generally sufficient. According to the 2007 to 2008 National Health and Nutrition Examination Survey (NHANES), the mean intake of vitamin B_{12} for the United States population is 5.2 mcg/day, which is well above the 2.4-mcg recommended daily allowance for adults. Yet vitamin B_{12} deficiency affects between 1.5% and 15% of the United States population. Malabsorption of vitamin B_{12} is especially common in older people due to atrophic gastritis and subsequent reduced levels of gastric acid secretion, but it is also noted following gastric surgical procedures, in those with GI disorders such as Crohn's and celiac disease, and in patients with pernicious anemia. In addition, prolonged acid suppression therapy has been recognized as a cause of decreased vitamin B$_{12}$ absorption, although the clinical significance of this finding is debated.

In addition to macrocytic anemia, permanent neurologic damage may result if vitamin B$_{12}$ deficiency is not corrected. Although cognitive decline has been reported in vitamin B$_{12}$–deficient patients, supplementation in nondeficient patients with dementia or Alzheimer's disease has not improved cognitive function. A link between low vitamin B$_{12}$ concentrations and cardiovascular disease also has been suggested due to the effects of the nutrient on homocysteine metabolism. Elevated homocysteine concentrations are associated with an increased risk of stroke and coronary heart disease and are noted in vitamin B$_{12}$–deficient states. Despite reductions in homocysteine levels following administration of vitamin and mineral supplements that included vitamin B$_{12}$, differences in cardiovascular outcomes following long-term use of vitamin B$_{12}$ have not been documented. To date, data from large clinical trials do not support the use of vitamin B$_{12}$ supplements to protect against cardiovascular events.

CASE SUMMARY

- The patient's clinical picture is consistent with vitamin B$_{12}$ deficiency anemia likely resulting from inadequate dietary intake and malabsorption due to Crohn's disease involving the ileum.

- Therapy with vitamin B$_{12}$ should be initiated, with parenteral therapy more reliably correcting the deficiency than oral therapy in this patient.

- Clinical symptoms should improve within days to weeks of vitamin B$_{12}$ supplementation. CBC and serum cyanocobalamin concentrations should be obtained in 1 month to evaluate the efficacy of therapy.

For more information on the care plan and facilitator's guide please visit http://www.mhpharmacotherapy.com

74 Folic Acid Deficiency Anemia

Janice L. Stumpf

PATIENT PRESENTATION

Chief Complaint

"Ah, man, I'm so tired."

History of Present Illness

Shawn Johnson is a 19-year-old thin, African-American male brought to the emergency department by his college roommates due to increasing fatigue over the past 3 days. He doesn't own a thermometer but reports feeling hot and having shaking chills. He notes that he had a sore throat followed by runny nose, both of which have resolved. He has not had vomiting or diarrhea. He did not receive a flu vaccine this season. A rapid diagnostic test reveals influenza A virus infection.

Past Medical History

Sickle cell disease

Pain—chronic, intermittent, due to sickle cell crises

S/P splenectomy—age 10 years

H/O otitis media

Family History

Sickle cell disease: father, uncle

Sickle cell trait: mother, sister

Social History

Sophomore in college

Tobacco/Alcohol/Substance Use

Nonsmoker. Alcohol: 2-3 beers per day on weekends. No illicit drug use reported.

Allergies/Intolerances/Adverse Drug Events

Codeine: stomach upset

Meperidine: seizure

Ampicillin: hives and shortness of breath

Medications (Current)

Hydroxyurea 2000 mg orally once daily × 5 years

Oxycodone/acetaminophen 5 mg/325 mg as needed for pain

Review of Systems

Complains of fatigue for several months, which has increased over the past few days so that it is now difficult to walk the 15 minutes to class from his campus apartment. Has had fever for 2 days, with shaking chills. He reports no pain.

Physical Examination

▶ General

Thin, very sleepy, African-American male who appears dehydrated. A&O × 3.

▶ Vital Signs

BP 116/70 mm Hg, P 90, RR 18, T 38.8°C

Weight 135.6 lb. (61.6 kg)

Height 70 in. (177.8 cm)

▶ Skin

Cold extremities. Dry skin. Pale nail beds.

▶ HEENT

PERRLA. Yellow sclerae. Right tympanic membrane mildly inflamed but no effusion. Dry and pale mucosa.

▶ Neck and Lymph Nodes

Normal

▶ Chest

Normal breath sounds bilaterally. No rales, rhonchi or wheezing.

▶ Cardiovascular

RRR; normal S_1, S_2; (−) S_3 or S_4

▶ Abdomen

Asplenic. Not tender; no distention; no rebound

▶ Neurology

Deep tendon reflexes intact.

▶ Extremities

Cold to touch; palpable pulses

▶ *Genitourinary/Rectal*

Normal

Laboratory and Diagnostic Tests

	Conventional Units	SI Units
Na	145 mEq/L	145 mmol/L
K	4.1 mEq/L	4.1 mmol/L
Cl	102 mEq/L	102 mmol/L
CO_2	31 mEq/L	31 mmol/L
BUN	24 mg/dL	8.6 mmol/L
SCr	1.2 mg/dL	106 μmol/L
Glu	80 mg/dL	4.4 mmol/L
Ca	8.8 mg/dL	2.20 mmol/L
Phosphate	2.4 mg/dL	0.78 mmol/L
Albumin	2.8 g/dL	28 g/L
AST	40 IU/L	0.67 μkat/L
ALT	50 IU/L	0.83 μkat/L
Alk phos	70 IU/L	1.17 μkat/L
Bilirubin	1.2 mg/dL	20.5 μmol/L
WBC	$18 \times 10^3/mm^3$	$18 \times 10^9/L$
Hgb	10.5 g/dL	105 g/L; 6.51 mmol/L
Hct	30.2%	0.302
Plt	$154 \times 10^3/μL$	$154 \times 10^9/L$
Reticulocytes	3%	0.03
RBC	$2.97 \times 10^6/μL$	$2.97 \times 10^{12}/L$
MCV	101.7 μm³	101.7 fL
MCH	28.2 pg/cell	
MCHC	34.7 g/dL	347 g/L
RDW	24%	0.240
Plasma folate	2.8 ng/mL	6.3 nmol/L
Vitamin B_{12}	280 pg/mL	207 pmol/L

Peripheral blood smear: mild hemolysis, sickled erythrocytes and macrocytic red blood cells.

Assessment

Lethargic 19-year-old male with sickle cell disease who now presents with increasing fatigue, fever, and influenza virus infection confirmed with rapid diagnostic testing.

Student Work-Up

Missing Information/Inadequate Data

Evaluate: Patient database

Drug therapy problems

Care plan (by problem)

TARGETED QUESTIONS

1. What signs and symptoms of anemia does the patient have?

   Hint: See p. 995 and Table 66-2 in PPP

2. What is the likely cause of the patient's anemia?

   Hint: See p. 995 in PPP

3. How should the patient's anemia be managed?

   Hint: See p. 999 and Table 66-3 in PPP

4. How soon after initiating the therapy should the anemia resolve?

   Hint: See p. 999 in PPP

FOLLOW-UP

The patient returns to the emergency department in a week with right ear pain and recurrent fever. He is diagnosed with otitis media and provided a prescription for trimethoprim-sulfamethoxazole DS tablets (160 mg/800 mg) orally twice daily for 10 days.

What impact may the patient's antimicrobial therapy have on his folic acid deficiency anemia?

Hint: Use of trimethoprim-sulfamethoxazole is contra-indicated in patients with pre-existing megaloblastic anemia due to folic acid deficiency. Therefore, a different antibacterial should be selected for this patient. Trimethoprim and sulfamethoxazole inhibit successive enzymes in the folic acid pathway, thereby interfering with folic acid biosynthesis and subsequent bacterial growth. Although more selective for bacterial than mammalian cells, trimethoprim-sulfamethoxazole, especially in high doses for prolonged durations, has been reported to induce folic acid deficiency in patients at risk, including the elderly and those with malnutrition or chronic alcoholism. Anemia induced by trimethoprim-sulfamethoxaole may respond to folinic acid (leukovorin calcium) therapy. Although theoretically possible, there is no evidence that concomitant supplementation with usual doses of folic acid reduces the antibacterial efficacy of trimethoprim-sulfamethoxazole

🌐 GLOBAL PERSPECTIVE

Folic acid deficiency develops in all populations in which malnutrition is apparent; therefore macrocytic anemia is a global health concern. Anemia affects an estimated 2 billion individuals, nearly 30% of the world's population. The primary cause of anemia worldwide is iron deficiency, although mixed anemias resulting from concurrent deficiencies in folic acid and vitamin B_{12} may also be noted.

Because of the association between low folic acid levels during pregnancy and neural tube birth defects, in 1998, the FDA mandated addition of folic acid to many grain products, including bread, pasta, and cereals. In addition to the U.S., 75 other countries require fortification of milled wheat flour with folic acid. The folic acid food fortification program as well as increased awareness regarding the need for prenatal folic acid supplementation has reduced the incidence of neural tube defects by 30% to 50%.

The effect of folic acid supplementation on cancer is unclear. Low folate diets have been associated with an increased risk of breast, pancreatic, and colon cancer. However, the incidence of some cancers has increased since folic acid fortification efforts, and recent data suggest that high folic acid ingestion may increase the risk of colon, lung, breast, and prostate cancers.

In addition, low dietary folate intake been associated with an increase in the risk of coronary events, perhaps due to increases in homocysteine concentrations. Homocysteine is an amino acid that, when elevated, has been associated with coronary heart disease and strokes. Although folic acid supplementation appears to reduce homocysteine levels to normal, randomized studies of up to 2 years have not documented a concurrent decreased risk of cardiovascular events. Observational studies with longer treatment durations are ongoing.

CASE SUMMARY

- The patient's clinical picture is consistent with macrocytic anemia due to folic acid deficiency. The anemia likely developed as a consequence of poor dietary intake and increased demand for folic acid in the setting of red blood cell hemolysis and subsequent increased erythropoiesis in this patient with underlying sickle cell disease.

- Therapy with folic acid 1 mg po daily should be initiated and, in light of his sickle cell disease, should be continued indefinitely.

- Clinical symptoms should improve within days of initiating folic acid supplementation. CBC and plasma folate concentrations should be obtained in 2 months to assess response to therapy.

For more information on the care plan and facilitator's guide please visit http://www.mhpharmacotherapy.com

75 Sickle Cell Disease

Tracy M. Hagemann

PATIENT PRESENTATION

Chief Complaint
"I'm here for my 12 month follow-up after my bone infection."

History of Present Illness
SN is a 21-year-old female with sickle cell disease (Hb SS), who presents to clinic for follow-up post-osteomyelitis infection 1 year ago. Prior to the osteomyelitis, she had been previously healthy with only 1 vaso-occlusive crisis since starting hydroxyurea 3 years ago. She has a history of being adherent with her clinic appointments, but missed her last regular appointment 6 weeks ago due to being on vacation. Typically she is seen in clinic every 3 months for routine monitoring. She states that she takes her medications daily as prescribed and rarely misses doses, however she ran out of refills for her oral contraceptive 2 months ago. She has not required her pain medications in several months. She denies any feelings of dizziness or lightheadedness, but does feel fatigued.

Past Medical History
Sickle cell anemia (Hb SS) with many pain crises in the past; last pain crisis at age 19

Salmonella osteomyelitis of left tibia 1 year ago – surgical debridement and completed 6 weeks of intravenous antibiotic treatment

Cholecystectomy

Family History
Father has sickle cell trait (SCT), and is alive at age 42, with a history of hyperlipidemia and hypertension. Mother is alive at age 38 and has SCT and is prediabetic. Brother is alive at 17 and has SCT and asthma.

Social History
She is in her junior year at the local university majoring in elementary education. She uses public transportation to get to school and work. Employed part-time at a children's daycare facility. Just started dating a new boyfriend.

Tobacco/Alcohol/Substance Use
(–) alcohol; (–) tobacco or illicit drug use.

Allergies/Intolerances/Adverse Drug Events
No known drug allergies

Medications (Current)
Hydrocodone/Acetaminophen 7.5/325 mg one tablet every 6 hours prn pain

Hydroxyurea 500 mg four capsules once daily

Ibuprofen 600 mg po every 8 hours prn

Ortho-TriCyclen one tablet daily - currently not taking, ran out of refills

Review of Systems
Occasional sickle cell related pain relieved with hydrocodone/acetaminophen and ibuprofen. (–) tinnitus, vertigo, dizziness, lightheadedness; (+) fatigue.

Physical Examination

▶ *General*

Well-appearing, young African-American female in no distress

▶ *Vital Signs*

BP 120/65 mm Hg, P 60, RR 17, T 37.5°C

Weight 123 lb. (56 kg)

Height 64 in. (162 cm)

Pain 2/10

▶ *HEENT*

PERRLA, atraumatic, normocephalic. No lymphadenopathy

▶ *Chest*

Clear to auscultation

▶ *Cardiovascular*

RRR, no m/g/r

▶ *Abdomen*

Not tender/not distended; palpable liver

▶ *Extremities*

No edema, (–) pedal pulses, small scar on LLE, nontender

▶ *Genitourinary*

Examination deferred

▶ *Rectal*

Examination deferred

Laboratory Tests

Current

	Conventional Units	SI Units
Na	139 mEq/L	139 mmol/L
K	3.6 mEq/L	3.6 mmol/L
BUN	18 mg/dL	6.4 mmol/L
SCr	0.6 mg/dL	53 μmol/L
Hgb	7.3 g/dL	73 g/L; 4.53 mmol/L
Hct	31%	0.31
WBC	7×10^3/mm^3	7×10^9/L
Total bilirubin	0.4 mg/dL	6.8 μmol/L
AST	35 IU/L	0.58 μkat/L
ALT	48 IU/L	0.80 μkat/L
Reticulocytes	72,000/mm^3	—

Labs From Six months Ago

	Conventional Units	SI Units
Na	142 mEq/L	142 mmol/L
K	4.1 mEq/L	4.1 mmol/L
SCr	19 mg/dL	6.8 mmol/L
BUN	0.8 mg/dL	71 μmol/L
Hgb	9.4 g/dL	94 g/L; 5.83 mmol/L
Hct	34%	0.34
WBC	8×10^3/mm^3	8×10^9/L
Total bilirubin	0.4 mg/dL	6.8 μmol/L
AST	34 IU/L	0.57 μkat/L
ALT	50 IU/L	0.84 μkat/L
Reticulocytes	95,000/mm^3	—

Chest x-ray: Clear with no evidence of acute chest syndrome or infiltrates

Assessment

Twenty-one year old female with SCD, controlled pain, here for a routine monitoring visit. SCD managed on hydroxyurea, but laboratory work indicates myelosuppression.

Student Work-Up

Missing Information/Inadequate Data

Evaluate:
Patient database
Drug therapy problems
Care plan (by problem)

TARGETED QUESTIONS

1. What medication-related complications does the patient have?

   Hint: See pp. 1023-1024 in PPP

2. What modifications should be made to her hydroxyurea therapy?

   Hint: See pp. 1022-1023 in PPP

3. How should the patient's hydroxyurea therapy be monitored?

   Hint: See p. 1023 in PPP

4. What additional therapy or medications does she require, if any?

   Hint: See pp. 1021-1022 and Table 68-1 in PPP

5. What additional vaccinations are required for this patient? Are there any vaccines recommended for her, based on her history?

   Hint: See pp. 1021-1022 and Table 68-1 in PPP

FOLLOW-UP

SN fully recovered from her hydroxyurea toxicity and was restarted at 1800 mg daily. After 12 weeks at this dose, her dose was further increased to her original dose of 2000 mg daily, however after 2 weeks at this higher dose, she again developed toxicity. Her treatment was stopped and she recovered her counts to baseline.

Should she continue on hydroxyurea? What changes do you recommend to her medication regimen today?

Hint: See pp. 1023-1024 in PPP

⊙ GLOBAL PERSPECTIVE

Sickle cell disease (SCD) is an inherited group of red blood cell disorders that affects millions worldwide and is most common among those whose ancestry includes sub-Saharan Africa, regions in the Western Hemisphere (South America, the Caribbean, and Central America), Saudi Arabia, India and Mediterranean countries such as Turkey. Because of population migration, SCD is present in most countries. SCD is a significant cause of morbidity and mortality. The World Health Organization estimates that SCD contributes to 5% of the deaths of children younger than 5 years of age in some African countries. Many young adults with SCD are at risk for premature death. Each year, more than 300,000 babies with severe forms of SCD are born worldwide, with the majority in low- and middle-income countries. The most cost-effective strategy for reducing the burden of SCD worldwide is to utilize both disease management with prevention programs, such as genetic counseling. Barriers include inequitable access to health services, lack of research initiatives and lack of awareness of the international community of the global burden of SCD and related disorders.

REFERENCE

1. World Health Organization. http://www.afro.who.int/en/health-topics/topics/4405-sickle-cell-disease.html Accessed April 24, 2015.

CASE SUMMARY

- The patient has been well-controlled for 3 years on hydroxyurea therapy with good control of complications overall. However, today her laboratory work shows significant myelosuppression due to hydroxyurea toxicity. Her hydroxyurea therapy should be temporarily discontinued and she should be followed in clinic every 2 weeks for blood work to monitor her recovery. After 12 weeks of monitoring, if no further toxicity is seen, she should have her hydroxyurea restarted at a lower dose (2.5-5 mg/kg/day less than the dose at which she became toxic) and monitored every 2-4 weeks with dose increases up to 35 mg/kg/day, if tolerated.

- Because she is to be continued on hydroxyurea and is of child-bearing age with a new boyfriend, she should be counseled on the importance of contraception and should have an oral contraceptive refilled at this time. If in the future, she is nonadherent to this medication, a longer-acting contraceptive such as Depo-Provera may be considered. She should also be counseled that prescription contraceptives do not protect against sexually transmitted diseases and so she and her partner should use condoms. She may also want to consider receiving the HPV vaccine since she is in the target group of 9-26 years of age.

- She should be prescribed folic acid. Since SCD and hydroxyurea may both lead to folate deficiency, and hydroxyurea may mask the symptoms of folate deficiency, this is an important medication for her to receive.

- Her immunization history should be reviewed. She should receive a dose of Prevnar13 to help protect against invasive pneumococcal disease, but since she is currently neutropenic, should wait until her blood counts recover. She should also consider a dose of Tdap based on her employment at the daycare. She should continue to receive annual flu vaccination.

For more information on the care plan and facilitator's guide please visit http://www.mhpharmacotherapy.com

76 Bacterial Meningitis

April Miller Quidley   Phillip L. Mohorn

PATIENT PRESENTATION

Chief Complaint

The patient is very somnolent and unable to provide a history. Her history is from her mother, who reports that the patient complained of generalized body aches, fevers, hearing loss, somnolence, and a severe pounding headache for several days prior to presentation.

History of Present Illness

Jodi Smith is a 20-year-old female college student, who presents to the emergency department (ED) with a 3-day history of generalized body aches, fevers, vomiting and diarrhea, in addition to severe headache, neck stiffness, and bilateral hearing loss beginning yesterday. The patient's mother is at the bedside and provided most of the history. She states that her daughter came home approximately 3 days ago, in distress related to generalized body aches. She was in her normal state of health prior to that time. None of her friends at college has reported any signs or symptoms of illness, and she works at a daycare center.

Past Medical History

Sickle cell disease, several severe pain crises a year since age 15 years, no history of acute chest syndrome or cerebrovascular accident (CVA)

Bipolar I disorder

Family History

Father has hypertension and the sickle cell trait. Mother has type 2 diabetes and the sickle cell trait. She has no siblings.

Social/Work History

The patient is a junior in college and lives in an apartment with one other person. She has no other health complaints. She has been working at a daycare center since she started college.

Tobacco/Alcohol/Substance Abuse

Unable to fully assess due to the patient's mental status; mother reports no known tobacco or illicit drug use.

Allergies/Intolerances/Adverse Event History

No known allergies or intolerances according to the patient's mother

Medications

▶ *Inpatient*

0.9% sodium chloride IV at 125 mL/h

▶ *Home*

Morphine 10 mg po every 4 hours as needed for pain (only uses during acute pain crises)

Hydroxyurea 1000 mg po daily

Divalproex sodium ER 1500 mg po daily

▶ *Review of Systems*

Positive for fevers, bilateral headache, neck stiffness, anorexia, nausea, vomiting, diarrhea. No vision changes. Hearing loss as above. No chest pain, shortness of breath or rash.

Physical Examination

▶ *General*

The patient is an ill-appearing female patient. She is somnolent but easily arousable. She is mildly diaphoretic.

▶ *Vital Signs*

BP 102/74 mm Hg, P 114, RR 20, T 38.8°C

Weight 123 lb. (56 kg)

Height 61 in. (155 cm)

Reports moderate neck pain

▶ *Skin*

Patient appears diaphoretic; no ecchymoses, rashes, or lesions noted

▶ *HEENT*

PERRLA; patient has apparent bilateral hearing loss and does not respond to auditory stimuli; mucous membranes are slightly dry

▶ *Neck and Lymph Nodes*

(+) Nuchal rigidity; (−) Kernig's sign; (−) Brudzinski's sign

▶ **Chest**

Clear to auscultation bilaterally

▶ **Breasts**

Examination deferred

▶ **Cardiovascular**

Sinus tachycardia

▶ **Abdomen**

Nontender; nondistended; no hepatomegaly or splenomegaly noted

▶ **Neurology**

Hearing loss; no other focal neurologic deficits noted; moves extremities equally bilaterally

▶ **Genitourinary**

Examination deferred

▶ **Rectal**

Examination deferred

Laboratory and Diagnostic Tests

Obtained in ED

	Conventional Units	SI Units
Na	138 mEq/L	138 mmol/L
K	4.7 mEq/L	4.7 mmol/L
Cl	103 mEq/L	103 mmol/L
CO_2	23 mEq/L	23 mmol/L
BUN	10 mg/dL	3.57 mmol/L
SCr	0.5 mg/dL	44.2 µmol/L
Glu	135 mg/dL	7.49 mmol/L
Ca	8.5 mg/dL	2.12 mmol/L
Mg	2.4 mEq/L	1.2 mmol/L
Phosphate	3.1 mg/dL	1 mmol/L
Hgb	10.3 g/dL	103 g/L; 6.39 mmol/L
Hct	27.9%	0.279
WBC	$20 \times 10^3/mm^3$	$20 \times 10^9/L$
Plt	$192 \times 10^3/mm^3$	$192 \times 10^9/L$
Albumin	3.8 g/dL	38 g/L
Valproic Acid	75 mg/L	520 µmol/L
CSF Studies		
WBC	$8.2 \times 10^3/mm^3$	$8.2 \times 10^9/L$
WBC differential		
Monos	10%	0.10
PMNs	88%	0.88
Lymphs	2%	0.02
Protein	142 mg/dL	1420 mg/L
Glu	54 mg/dL	3 mmol/L

▶ **Cultures**

Blood cultures × 2: Pending
  Cerebrospinal fluid (CSF) Opening pressure: 28 mm Hg
  CSF Gram stain: Gram-positive diplococci

▶ **Radiology**

Computed Tomography Scan of Head: No acute abnormalities

Assessment

Twenty-year-old female with signs, symptoms, and laboratory/diagnostic tests consistent with bacterial meningitis

Student Work-Up

Missing Information/Inadequate Data

Evaluate: Patient database

Drug therapy problems

Care plan (by problem)

Missing information:

Pending culture data, baseline hearing tests

TARGETED QUESTIONS

1. Which symptoms in this patient's history suggest the diagnosis of bacterial meningitis?

   Hint: See p. 1051 in PPP

2. What do this patient's cerebrospinal fluid (CSF) findings indicate?

   Hint: See Table 70-2 in PPP

3. What in this patient's history may indicate the causative organism of bacterial meningitis?

   Hint: See Table 70-1 in PPP

4. Why should empiric antibiotic therapy in bacterial meningitis include broad-spectrum coverage with more than one agent?

   Hint: See p. 1052 in PPP

5. What route(s) of antibiotic administration is (are) appropriate in bacterial meningitis?

   Hint: See p. 1050 in PPP

6. What vaccination(s) should be administered to help prevent invasive *Streptococcus pneumoniae* meningitis?

   Hint: See p. 1058 in PPP

FOLLOW-UP

Twenty-four hours later, CSF cultures return and are positive for *S. pneumoniae*. The patient continues to receive empiric antibiotics (as recommended in your Care Plan).

Should your antibiotic regimen be altered? If so, how? Also, what (if any) prophylaxis would you recommend for this patient's contacts?

Hint: See p. 1058 and Table 70-3 in PPP

☉ GLOBAL PERSPECTIVE

Worldwide, approximately 1.2 million cases of bacterial meningitis occur annually and result in 135,000 deaths. Vaccination has changed the microbiology and predominant causative organisms in the United States. Both *Haemophilus influenzae* and pneumococcal vaccination have decreased the incidence of infections secondary to these organisms in the United States. Due to limited vaccine availability and cost in developing countries, the incidence of disease secondary to these organisms has not decreased significantly. Likewise, polio and mumps vaccination in the United States has virtually eliminated these organisms as a cause of viral encephalitis. However, these remain important causative agents to consider in developing countries.

CASE SUMMARY

- The patient's clinical picture including nuchal rigidity, altered mental status, and hearing loss is consistent with a severe case of bacterial meningitis. Prompt initiation of broad-spectrum antimicrobial therapy is essential to ensure optimal patient outcomes.

- Initial information including CSF studies and culture data are key to guiding the clinician toward appropriate empiric therapy and narrowing therapy to target-specific pathogens.

- The patient's social situation and contacts are important to consider in some cases to determine prophylaxis of close contacts.

For more information on the care plan and facilitator's guide please visit http://www.mhpharmacotherapy.com

77 Pneumonia

Diane M. Cappelletty

PATIENT PRESENTATION

Chief Complaint

Found by her husband having a seizure. In the prior 5 days she had been babysitting her 4 year old grandson who was sick with an upper respiratory infection and otitis media. She had been complaining of being tired, short of breath, coughing.

History of Present Illness

Cindy Milner is a 57-year-old woman who presents to the emergency department with a seizure. The seizure was treated and stopped by the paramedics. She is conscious but is groggy. She has some mild-to-moderate chest discomfort, but denies any sharp pains or heaviness in her chest. She does not have nausea, vomiting, or diarrhea.

Past Medical History

Chronic obstructive pulmonary disease (COPD) (15 years)

Tonic-clonic seizures (20 years)

Hypertension (HTN) (10 years)

Family History

Father died of lung cancer at age 55. Mother age 79 has HTN, hypothyroidism, and resides in a senior center. She has one brother who has COPD and HTN.

Social History

She lives with her husband and has one daughter. She does not work.

Tobacco/Alcohol/Substance Use

Social drinker; + tobacco history 1 ppd × 30 years, no illicit drug use

Allergies/Intolerances/Adverse Drug Events

Sulfa

Medications (Current)

Lisinopril (Prinivil) 20 mg po daily

Carbamazepine-XR 200mg po twice daily

Fluticasone/Salmeterol DPI (Advair) 250 mcg/50 mcg one inhalation twice daily

Albuterol 1-2 puffs every 4-6 hours as needed for shortness of breath (SOB)

Acetaminophen 500 mg po as needed for headache

Review of Systems

Occasional headaches relieved with acetaminophen; occasional tinnitus; (–) vertigo; this is the first seizure in the past year, (–) syncope, or loss of consciousness; mild pain/discomfort in her chest; (+) SOB; (–) nausea, vomiting, or diarrhea.

Physical Examination

▶ **General**

Breathing fast, with increased work of breathing, appears in moderate respiratory distress

▶ **Vital Signs**

BP 108/75 mm Hg, P 82, RR 18, T 38.8°C, pulse oximetry 87% (0.87) on room air

Weight 185 lb. (84.1 kg)

Height 65 in. (165 cm)

▶ **Skin**

Normal; (–) rashes or lesions

▶ **HEENT**

PERRLA, EOMI; trace periorbital edema; (–) sinus tenderness; TMs appear normal

▶ **Neck and Lymph Nodes**

Negative for lymphadenopathy

▶ **Chest**

Wheezing bilaterally, worse on the right side; decreased breath sounds over the upper and lower right lobe.

▶ **Cardiovascular**

RRR; normal S_1, S_2; (–) S_3 or S_4

▶ **Abdomen**

Not tender/not distended

▶ **Neurology**

Recent tonic-clonic seizure; deep tendon reflexes normal

▶ *Radiologic Studies*

Chest x-ray: right upper and lower lobe infiltrates (lower lobe infiltrate is more defined)

Laboratory Tests

▶ *Sputum Culture*

Pending; Gram stain: moderate WBCs, rare squamous epithelial cells, no organisms seen

▶ *Blood Culture*

Pending

Assessment

Fifty-seven-year-old woman post tonic-clonic seizure with signs, symptoms, and laboratory tests consistent with mild-moderate community-acquired pneumonia and possible aspiration pneumonia.

Student Work-Up

Missing Information/Inadequate Data

Evaluate:	Patient database
	Drug therapy problems
	Care plan (by problem)

TARGETED QUESTIONS

1. What signs, symptoms, and diagnostic tests support the diagnosis of pneumonia in the patient?

   Hint: See pp. 1067-1069 in PPP

2. What are the organisms most likely causing pneumonia and what resistance issues are associated with these organisms?

   Hint: See Table 71-1 and p. 1066 in PPP

3. What patient factors need to be considered prior to selecting an empiric treatment regimen?

   Hint: See p. 1067 in PPP

4. What therapeutic regimen would you select (including the duration of therapy)?

   Hint: See pp. 1071-1075 in PPP

5. How would you monitor the patient?

   Hint: See p. 1074 in PPP

6. Should the patient be vaccinated, and if so, what vaccinations should she receive?

   Hint: See pp. 1074-1075 in PPP

7. What would happen to the therapeutic regimen or monitoring for each of the following situations:

   (a) What if the patient had risk factors for pseudomonas or MRSA?

   Hint: See pp. 1071-1075 in PPP

   (b) What if the patient had a β-lactam allergy (rash vs. hives/tongue swelling)?

   Hint: See pp. 1071-1075 in PPP

   (c) What if the patient had a condition that required warfarin therapy?

☉ GLOBAL PERSPECTIVE

Viral pneumonia (specifically influenza) is of much greater concern for global spread causing pandemics than is bacterial pneumonia. Not all patients infected with influenza develop pneumonia, but those that do have a greater mortality risk than those without pneumonia. Vaccination against influenza can prevent the disease or minimize symptomatology if the disease is contracted. The polysaccharide vaccine against *Streptococcus pneumoniae* covers 85-90% of the isolates responsible for causing disease in human beings. A conjugated pneumococcal vaccine was recently approved for adults 50 years of age and older, which may provide an improved immune response.

CASE SUMMARY

- Her clinical picture is consistent with mild-moderate community-acquired pneumonia and possible aspiration pneumonia.

- Her seizure history puts her at increased risk of aspiration pneumonia.

- She should receive the pneumococcal vaccine once and the influenza vaccine yearly.

For more information on the care plan and facilitator's guide please visit http://www.mhpharmacotherapy.com

78 Influenza

Heather L. Girand

PATIENT PRESENTATION

Chief Complaint
"I think I have strep throat and I feel miserable. I need antibiotics so that I can go to class this afternoon."

History of Present Illness
WD is a 19-year-old female who presents to the university health center with complaints of sore throat, malaise, headache, chills, myalgias, and cough. She reports that she began feeling ill last night around 11:00 p.m. when she "wasn't quite right" and felt achy. She also had a headache, so she took some ibuprofen and went to bed. She awoke at 2:00 a.m. with worsening muscle aches, so she took more ibuprofen and went back to sleep. At 4:30 a.m., she woke up with a sore throat, chills, and a nonproductive cough. She took more ibuprofen but it did not provide much relief. She arrived at the health center at 8:00 a.m. so that she could be the "first patient in and out" with the hope of making it to her afternoon class. She reports that she hasn't eaten anything since last night's dinner at 8:00 p.m.

Past Medical History
Type 1 diabetes mellitus (T1DM) (diagnosed at 12 years of age)

Asthma (diagnosed "in elementary school")

Concussion (3 years ago)

Family History
Father has hypertension. Mother has hypothyroidism and asthma. Has two younger siblings who are both healthy.

Social History
Freshman in her second semester at the university; lives in a dormitory with two other roommates. One roommate had strep throat last week. Doesn't smoke or report using illicit drugs. Occasional alcohol intake ("1-2 beers a week"). Sexually active with one male partner. Immunizations not up-to-date; hasn't had "any shots for at least 5 years" except for influenza vaccine which she received last year (hasn't received it this season). Has prescription insurance through father's health plan.

Allergies/Intolerances/Adverse Drug Events
Erythromycin – abdominal cramping and diarrhea ("about 5 years ago")

Medication History

▶ Current
Insulin glargine 20 units subcutaneously at bedtime (usually around 11:00 p.m.)

Insulin aspart 1 unit subcutaneously for every 15 g of carbohydrate

Insulin aspart 1 unit subcutaneously for every 45 mg/dL above goal blood sugar

Albuterol MDI 2 puffs every 4-6 hours as needed

Ortho Tri Cyclen 1 tablet daily (has been taking daily without interruption for the past month "to avoid periods" for upcoming spring break trip in 3 weeks)

Ibuprofen 200 mg; took 3 tablets last night (at 11:00 p.m.), 3 tablets at 2:00 a.m. and 3 tablets at 4:30 a.m.

▶ Prior
None for this illness

Review of Systems
(+) Chills, sore throat, headache, and myalgias, (–) fatigue, sneezing, nausea, vomiting, diarrhea, or constipation, (+) intermittent dry cough; (–) wheezing; (–) recent change in appetite or urinary frequency.

Physical Examination

▶ General
Slender, mixed-race female in mild distress

▶ Vital Signs
BP 122/65 mm Hg, P 88, RR 15, T 103.2°F (39.6°C)

Weight 121 lb. (55 kg)

Height 66 in. (167.6 cm)

Pain 5/10

▶ **Skin**

Flushed and warm

▶ **HEENT**

PERRLA, EOMI; (–) conjunctivitis or drainage from eyes; (–) TM abnormalities or otorrhea; normal appearing nasal mucosa with some clear rhinorrhea present; (+) erythematous pharynx; (–) tonsillar enlargement or exudate; mucus membranes moist

▶ **Neck and Lymph Nodes**

(+) nontender cervical lymphadenopathy; (–) neck stiffness or pain

▶ **Chest**

Breath sounds heard in all lung fields; (–) crackles; (+) mild intermittent expiratory wheezes; (+) intermittent nonproductive cough

▶ **Cardiovascular**

RRR, normal S_1 and S_2

▶ **Abdomen**

(+) bowel sounds; not tender or distended; (–) masses

▶ **Neurology**

Grossly intact without focal deficits; deep tendon reflexes normal

▶ **Extremities**

No swelling or edema noted

▶ **Genitourinary**

Examination deferred

▶ **Rectal**

Examination deferred

Laboratory Tests

Rapid streptococcal antigen test (–)

Nasopharyngeal swab (+) for influenza A virus

POC glucose (fasting): 180 mg/dL (10 mmol/L)

Assessment

Nineteen-year-old woman with underlying asthma and type 1 diabetes who has signs and symptoms consistent with influenza infection

---

Student Work-Up

Missing Information/Inadequate Data

Evaluate: Patient database

                Drug therapy problems

                Care plan (by problem)

Additional information:

1. What vaccines has she received and when were they administered?

2. How often does she need to use albuterol? How often does she have asthma symptoms? Does her asthma interfere with her ability to exercise or perform other activities? How often does she have exacerbations that require medical care or corticosteroids? Does she have an asthma action plan?

3. Does the patient have any sick contacts with similar symptoms?

4. How controlled is her diabetes? What is her hemoglobin A1C and when was it last measured? How does she manage sick days?

TARGETED QUESTIONS

1. What signs and symptoms of influenza does this patient have?

   Hint: Symptoms of influenza are similar to those of the common cold (fatigue, headache, cough, fever), but it is typical to have higher fevers and muscle aches with influenza. See p. 1088 in PPP

2. What treatments could be considered for this patient?

   Hint: Symptomatic therapy is recommended for viral upper respiratory tract infections. Antiviral therapy may reduce the duration of symptoms if initiated within 48 hours of illness onset. See pp. 1072 and 1087-1089 and Table 72-6 in PPP

3. What counseling points would you discuss with this patient?

   Hint: Many of the same principles that pertain to the common cold also apply to influenza. See pp. 1087-1090 in PPP

4. How should you address this patient's request for antibiotics to treat this infection?

   Hint: Most cases of pharyngitis are viral and this patient has confirmed influenza A infection. Her rapid streptococcal antigen detection test is negative, so it is unlikely that she also has streptococcal pharyngitis. Therefore, antibiotics are not indicated. See pp. 1084-1085 in PPP and Figure 72-4

5. Is this patient a candidate for the influenza vaccine?

   Hint: Documented influenza infection does not provide immunity to other influenza subtypes; therefore, if a patient is at risk for influenza and is infected in a particular season, it is recommended to vaccinate with the seasonal influenza vaccine to protect against the remaining subtypes. See pp. 1074-1075 and 1257 in PPP

6. What if this patient has an allergy to eggs?

   Hint: Most patients with egg allergies can still safely receive influenza vaccines, depending on the specific allergic reaction. Patients with severe egg allergies (i.e., anaphylaxis) should not be vaccinated with most influenza vaccines because they contain small amounts of egg protein; however, the recombinant influenza vaccine does not contain egg protein and can be given to patients with severe egg allergies. See p. 1257 and Table 86-1 in PPP

7. What if this patient had evidence of pneumonia at the time of presentation?

   Hint: See pp. 1070-1071 and Table 71-2 in PPP

☉ GLOBAL PERSPECTIVE

The global impact of influenza on morbidity and mortality is notable with more than 1 million deaths occurring annually. Influenza infection rates peak in cold winter months in the Northern Hemisphere, and epidemics in the Southern Hemisphere usually occur 6 months before or after those in the Northern Hemisphere. There is also a high background rate of infection in tropical climates. Poor outcome is associated with secondary bacterial pneumonia or infection with specific influenza strains (e.g., the recent H5N1 or avian influenza). Similar to the United States, morbidity and mortality is higher in the age extremes, pregnancy, and in those with cardiopulmonary or other chronic illnesses. Vaccination can limit the spread of infection, but it is not as effective in preventing illness in the elderly. Limited resources in developing countries limit the impact of vaccination on the spread of influenza. Educational efforts should focus on hand hygiene, isolation of those who are ill, and other infection control measures where possible.

CASE SUMMARY

- This patient's clinical picture is consistent with influenza infection and not streptococcal pharyngitis. Antibiotic therapy is not indicated, but antiviral therapy with oseltamivir should be used because the patient is presenting within the first 48 hours of illness and she has underlying medical conditions that increase her risk for severity (diabetes and asthma).

- Nonprescription medications can be used to relieve the symptoms and discomfort that are present. Single-ingredient products that target the patient's symptoms are preferred. Analgesics such as acetaminophen or ibuprofen can be used to treat her fever and discomfort.

- If her symptoms do not improve within 7-10 days or if she develops shortness of breath, difficulty breathing, dehydration, confusion, or other signs of worsening illness, she should seek medical attention immediately.

- She is a candidate for annual influenza vaccination, and she should receive the inactivated injectable influenza vaccine after this acute infection resolves.

KEY REFERENCES/READINGS

1. Influenza Antiviral Medications: Summary for Clinicians. 2015. CDC Influenza (Flu): United States. Available at: www.cdc.gov/flu/professionals/antivirals/summary-clinicians.htm. Accessed June 18, 2015.

For more information on the care plan and facilitator's guide please visit http://www.mhpharmacotherapy.com

79 Upper Respiratory Infection

Heather L. Girand

PATIENT PRESENTATION

Chief Complaint

"I thought my son had a cold, but today he woke up with a high fever, and his left eye was crusty and stuck shut."

History of Present Illness

JJ is a 3-year-old boy who presents with his mother to the family medicine clinic with complaints of fever, eye discharge, increased nasal congestion and discharge, poor appetite, and irritability. JJ has had nasal congestion, a runny nose, and intermittent sneezing for the "past few months" (mother is not sure exactly when these symptoms first appeared). Then, he developed increased nasal congestion about 1 week ago and has been taking more naps than usual over the past 3 days. His appetite has also diminished over the past couple of days. This morning, he awoke at 4:30 a.m., crying and irritable. His left eye was matted shut and there was thick nasal discharge coming from his left nostril. He also had a temperature of 102.3°F (39.1°C). His mother gave him some nonprescription cold medicines over the past 2 days but they did not seem to help his symptoms and made him "loopy."

Past Medical History

Upper respiratory tract infections 2-3 times each year

Acute otitis media (18 months of age)

MRSA (methicillin-resistant *Staphylococcus aureus*) abscess and cellulitis (13 months of age)

RSV (respiratory syncytial virus) bronchiolitis (6 months of age)

Gastroesophageal reflux (diagnosed at 3 months of age)

Family History

Father has exercise-induced asthma, dyslipidemia, and seasonal allergies. Mother has perennial allergic rhinitis and eczema. He has a 5-year-old sister with autism spectrum disorder (ASD) and asthma.

Social History

Lives with parents and sister. Attends daycare 4 days per week. Has one dog. Mother is a current cigarette smoker but reportedly smokes outside only. Immunizations not up-to-date; parents are "anti-vaccines" after their daughter developed ASD at 2 years of age.

Allergies/Intolerances/Adverse Drug Events

Trimethoprim-sulfamethoxazole

Amoxicillin

Medication History

▶ Current

Diphenhydramine 12.5 mg/5 mL 1 teaspoon po every 6 hours as needed

Children's Robitussin Cough and Cold CF (dextromethorphan 10 mg/10 mL; guaifenesin 100 mg/10 mL; phenylephrine 5 mg/10 mL) 1 teaspoon po every 4 hours as needed

▶ Prior

None for this illness

Review of Systems

(+) Fatigue, fever, nasal congestion, thick nasal discharge, (+) left eye discharge; (−) sneezing, neck stiffness, or photophobia; (+) intermittent dry cough; (−) wheezing; (+) reduced appetite; (−) nausea, vomiting, constipation, or diarrhea; (−) change in urinary frequency.

Physical Examination

▶ General

Slightly irritable young Caucasian male in mild distress

▶ Vital Signs

BP 110/65 mm Hg, P 118, RR 22, T 102.5°F (39.2°C)

Weight 31 lb. (14.1 kg)

Height 38.5 in. (97.8 cm)

Pain 4/10 (Faces scale)

► **Skin**

Three small bruises on bilateral shins; no abrasions or other abnormalities

► **HEENT**

PERRLA, EOMI; (+) conjunctivitis and purulent discharge from left eye; right eye normal appearing; dark circles under eyes bilaterally; (+) erythematous left TM with severe bulging and limited mobility; unable to visualize right TM because of cerumen; (−) otorrhea; (+) inflamed nasal mucosa with purulent discharge bilaterally; oropharyngeal cobblestone appearance with presence of thick, postnasal discharge; (−) tonsillar exudate; (+) foul-smelling breath; mucus membranes moist

► **Neck and Lymph Nodes**

(+) nontender cervical lymphadenopathy; (−) neck stiffness or pain

► **Chest**

CTA bilaterally; good air exchange; (−) wheezes; (+) intermittent nonproductive cough

► **Cardiovascular**

Tachycardic, regular rhythm, normal S_1 and S_2

► **Abdomen**

Not tender or distended; (−) masses

► **Neurology**

Grossly intact; deep tendon reflexes normal

► **Extremities**

No swelling or edema noted

► **Genitourinary**

Examination deferred

► **Rectal**

Examination deferred

Laboratory Tests

None performed

Assessment

Three-year-old boy with signs and symptoms consistent with acute otitis media, conjunctivitis, and bacterial rhinosinusitis; concurrent allergic rhinitis also likely

Student Work-Up

Missing Information/Inadequate Data

Evaluate: Patient database

Drug therapy problems

Care plan (by problem)

Additional information

1. Medication allergy/intolerance information: date and description of reactions.

2. Nonprescription medication information: how many doses of each medication were given? When were the last doses given? Were these medications self-prescribed or recommended by a healthcare provider?

3. Does the patient have any sick contacts with similar symptoms?

4. What, if any, vaccines have been given and when were they administered?

5. Does the patient have prescription insurance?

6. Does the patient have current or recent symptoms of gastroesophageal reflux?

TARGETED QUESTIONS

1. What signs and symptoms of acute bacterial rhinosinusitis (ABRS) does this patient have?

   Hint: See p. 1082 in PPP

2. What signs and symptoms of acute otitis media (AOM) does this patient have?

   Hint: See p. 1079 in PPP

3. Should this patient be treated with an antibiotic? If yes, what is the drug of choice for this patient?

   Hint: See pp. 1078-1080 and 1082-1083 in PPP

4. What counseling points regarding antibiotic treatment would you discuss with this patient's mother?

   Hint: See pp. 1080-1081 and 1083 in PPP

5. What adjunctive treatments could be considered for this patient?

   Hint: A viral upper respiratory tract infection may have preceded AOM and ABRS, and concurrent allergic rhinitis is a likely contributor to the development of these infections in this patient. Nonprescription medication use should be limited in young children with viral upper respiratory tract infections. See pp. 1087 and 1089 in PPP

FOLLOW-UP

Two days later, the patient's mother calls the family medicine clinic because her son is experiencing "diarrhea." She is worried that he is allergic to the antibiotic that was prescribed. His stools are described as "loose" but some are formed and some are watery in nature. He has not missed any doses of the antibiotic and the last dose that he received was this morning at 8 a.m. She reports that his other symptoms are improving and he has been afebrile for 24 hours. He is eating and drinking normal amounts.

What actions, if any, would you take?

⊙ GLOBAL PERSPECTIVE

AOM is a common childhood infection worldwide with an increased incidence in high-risk populations, such as American and Canadian Indians, Inuit, and aboriginal Australians. Complications such as mastoiditis and hearing impairment are more common in these high-risk groups, in children with lower socioeconomic status or who live in crowded conditions, and in developing countries. ABRS is also common worldwide and associated with allergic rhinitis, asthma, cystic fibrosis, gastroesophageal reflux, and immunodeficiencies. Geographic differences in bacterial causes, microbial resistance patterns, and access to pneumococcal conjugate vaccines affect treatment choices that are based on likely etiologies of these infections. Watchful waiting may be an appropriate option for many children with AOM and patients with uncomplicated ABRS in the developed world, but this approach requires close access to medical follow-up care. Risk factor reduction is an important educational target for developing countries and other high-risk groups that may lack access to modern medical care.

CASE SUMMARY

- This patient's clinical picture is consistent with AOM with concurrent conjunctivitis and ABRS. Antibiotic therapy is indicated because of infection severity and clinical course that are suggestive of a bacterial cause.

- Antibiotic selection is nearly always empiric and should target probable infecting organisms. Amoxicillin-clavulanate is an appropriate first-line antibiotic because *Haemophilus influenzae* is a common cause of AOM when purulent conjunctivitis is present; addition of clavulanate to amoxicillin expands the spectrum of activity to include beta-lactamase producing organisms. High dose (90 mg/kg/day divided twice daily) is preferred in order to overcome possible penicillin resistance in pneumococci in patients who are at risk for resistant infections (daycare attendance; severe infection characterized by high fever). If he is unable to tolerate this antibiotic because of an allergy, alternative choices to consider are cefdinir, cefpodoxime, or cefuroxime.

- Nonprescription medications such as single-ingredient acetaminophen or ibuprofen could be considered for pain and fever control; other nonprescription cough and cold medications should be discouraged because of a lack of data supporting their safety and efficacy in young children.

- A nonprescription intranasal corticosteroid (such as triamcinolone) and/or an oral antihistamine (such as loratadine, cetirizine, or fexofenadine) should be considered for this child to manage his allergic rhinitis. Allergic rhinitis is associated with an increased risk of AOM and ABRS.

KEY REFERENCES/READINGS

1. Rosenfeld RM, Piccirillo JF, Chandrasekhar SS, et al. Clinical practice guideline (update): adult sinusitis. Otolaryngol Head Neck Surg. 2015;152(2 Suppl):S1-39.
2. Seidman MD, Gurgel RK, Lin SY, et al. Clinical practice guideline: allergic rhinitis. Otolaryngol Head Neck Surg. 2015;152(1 Suppl):S1-S43.

For more information on the care plan and facilitator's guide please visit http://www.mhpharmacotherapy.com

80 Cellulitis

Christy M. Weiland

PATIENT PRESENTATION

Chief Complaint

Patient reports "I missed golf yesterday because I am having trouble with my arm. I have this sore on it."

History of Present Illness

Mr. Gene Phillips is a 69-year-old man who presents to his primary care physician complaining of an open lesion on his arm and the inability to play golf. His wife reports him not feeling well the last few days and being really tired. Mr. Phillips does not recall how or when the sore appeared however probably in the last week. It has become more red and sensitive over the last two days. He says he has never had a sore on his arm in the past; however, he gets sores on his leg that take a while to heal. Mr. Phillips is most concerned about feeling better so he can go play golf.

Past Medical History (PMH)

Chronic obstructive pulmonary disease (COPD)(diagnosed 10 years ago)has had one exacerbation in the past year which he was hospitalized for two months ago

Peripheral vascular disease (PVD)(diagnosed 5 years ago)

Hypothyroidism (diagnosed 7 years ago)

Coronary artery disease (CAD) (diagnosed 5 years ago) had a drug eluting stent placed 7 months ago and has had no chest pain since

Gastric esophageal reflux disease (GERD)

Family History

Unknown. He was adopted when he was 2 years old

Social/Work History

Retired electrical engineer

Married and lives with his wife at an assisted living facility

Tobacco/Alcohol/Substance Use

Previous smoker; quit when he was 30 (approximately 10 pack year history)

Drinks alcohol socially

Denies any substance abuse

Allergy/Intolerance/Adverse Event History

Oxycodone (nausea)

Sulfa drugs (unknown reaction)

Medication History

▶ *Current Medications*

Albuterol HFA 2 puffs inhaled q 6 hrs prn sob

Aspirin EC 81 mg po q day

Atorvastatin 20 mg po q day

Clopidogrel 75 mg po q day

Fluticasone/salmeterol (Advair Diskus) 250/50 mg inhale bid

Levothyroxine 100 mcg po q AM

Lisinopril 2.5 mg po q day

Ranitidine 75 mg po q day

Diphenhydramine 50 mg po q hs prn sleep

▶ *Prior Medication Use*

Completed prednisone taper 3 weeks ago

Review of Systems

(+) fever, denies chills, nausea or vomiting. He endorses pain at the lesion site on right forearm with noted erythema. Symptoms have been present for 2 days, duration of lesion is unknown.

Physical Exam

▶ *General*

Well-nourished man who appears lethargic with no acute distress

▶ *Vital Signs*

HR 112 bpm, BP 110/68 mmHg, RR 14, Temp 38.8°C

Pain 3/10

▶ *Skin*

Open lesion on right anterior forearm. One recent abrasion seems to be healing well on left lower extremity. Discoloration of skin throughout extremities. All other skin intact.

▶ **HEENT**

Dry mucus membranes. Pupils are equal, round and reactive to light.

▶ **Cardiovascular**

Sinus tachycardia, no murmurs

▶ **Abdomen**

Soft, nontender

▶ **Extremities**

Right forearm lesion noted above. It is erythemiditis, blanching and tender to touch. Lesion is two inches in length with purulent drainage.

Laboratory and Other Diagnostic Tests

	Conventional Units	SI Units
Na	135 mEq/L	135 mmol/L
K	4 mEq/L	4 mmol/L
Cl	108 mEq/L	108 mmol/L
CO_2	22 mEq/L	22 mmol/L
BUN	14 mg/dL	5 mmol/L
SCr	0.9 mg/dL	79 μmol/L
CrCl	100 mL/min	1.67 mL/s
Glu	107 mg/dL	5.9 mmol/L
WBC	$16.2 \times 10^3/mm^3$	$16.2 \times 10^9/L$
Plt	$160 \times 10^3/mm^3$	$160 \times 10^9/L$

Assessment

Mr. Phillips is a pleasant 69-year-old man who requires inpatient therapy due to cellulitis of the right upper extremity complicated by SIRS (systemic inflammatory response syndrome).

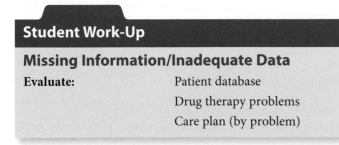

Student Work-Up

Missing Information/Inadequate Data

Evaluate: Patient database

Drug therapy problems

Care plan (by problem)

TARGETED QUESTIONS

1. Which signs and symptoms indicated Mr. Phillips is a candidate for inpatient therapy?

   Hint: Infections initially present with localized symptoms where the infection has started, such as the area of the broken skin barrier, and if worsens can lead to systemic symptoms. To assess the severity of an infection this must be considered

2. Does Mr. Phillips have any risk factors for multidrug resistant organisms? If so describe them.

   Hint: When treating a bacterial infection, it is essential to consider which organisms are potential pathogens so that drug therapy selected is appropriate. Considerations such as infection location, patient's immune system, as well as which organisms a patient may have exposure to are important factors. For example, residents of a skilled nursing facility or long-term care facility are considered to be at risk of multidrug resistant organisms. See p. 1094 in PPP

3. Which organisms should be considered as potential pathogens as a source for this infection?

   Hint: See p. 1096 in PPP

4. Describe an appropriate empiric inpatient therapy regimen for Mr. Phillips' infection?

   Hint: See pp. 1094 and 1097 in PPP

5. Appropriate antibiotic therapy was initiated based on your recommendation. What indicators would determine when it is appropriate to (1) de-escalate therapy or (2) change from an IV to a by-mouth regimen.

   Hint: Many times cultures are used to de-escalate antibiotic therapy; however, in cellulitis, unless there is an abscess or incision and drainage, a culture of the infection is not recommended. Cultures from punch biopsy yield an organism in less than a third of the cases because the concentration of bacteria in the tissues is usually quite low. Additionally, there is a risk of contamination with skin normal flora. In this scenario, due to the systemic symptoms of infection blood cultures are warranted; however, other indicators besides cultures will need to be used to tailor therapy. See p. 1096 in PPP

FOLLOW-UP

Thirty-six hours after appropriate empiric antibiotics were initiated, the patient's SIRS symptoms resolved. He was continued on the therapy for a total of 4 days and then narrowed antibiotics to po cephalexin. In addition to the cephalexin, the team would like to continue MRSA coverage due to a positive nasal MRSA swab performed at the hospital indicating he is colonized with MRSA. What additionally therapy is appropriate for MRSA coverage?

🌐 GLOBAL PERSPECTIVE

Skin and soft tissue infections are prevalent across the world. Skin problems including cellulitis are estimated to be the second most common diagnosis in returning travelers from international travel. Tropical locations with high humidity are considered high-risk areas and very common specifically returning from Sub-Saharan Africa and Southeast Asia. Organisms associated with skin and soft tissue infections are fairly consistent across the world with *Staphylococcus aureus* being the most predominant and methicillin resistance being about one-third of the isolates. The tropical conditions both heat and humidity make organisms such as MRSA and PantoneValentine leukocidin toxin-associated *Staphylcoccus aureus* infections much more common, which are correlated to more severe tissue destruction.

- MRSA should be considered in populations that have potential exposure to MRSA, immunocompromised individuals, or other comorbidities that increase the risk.

For more information on the care plan and facilitator's guide please visit http://www.mhpharmacotherapy.com

CASE SUMMARY

- Symptoms for cellulitis usually are localized with a break in the skin barrier, but can lead to a systemic infection.
- The majority of cellulitis infections are due to streptococcal organisms.

81 Diabetic Foot Infection

Christy M. Weiland

PATIENT PRESENTATION

Chief Complaint

"I was just in here 2 weeks ago and you guys said that my foot was fine, but it is getting worse and hurts to walk on it."

History of Present Illness

Mr. Mark Summers' is a 65-year-old man who has had diabetes mellitus (DM) for 23 years. It is intermittently controlled with hemoglobin A1c between 7-10 the last few years. It seems to vary based on his work schedule. He came in 2 weeks ago with an open lesion on his foot (4 cm in length) it was noted to be dry and noninfected. He was instructed to change socks twice daily keeping the area free of moisture, but keep the skin well hydrated. He reports the last week it has increased in pain and is now having trouble walking on it. The lesion has been weeping fluid for 4 days now. Of note, he has had two previous foot infections in the last 2 years, one included a hospitalization.

Past Medical History (PMH)

Diabetes mellutis 2 (diagnosed 23 years ago)

Hypertension (HTN)

Coronary artery disease; had one drug eluting stent placed 2 years ago

Erectile dysfunction

Atrial fibrillation (diagnosed 4 years ago)

Peripheral neuropathy (unknown diagnosis date)

Previous history of MRSA (methicillin-resistant Staphylococcus aureus)

Family History

Mom: died of colon cancer at age 84

Dad: died of myocardial infarction at age 78

Social/Work History

Long-haul truck driver for 30 years

Tobacco/Alcohol/Substance Use

Endorses a glass of whiskey on the weekends

Allergy/Intolerance/Adverse Event History

NKDA

Medication History (Current)

Aspirin 81 mg po q AM

Clopidogrel 75 mg po q PM

Glargine 76 units subcutaneous q AM

Hydrochlorothiazide 25 mg po q AM

Lispro insulin 22 units subcutaneous with each meal

Metoprolol succinate 25 mg po q AM

Review of Systems

(−) fever, chills, nausea or vomiting. He endorses pain at the site of the lesion and surrounding area. This has been worsening over 4 days.

Physical Exam

▶ *General*

Well-nourished gentleman in no acute distress.

▶ *Vital Signs*

BP 152/82 mm Hg, HR 65 bpm, RR 12, T 37.3°C

Pain 7/10

▶ *Skin*

Open lesion about 4 cm on left inferior aspect of foot, inflamed area surrounding is minimal. Small amount of purulent, copious, foul smelling weeping fluid, dehydrated, Noted, thickened, worn skin.

▶ *Cardiovascular*

NSR

▶ *Extremities*

No other noted lesions. Lower extremities cold to the touch. Noted neuropathy on lower extremities.

Laboratory and Other Diagnostic Tests

	Conventional Units	SI Units
Hemoglobin A1c	8.9	0.089
Fasting blood sugar reported by patient	196 mg/dL	10.8 mmol/L

Assessment

Mr. Summers, a 65-year-old with long-standing, mostly uncontrolled diabetes with complications including microvascular disease and now with a diabetic foot infection.

Student Work-Up

Missing Information/Inadequate Data

Evaluate: Patient database

Drug therapy problems

Care plan (by problem)

TARGETED QUESTIONS

1. What risk factor(s) does this patient have for a diabetic foot infection?

   Hint: See pp. 1098-1099 in PPP

2. List the most likely organism(s) that is/are contributing to the diabetic foot infection.

   Hint: When considering potential pathogens make sure to consider the patient's history as well as physical exam. See p. 1098 in PPP

3. What recommendations are appropriate for prevention of another diabetic foot infection?

   Hint: Consider assisting patients in overcoming very specific barriers to controlling blood glucose or foot care. What are Mr. Summers' potential barriers?

4. Classify Mr. Summers' ulcer based on the PEDIS scale and describe what it signifies.

   Hint: See Table 73-5 in PPP

5. Create a treatment plan for Mr. Summers' infection including nonpharmacologic and pharmacologic therapy.

   Hint: While pharmacist do not diagnose, it is essential to be able to classify disease states to assist with therapy plans. Question 4 is necessary to answer this question. See Table 73-6 in PPP

FOLLOW-UP

After presenting your recommendation to the physician, she prescribed the antibiotic(s) and the patient was told to follow up in 1 week. Two days later, the patient called and reported a diffuse, nonraised rash after taking the antibiotic. He took diphenhydramine but is still itching. He does not want to take the antibiotic anymore and wants to know if that is alright.

Determine an alternative therapy that the physician can prescribe for Mr. Summers since he has an allergic reaction to the current antibiotic.

Hint: See pp. 1100-1101 in PPP

🌐 GLOBAL PERSPECTIVE

India is known for having the largest number of persons with diabetes in the world. Type 2 diabetes prevalence is growing more rapidly in this area due to marked demographic and socioeconomic changes in the region. Currently it is predicted that 41 million have diabetes and by 2025 that number is expected to be 66 million. A program called "Step-by-Step Improving Diabetes Foot care in the developing world" was started in India. Teams of physicians and nurses were trained in a 2-day course about basic foot care and how to educate patients, as well as give the teams hands-on experience in treatment of trivial foot lesions. The health care providers were then encouraged to set up model diabetic foot clinics where they would be able to prevent trivial foot lesions becoming catastrophe. One hundred clinics were set up and then surveyed in years 1 and 2 after the training. It was estimated that in the first year at least 900 lower limbs and in the second year 1943 limbs were saved.

CASE SUMMARY

- Diabetic foot infection is a complication of diabetes and is typically preventable with blood sugar control, appropriate foot hygiene including proper fitting shoes, and monitoring of feet.
- Diabetic foot infections are classified based on the severity of the infection that then drives appropriate therapy for the infection.
- Patient education has a large role in treating a diabetic foot infection and can prevent further infections.

KEY REFERENCE/READINGS

1. Bakker K, Abbas ZG, & Pendsey SP. (2006). Step by step, improving diabetic foot care in the developing world. A pilot study for India, Bangladesh, Sri Lanka and Tanzania. Pract Diab Int. 23:365-369.

For more information on the care plan and facilitator's guide please visit http://www.mhpharmacotherapy.com

82 Infective Endocarditis

Ronda L. Akins   Katie E. Barber

PATIENT PRESENTATION

Chief Complaint

"The infection on my groin still hurts and I think it is getting worse despite me taking all of my antibiotics. I've also had a fever for the past couple of days. I don't feel very well, my leg feels like it is more swollen, my stomach hurts, and I am really tired all the time."

History of Present Illness

AS is a 24-year-old African-American female who presents to the emergency department (ED) with complaints of periodic fevers [101-103°F (38.3-39.4°C)], chills, fatigue, and abdominal pain for the past 2 days, as well as left groin erythema and edema for the past 1-2 weeks. She previously presented to the ED 5 days ago and was subsequently diagnosed with cellulitis over the area of a nicked shaving wound. Other than 5 days ago, she has not been admitted to the hospital since birth. During that ED visit, there was slight drainage from the area that was collected and sent for culture and sensitivity. The patient was treated with a single intravenous dose of vancomycin 1000 mg and sent home with a prescription for 10 days of oral clindamycin therapy for which she states 100% adherence. Since the initial presentation, the cellulitis has spread extending down the upper leg with increased edema and fluctuance over the wound. She reports taking ibuprofen and acetaminophen for increased pain and swelling, as well as fever over the past few days.

Past Medical History

Migraine headaches (2 years); typically has 1-2 per month often around menses

Cellulitis left upper leg (5 days prior to this admission)

Several boils (armpits and buttocks) over the past 6 months treated with topical antibiotic ointment at home

Family History

Father and mother are both alive. Father is 48 and has a history of asthma and diabetes. Mother is 46 and has dyslipidemia. She has one older and one younger sibling: one sister aged 18 and one brother aged 26; both are healthy.

Social History

She is unmarried with no children. She lives with her boyfriend and is employed as an elementary school teacher.

Tobacco/Alcohol/Substance Use

Admits to tobacco use (1/2 ppd × 5 years) and drinks alcohol on occasion (3-4 drinks per week). She denies illicit drug usage.

Allergies/Intolerances/Adverse Drug Events

Sulfa (unknown reaction)

Medications (Current)

Clindamycin po × 5 days

Yaz 1 tablet po daily (started birth control 6 years ago)

Fioricet 1 tablet po q 4-6 h prn migraine headaches

Acetaminophen 500 mg (2 tablets) po q 6 h prn pain/fever × 2 weeks

Ibuprofen po prn pain/fever × 2 weeks and prn headaches

Review of Systems

Purulent cellulitis and suspected abscess in upper left leg/groin area; no other significant medical problems.

Physical Examination

▶ *General*

Physically fit, well-appearing, African-American female in moderate acute distress

▶ *Vital Signs*

BP 124/76 mm Hg, P 95, RR 24, T 39.5°C

Weight 120 lb. (54.5 kg)

Height 63 in. (160 cm)

Complains of significant upper left leg/groin pain and swelling

▶ *Skin*

Erythema, edema, and fluctuance around groin area; (+) petechial rash on trunk, (+) Janeway lesions noted on the patient's right hand (one lesion on the thumb and one between the little and ring finger)

▶ *HEENT*

PERRLA, EOMI; no scleral icterus, (+) petechia on palate, (−) Roth's spots, dry mucus membranes, no exudates noted in throat

▶ **Neck and Lymph Nodes**

Supple; (–) lymphadenopathy

▶ **Chest**

Clear to auscultation bilaterally

▶ **Cardiovascular**

RRR, (+) murmur noted (no previous history of murmur)

▶ **Abdomen**

Soft, nondistended, nontender; (+) bowel sounds; (–) organomegaly

▶ **Neurology**

Grossly intact; AAO × 3; (–) focal or sensory deficit noted

▶ **Extremities**

Localized 2+ edema, erythema and fluctuance over the upper left leg/groin with a small focal lesion; pulses are 2+ and equal bilaterally. No clubbing or cyanosis of the fingers noted. No splinter hemorrhages noted.

Laboratory Tests on Admission

	Conventional Units	SI Units
Na	137 mEq/L	137 mmol/L
K	4.8 mEq/L	4.8 mmol/L
Cl	103 mEq/L	103 mmol/L
CO_2	24 mEq/L	24 mmol/L
BUN	16 mg/dL	5.71 mmol/L urea
SCr	0.9 mg/dL	79.56 µmol/L
Glucose	100 mg/dL	5.55 mmol/L
Ca	9.2 mg/dL	2.3 mmol/L
Mg	2.0 mg/dL	0.82 mmol/L
PO_4	3.1 mg/dL	1.00 mmol/L
Hct	39.2%	0.39 (fraction)
WBC	$21.4 \times 10^3/\mu L$	$21.4 \times 10^9/L$
WBC differential percent	85/0/0/9/6	85/0/0/9/6
Platelets	$320 \times 10^3/\mu L$	$320 \times 10^9/L$
Albumin	4.1 g/dL	41 g/L
AST	42 IU/L	0.70 µkat/L
ALT	19 U/L	0.32 µkat/L
Alk phos	85 IU/L	1.42 µkat/L

▶ **Cultures**

Blood cultures taken on admission; results pending

Wound culture (pus/drainage) from upper leg/groin taken 5 days prior to this admission in the ED –

Staphylococcus aureus; see culture and susceptibilities table for results.

Assessment

A 24-year-old female with signs, symptoms, and laboratory tests consistent with upper left leg/groin cellulitis/abscess and suspected endocarditis to be admitted for IV antibiotics (vancomycin plus piperacillin/tazobactam).

Student Work-Up

Missing Information/Inadequate Data

Evaluate:
Patient database
Drug therapy problems
Care plan (by problem)

TARGETED QUESTIONS

1. What signs and symptoms of IE are present on admission for this patient based on Duke classification, including the specific "type" clinical diagnosis category?

   Hint: See p. 1109 and Table 74-2 in PPP

2. Is the initial empiric antibiotic therapy (vancomycin plus piperacillin/tazobactam) appropriate treatment for this patient?

   Hint: See pp. 1111-1113 in PPP and refer to the following reference for additional information:

   Baddour LM, et al. Circulation 2015;132:1435-1486 (specifically culture negative section)

3. Are there any potential concerns with the dual broad-spectrum therapeutic regimen in this patient?

   Hint: Refer to the following reference for additional information:

   Burgess LD, et al. Pharmacother. 2014;34(7):670-676

FOLLOW-UP

After the patient was admitted to the hospital for initiation of broad-spectrum antibiotics, additional tests were performed to assist in the diagnosis of IE with the following clinical course.

Laboratory Tests After Admission

▶ **Cultures**

Day 1 (admission blood cultures × 2): no growth

Day 2 (pus/drainage of left groin abscess): *Staphylococcus aureus*; see culture and susceptibilities table for results

Day 5 (blood cultures × 2): no growth

Day 9 (blood cultures × 2): no growth

Culture and Susceptibility Results

	Wound (Left Groin) Initial ED visit	Blood × 2 (both drawn peripherally) Day 1 (on admission)	Aspirate (Left Groin abscess) Day 2	Blood × 2 (peripheral draw × 1 and through PICC line × 1) Day 5	Blood × 2 (peripheral draw × 1 and through PICC line × 1) Day 9
Gram stain	Gram-positive cocci in clusters		Gram-positive cocci in clusters		
Organism	*S. aureus* MIC (mg/L)	No growth (final)	*S. aureus* MIC (mg/L)	No growth (final)	No growth (final)
Clindamycin	≤0.5 (S)		≤0.5 (S)		
Daptomycin	0.25 (S)		0.25 (S)		
Erythromycin	>4 (R)		>4 (R)		
Gentamicin	>8 (R)		>8 (R)		
Moxifloxacin	>4 (R)		>4 (R)		
Linezolid	0.5 (S)		0.5 (S)		
Oxacillin	>2 (R)		>2 (R)		
Penicillin	>8 (R)		>8 (R)		
Rifampin	≤1 (S)		≤1 (S)		
Quinupristin/Dalfopristin	≤0.5 (S)		≤0.5 (S)		
Tetracycline	≤1 (S)		≤1 (S)		
Trimethoprim/ Sulfamethoxazole	≤2/38 (S)		≤2/38 (S)		
Vancomycin	0.5 (S)		1 (S)		

► **Imaging**

Day 2: CT of the left groin showed a 3 × 4 cm (1.2 × 1.6 in.) abscess. Surgery drains abscess and sends aspirate for culture.

Day 3: TTE had poor visualization of the valves; results inconclusive.

Day 5: TEE shows a vegetation [1.4 × 0.9 cm (0.55 × 0.35 in.)] on the atrial aspect of the mitral valve.

Pertinent Labs During Admission

Laboratory Tests	Conventional Units	SI Units
Day 1:		
SCr	0.9 mg/dL	68.67 μmol/L
WBC	21.4 × 10³/μL	21.4 × 10⁹/L
Day 3:		
SCr	1.2 mg/dL	91.56 μmol/L
WBC	23.4 × 10³/μL	23.4 × 10⁹/L
Vancomycin peak (drawn at 1140)	45.6 mg/L	31.5 μmol/L
Vancomycin trough (drawn at 0815)	12.7 mg/L	8.8 μmol/L

Day 5:		
SCr	0.9 mg/dL	68.67 μmol/L
WBC	16.2 × 10³/μL	16.2 × 10⁹/L
Vancomycin peak (drawn at 1140)	34.2 mg/L	23.6 μmol/L
Vancomycin trough (drawn at 0815)	17.1 mg/L	11.8 μmol/L
Day 9:		
SCr	0.8 mg/dL	61.04 μmol/L
WBC	10.2 × 10³/μL	10.2 × 10⁹/L
Day 14:		
SCr	0.8 mg/dL	61.04 μmol/L
WBC	8.9 × 10³/μL	8.9 × 10⁹/L

Hospital Course

The patient was placed on vancomycin 1000 mg IV q 12 h and piperacillin/tazobactam 3.375 g IV q 6 h for broad coverage of IE and left upper leg/groin cellulitis/abscess. She continues to have intermittent febrile episodes [day 3 – spikes up to 40.0°C (104.0°F)] despite therapy. On hospital day 3, peaks and troughs were drawn and reported for vancomycin (see pertinent laboratory during admission table). Vancomycin dose was then increased to 750 mg q 8 h. On hospital day 5, blood cultures finalized as negative so repeat cultures were obtained, particularly after the TEE was noted positive for a vegetation. Additionally, left groin abscess cultures revealed methicillin-resistant *S. aureus* with the same susceptibility pattern as the culture obtained in the emergency department on her previous visit. Repeat blood cultures continued to remain negative. On hospital day 9, cultures remained negative and no additional sources of infection, other than the skin/soft tissue site, were identified. At that time, the team decided that the likely cause for the infective endocarditis was a disseminated MRSA infection originating as a skin infection. Therefore, piperacillin/tazobactam was discontinued. On hospital day 14, after continued improvement and repeat negative blood cultures, the patient was sent home on outpatient IV vancomycin therapy for the remaining 4 weeks of her 6 weeks course.

FOLLOW-UP TARGETED QUESTIONS

4. How often are blood cultures positive in IE? Why are this patient's cultures negative? How should this patient be monitored for resolution of infection/adverse drug effects? Include additional tests, procedures, etc.

   Hint: See pp. 1112 and 1120 in PPP and refer to the following reference for additional information:

   Baddour LM, et al. Circulation 2015;132:1435-1486

5. What should you recommend after reviewing this patient's antibiotic profile including vancomycin concentrations?

   Hint: See p. 1121 in PPP and refer to the following reference to provide updated dosing strategy for vancomycin:

   Rybak M, Lomaestro B, et al. Am J Health-Syst Pharm. 2009;66:82-98

6. Should this patient receive IE prophylaxis for future dental visits? Include type of dental procedure, rationale for prophylaxis, and regimen if appropriate.

   Hint: See p. 1120 and Tables 74-8 and 74-9 in PPP

☉ GLOBAL PERSPECTIVE

IE is an infection typically involving the heart valves and nearby endocardial tissue. This disease state often has an aggressive clinical course with numerous complications and high mortality rates. Incidence of IE appears to be similar throughout developed countries. There is significant variability in patient presentation from subacute illness to severe sepsis. Select patient populations (i.e., IV drug abusers, diabetics, elderly) have an increased risk of developing IE with less common and/or resistant pathogens. Regardless of type of patient or pathogen, IE is often difficult to diagnose and treat. In underdeveloped countries, the mortality rates are often higher secondary to the problematic nature of this infection. Additionally, treatment should be carefully monitored to ensure therapeutic response and minimization of disease complications or drug toxicity. Patient follow-up is crucial to appropriately assess for a curative outcome.

CASE SUMMARY

- Despite negative cultures throughout the hospital admission, her clinical presentation, as well as echocardiographic results, are consistent with IE requiring appropriate antibiotic therapy.

- Initial empiric antibiotics, per IE treatment guidelines, should be targeted against likely causative organisms for IE, including coverage for possible culture negative organisms or rationale for negative blood cultures can not be determined.

- Monitoring of clinical response is crucial to assess appropriate antibiotic therapy and re-assessment is required if satisfactory outcome is not achieved. De-escalation of therapy should be based on appropriate findings such as microbiological data, response to therapy, and clinical judgment regarding source of IE (if able to determine).

For more information on the care plan and facilitator's guide please visit http://www.mhpharmacotherapy.com

83 Tuberculosis

John Leander Po

PATIENT PRESENTATION

Chief Complaint

"Having had a dry cough for the last 8 weeks, I experienced sharp chest pain on the right side that started 2 days ago. This happened while having night sweats that required changing sheets, and an unintentional weight loss of 20 lb. (9 kg) over the past months."

History of Present Illness

CG is a 34-year-old Filipino Domestic female with a history significant for type II diabetes mellitus (DM) and hypertension (HTN) who initially presented to her primary care clinic with complaints of a dry cough, occasionally producing flecks of white thick sputum over the last 8 weeks. She had just arrived from the Philippines, with documentation showing a positive a Tuberculin Skin Test (TST) result of 12 mm, followed by a chest x-ray that was interpreted as within normal limits. The patient's symptoms were accompanied by intermittent drenching night sweats and an unintentional loss of 20 lb. (9 kg) over the last 2 months.

Additional questions revealed she was fatigued, having the sensation of feeling "feverish" and experiencing difficulty "catching her breath" after walking a short distance. Three days prior to admission, the patient experienced sudden onset of right pleuritic chest pain along the mid axillary line, just below the level of the right nipple. The pain was severe, and woke her up from sleep. It was exacerbated with inspiration, with no relieving factors. The pain did not improve when she tried over the counter ibuprofen.

Given the patient's symptoms, she was given a mask and was subsequently transported to the Emergency Department (ED).

Past Medical History

HTN (diagnosed 11 months ago)

Type 2 DM (diagnosed 24 months ago)

Immunized with Bacille-Calmet-Guerin (BCG) as a child

Family History

Mother (age 67) had TB at 15 years old for which she received therapy

Father died of metastatic lung cancer (age 66)

Sister (age 37) has Type II DM and HTN

Social History

The patient immigrated to the United States from the Philippines 10 weeks ago. She was to serve as a domestic servant in an affluent family with two children. She started work almost immediately after arriving to the United States.

Tobacco/Alcohol/Substance Use

Drinks a glass of wine daily. Denies any tobacco or illicit drug use.

Allergies/Intolerances/Adverse Drug Events

Levofloxacin (rash)

Medications (Current)

Lisinopril 20 mg by mouth daily

Metformin 500 mg by mouth twice daily

Glyburide 5 mg by mouth daily

Ibuprofen 200 mg by mouth prn pain

Review of Systems

Pertinent review of systems are as described in the history of present illness. The patient reports feeling occasionally feverish. Otherwise, the remaining review of systems are negative.

Physical Examination

▶ *General*

Pleasant, slightly overweight Filipino female in no acute distress

▶ *Vital Signs*

BP 145/83 mm Hg, P 88, RR –18, T 37.5°C

Weight 72.6 lb. (33 kg)

Height 59 in. (150 cm)

▶ *HEENT*

Normal cephalic, atraumatic; pupils equal and reactive to light and accommodation bilaterally; extraocular muscles intact; good dentition; moist mucous membranes with no ulcers; no phargeal discharge; no nares discharge; tracheal midline

▶ **Neck and Lymph Nodes**

1 cm nontender, unfixed, nodule on the right anterior cervical chain area. Otherwise, trachea mideline.

▶ **Chest**

No retractions or use of accessory muscles. Symmetrical expansion of the chest. Dullness to percussion, egophony and tactile fremitus noted in the right middle lung field. Bronchial breath sounds also noted in the right middle lung field. No rales or rhonchi.

▶ **Cardiovascular**

Regular rate and rhythm, normal S_1, S_2; no pedal edema

▶ **Abdomen**

Not tender/not distended; no organomegaly; no abdominal guarding or rebound. Normal bowel sounds.

▶ **Neurology**

Cranial nerves II-XII intact. No gross motor or sensoral deficits elicited. Normal patellar deep tendon reflexes bilaterally. Normal finger-to-nose tracing.

▶ **Genitourinary and Rectal**

Examination deferred

Laboratory Tests

On Admission

	Conventional Units	SI Units
Na	142 mEq/L	142 mmol/L
K	4.1 mEq/L	4.1 mmol/L
Cl	101 mEq/L	101 mmol/L
CO_2	26 mEq/L	26 mmol/L
BUN	20 mg/dL	7.1 mmol/L
SCr	0.7 mg/dL	62 μmol/L
Glu	153 mg/dL	8.5 mmol/L
AST	55 IU/L	0.92 μkat/L
ALT	61 IU/L	1.02 μkat/L
Total bilirubin	1 mg/dL	17.1 μmol/L
HbA1c	7.2%	0.072 (55 mmol/mol Hgb)
Hgb	13.5 g/dL	135 g/L
Hct	40%	0.40
WBC	$10.6 \times 10^3/mm^3$	$10.6 \times 10^9/L$
PMN	62%	0.62
Lymphocytes	34%	0.34
Monocytes	5%	0.05
Sputum culture	Normal respiratory flora	
	Acid-fast bacilli smear (+)	

▶ **Skin Test Results (From Immigration Papers)**

TST with purified protein derivative (PPD): 12 mm at 48 hours

▶ **Chest X-Ray**

Right middle and upper lobe infiltrate

1 cm cavitary lesion in the lower aspect of the right upper lobe

Assessment

Thirty-four-year-old Filipino Domestic female with a history significant for type II DM and HTN, presenting with signs, symptoms, labs, and radiologic features consistent with active tuberculosis disease, latent tuberculosis infection, and caseating sputum production.

Student Work-Up

Missing Information/Inadequate Data

Evaluate: Patient database

Drug therapy problems

Care plan (by problem)

TARGETED QUESTIONS

1. What factors does one need to consider when interpreting a Tuberculin Skin Test (TST), and what criteria is used to determine if a patient tests positive?

   Hint: See p. 1125 in PPP

2. What implications to the TST and Interferon Gamma Release Assay (IGRA) does prior vaccination with Bacille-Calmet-Guerin (BCG) with respect to affecting test results?

   Hint: See p. 1125 in PPP

3. In patients with laboratory-confirmed drug-susceptible active pulmonary *Mycobacterium tuberculosis* (MTB), what are the World Health Organization's recommended standard medication(s) and duration of treatment? How would this differ if the patient were HIV positive?

   Hint: See Tables 75-3 and 75-5 in PPP

4. The patient's liver function tests are slightly elevated. Why is this important and does it change the management of her TB infection?

   Hint: See p. 1131 in PPP

5. How does one monitor for clinical response to active TB therapy?

   Hint: See pp. 1131-1132 in PPP

FOLLOW-UP

Patient was placed in airborne isolation. Three induced sputum specimens were acid fast bacillus (AFB) stained, revealing organisms that were identified 6 weeks later (by culture and molecular typing) as *Mycobacterium tuberculosis* resistant to isoniazid (INH).

How does this information change your recommended drug combination and duration of drug therapy?

Hint: See p. 1127 in PPP

Based on the case, who else should be tested and evaluated for active TB?

Hint: See Table 75-2 in PPP

🌐 GLOBAL PERSPECTIVE

Though there is a cure for this preventable disease, *Mycobacterium tuberculosis* infects one-third of the world's population. TB is contagious, and can be spread from person to person through the air. Its nonspecific signs and symptoms like cough, fevers, and night sweats are mild on disease onset, and result in the delay of care while increasing the number of those who are infected. Without the appropriate treatment, up to two-thirds of those infected with TB will die. Overall, the highest incidents of active TB patients reside in India, Southeast Asia and Sub-Saharan Africa.

People infected with the Human Immunodeficiency Virus (HIV) are a particularly vulnerable population, resulting in significant morbidity and mortality, especially in working adults (25-44 years of age). The weakened immune system makes active TB infection severe and difficult to control. Africa accounts for approximately 80% of the HIV positive TB cases. The development of drug resistant TB is the result of drug mismanagement, especially when using poor-quality drugs, incorrectly prescribing habits by physicians, and when treatment is inconsistent and incomplete. The global development of multidrug resistant (MDR TB*) and extremely multidrug resistant (XDR TB) is multifactorial. These factors include patient nonadherence to weeks of therapy, the lack of qualified human resources, poor infection control practices, insufficient laboratory capacities, and weak surveillance systems.

CASE SUMMARY

- This case is clinically consistent with active pulmonary tuberculosis which is highly contagious; therapy should be initiated.
- First line recommendations for TB therapy involves 4 drugs: isoniazid (INH), rifampin (RIF), pyrazinamide (PZA) and ethambutol (EMB). However, the rise in multidrug resistance testing requires susceptibility testing results. Based on these results, the treatment regimen might need to be revised.
- Liver function tests should be monitored due to drug toxicity and pre-existing enzyme elevations.
- Close contacts should be treated with rifampin since INH-resistant strain was isolated from in the patient.

REFERENCES

1. World Health Organization. A global action framework for TB research in support of the third pillar of WHO's end TB strategy. 2015. http://www.who.int/tb/publications/global-framework-research/en/ Accessed January 3, 2016.
2. Centers for Disease Control and Prevention Division of Tuberculosis Elimination (DTBE). National action plan for combating multidrug-resistant tuberculosis. 2015. https://www.whitehouse.gov/sites/default/files/microsites/ostp/national_action_plan_for_tuberculosis_20151204_final.pdf Accessed January 12, 2016.

For more information on the care plan and facilitator's guide please visit http://www.mhpharmacotherapy.com

84 Clostridium Difficile Infection

Monica A. Donnelley   Brett H. Heintz
Jeremiah J. Duby

LEARNING OBJECTIVES

Identify the signs and symptoms of *Clostridium difficile* infection (CDI)

List the risk factors for CDI

Select an appropriate treatment and monitoring plan for antimicrobial therapy

Consider the role of adjunctive agents and supportive care

PATIENT PRESENTATION

Chief Complaint

New onset watery diarrhea and recurrence of leukocytosis.

History of Present Illness

Jim Larsen is an 86-year-old male who was recently admitted to the intensive care unit 10 days ago with a diagnosis of necrotizing fasciitis. Prior to admission, the patient was noted to have a round dark-red area on the under side of his right elbow. The area of redness expanded to encompass the whole elbow and to cover most of his right arm despite taking an outpatient prescription for levofloxacin and prednisone. JL presented to the emergency department (ED) with complaints of severe pain despite his use of oral analgesics and compliance with his antimicrobial and prednisone therapy. Urine output in the ED was noted to be zero and the patient reported he felt weak. He was taken to the OR and the diagnosis of necrotizing fasciitis was confirmed. The patient was empirically started on vancomycin, cefepime and clindamycin. Tissue cultures from the microbiology lab resulted in *Streptococcus pyogenes* (group A). The physician discontinued cefepime, started piperacillin/tazobactam and continued vancomycin and clindamycin. Now on hospital day 10, JL has numerous watery bowel movements, recurrence of leukocytosis, and presence of fever.

Past Medical History

Type 2 Diabetes Mellitus
Diabetic nephropathy
Diabetic retinopathy (blind in Right eye)
Hypertension

Surgical History

Right below knee amputation (BKA) (documented MRSA 2011)

Irrigation and debridement (I&D) wound upper extremity. Placement of wound vac right arm (04/09/2015)

Family History

Retired author

Social History

Married

Tobacco/Alcohol/Substance Use

Former passive smoker 1-2 cigarettes/week (quit date 05/23/1942)

Declines alcohol and/or illicit substance abuse

Sexually Active

Yes, female partner

Allergies

NKDA

Immunization History

Tdap (10/2000)
Influenza vaccine (10/2014)
Pneumococcal polysaccharide vaccine (PPSV23) (03/2015)

Medications (Current)

Hydrocodone-acetaminophen 10-325 mg 2 tablets po q 6 hours prn pain

Oxycodone-acetaminophen 5-325 mg 2 tablets po q 4 hours prn pain

Acetaminophen ES 500 mg by mouth q 4 hours prn pain

ASA 81 mg tablet po every day

Cholecalciferol 1000 units 1 tablet po every day

Nifedipine 30 mg CR 1 tablet po every day

Omeprazole 40 mg 1 capsule po once daily before meal

Triamterene 75 mg/hydrochlorothiazide 50 mg (Maxzide) 75-50 mg 1 tablet po every day

Metformin 1000 mg tablet po twice daily

Medications Added to Above List (On Admission)

Insulin aspart 18 units subcutaneous tid with meals

Insulin glargine 15 units subcutaneous units QHS

Cefepime 1 g IV q 8 hours

Vancomycin 1 g IV q 24 hours

Clindamycin 900 mg IV q 8 hours

Review of Systems

Constitutional: + **fever, + chills, fatigue, weakness**

Eyes: no changes in vision or eye pain. **Blind in right eye**

Ears, Nose, Mouth, Throat: no changes in hearing, congestion, or sore throat. **Deaf in right ear**

CV: no chest pain or palpitations

Resp: no shortness of breath or wheezing

GI: no abdominal pain, constipation, or diarrhea

GU: no hematuria, dysuria. **+ decrease in urinary frequency**

Musculoskeletal: no new myalgias or arthralgias. Reports tingling in lower extremities

Integumentary: no new rashes or moles

Neuro: no headaches

Allergy/Immunology: no congestion, rhinorrhea, or new allergies

▶ Vital Signs

Hospital Day 10:

BP 115/79 mm Hg, HR 80, RR 18, T 38.8°C

Weight 180.4 lbs (82 kg)

Height 69 in. (175.3 cm)

Elbow pain (3/10)

Physical Exam

▶ General

Elderly, ill-appearing man, lying in bed, moderately distressed

▶ Eyes

Right eye with fixed pupil, cloudy area over medial cornea. Left conjunctiva and cornea clear. Right pupil reactive to light with EOM intact. Sclerae normal.

▶ Ears

Almost no hearing on the left, hard of hearing on the right, TM pearly white

▶ Nose

Not examined

▶ Mouth

Dentures in place, no sign of lesions, normal mucosa and no erythema of posterior oropharynx.

▶ Neck

Neck supple. No adenopathy, thyroid symmetric, normal size.

▶ Heart

normal rate and regular rhythm, no murmurs, clicks, or gallops.

▶ Lungs

Breathing comfortably on room air, clear to auscultation, no wheezes or ronchi

▶ Abdomen

Soft, nontender, nondistended, nl bowel sounds, no masses or organomegally palpated.

▶ All 4 Extremities

RLE: warm, well perfused, amputated below the knee

LLE: warm, well perfused, 2+ DP pulse. LUE-unremarkable

RUE: Erythema from 6 cm distal to the shoulder to just pass the elbow, indurated around the elbow, no fluctuance noted, tender to palpation over entire erythematous area, able to passively range the elbow with pain. Grip strength 3/5 on right, 5/5 on left.

▶ Skin

Skin otherwise without rashes

▶ Rectal

not examined

▶ Neuro

A/O to person, date, location, and reason for visit. Able to answer direct questions, falling asleep between questions.

▶ Mental Status

Not examined

Laboratory Tests

Hospital Day 10

	Conventional Units	SI Units
WBC	$18.3 \times 10^3/mm^3$	$18.3 \times 109/L$
Hgb	12.1 g/dL	121 g/L; 7.5 mmol/L
Hct	36%	0.36
Plt	$224 \times 10^3/mm^3$	$224 \times 10^3/L$

Basic Metabolic Panel Hospital Day 10

	Conventional Units	SI Units
Na	134 mEq/L	134 mmol/L
K	4.1 mEq/L	4.1 mmol/L
Cl	98 mEq/L	98 mmol/L
CO_2	20 mEq/L	20 mmol/L
BUN	65 mg/dL	23.1 mmol/L
SCr	1.4 mg/dL (baseline 0.5 mg/dL)	123.8 µmol/L (baseline 44.2 µmol/L)
Glu	275 mg/dL	15.3 mmol/L
Ca	7.6 mg/dL	1.9 mmol/L
CRP	34.2 mg/L	
ESR	66 mm/hr	
Lactic acid	2.2 mg/dL	0.24 mmol/L
Hemoglobin	A1c 5.6%	0.056

Blood culture × 2 no growth to date

CXR: no consolidation

Humerus x-ray: soft tissue swelling with one focal area laterally at the level of humeral neck. No definite soft tissue emphysema. No acute fracture or dislocation

▶ Day 5 of Hospital Stay

Tissue culture from OR debridement *Streptococcus pyogenes* (group A)

Cefepime discontinued. Piperacilin/tazobactam 2.25 g q 6 h started

clindamycin and vancomycin continued

Procedures

Hospital day 2 irrigation and debridement (I&D) wound upper extremity. Placement wound vac right arm.

On hospital day 10, JL began having watery diarrhea, rise in serum creatinine from 0.5 to 1.8, and new leukocytosis following resolution of his initial leukocytosis. Watery stool was sent to the lab for toxin testing and PCR and the patient is found to be *C. difficile* positive. PCR testing reveal the strain is NAP1/B1/027 strain. The infectious diseases (ID) consult service agrees with the clinical pharmacist's recommendations to de-escalation the patient's antimicrobials and treat for a total duration of 14 days. Discontinue piperacillin/tazobactam, clindamycin, and vancomycin and start penicillin G 12 MU IV continuous infusion to end on hospital day 14. The patient's wound has been successfully irrigated and debrided.

Assessment

An 86-year-old man admitted for management of necrotizing fasciitis now presenting with signs, symptoms, and laboratory tests consistent with severe *Clostridium difficile* infection (CDI) that require therapy.

Student Work-Up

Missing Information/Inadequate Data

Evaluate: Patient database

Drug therapy problems

Care plan (by problem)

TARGETED QUESTIONS

1. What signs and symptoms of CDI does the patient have?
   Hint: See p. 1142 in PPP

2. What are the patient's risk factors for CDI?
   Hint: See pp. 1141-1142 in PPP

3. What antimicrobial agents are active against *C. difficile*?
   Hint: See p. 1141 in PPP

4. What antimicrobial agent(s) are most appropriate for the patient? (Please include dose, route, frequency, and duration of therapy.)
   Hint: See p. 1141 in PPP

5. List other pharmacologic and nonpharmacologic changes to the patient's therapy that may improve his outcome?
   Hint: See p. 1141 in PPP

FOLLOW-UP

The patient was discharged home on oral vancomycin 7 days ago and is clinically improving. His wife calls Dr. Ilsa Genevieve Luke to ask about fidaxomicin, she states she read online that it is a better treatment option for *C. difficile* infection. She would like her husband switched to this medication despite the cost.

What clinical and laboratory endpoints should be used to monitor the patient's progress?

Hint: See p. 1141 in PPP

Should Dr. Luke prescribe fidaxomicin for this patient? Is there a difference in recurrence rates between oral vancomycin and fidaxomicin?

Hint: See p. 1141 in PPP

What is the role, if any of probiotics in preventing recurrence of CDAD?

Hint: See p. 1142 in PPP

☉ GLOBAL PERSPECTIVE

Several outbreaks of *C. difficile* have been associated with highly virulent strain (NAP1/027) across the world, specifically first recognized in Canada and United Kingdom in 2003. Since this time, several other outbreaks have been associated with this strain of

C. difficile with high toxin production. Oral vancomycin therapy is currently recommended for severe *C. difficile* infection, but many patients may require surgical intervention. The availability of oral vancomycin therapy is limited in certain countries and the IV formulation of vancomycin administered orally is often prescribed.

CASE SUMMARY

- His current clinical picture is consistent with severe *C. difficile* infection.

- Oral vancomycin therapy would be a reasonable initial therapy for this patient with a dose of 500 mg po q 6 h in addition to metronidazole 500 mg IV q 8 h. The patient should be educated on appropriate use and potential GI side effects.

For more information on the care plan and facilitator's guide please visit http://www.mhpharmacotherapy.com

85 Intra-Abdominal Infection

Sarah M. Adriance   Brian L. Erstad

PATIENT PRESENTATION

Chief Complaint

"I have that pain in my abdomen again."

History of Present Illness

JK is 56-year-old male who presents with diffuse abdominal pain and a fever that was 101°F this morning at home. He increasingly has not been acting like himself per family member report, has eaten very little at meal times, and has also missed days of the medication he gets filled at the pharmacy.

Past Medical History

Alcoholic induced liver cirrhosis (diagnosed at age 49)

Spontaneous bacterial peritonitis (SBP) (approximately 1 year ago)

Surgical History

None

Family History

Father has hypertension and hyperlipidemia

Paternal grandfather died from myocardial infarction

Mother has hypothyroidism and breast cancer in remission

Social/Work History

Patient lives with sister and works as an electrician for a local company.

Tobacco/Alcohol/Substance Use

History of heavy alcohol consumption for 20 years, currently alcohol free. Last drink 1 year ago. No tobacco or illegal drug use.

Allergy/Intolerance/Adverse Event History

NKDA

Medication History (Current)

Disulfiram 250 mg daily

Spironolactone 200 mg daily

Furosemide 80 mg daily

Prior Medication Use

Spironolactone 100 mg daily

Furosemide 40 mg daily

Review of Systems

Patient's abdomen is bulging and tender; shifting dullness and tense ascites present. Persistent fever, malaise and decline in mental status has developed over previous 48 hours per family. Lower extremity edema present. An episode of SBP happened last year. Patient has never had any surgeries.

Physical Exam

▶ *General*

Caucasian male in moderate to severe acute distress with abdominal pain, swelling and mental status change from baseline.

Vital Signs

BP 102/60 mm Hg, P 103, RR 14, T 38.9°C

Weight 160 lb. (72.7 kg)

Height 74 in. (188 cm)

Abdominal Pain 9/10

▶ *Skin*

Mucous membrane color normal. No jaundice present

▶ *HEENT*

PERRLA, EOMI. No jaundice.

▶ *Neck and Lymph Nodes*

Supple; (–) lymphadenopathy

▶ *Chest*

Clear to auscultation

▶ *Cardiovascular*

RRR; normal S_1, S_2; (–) S_3 or S_4

▶ *Abdomen*

Bulging abdomen, tender upon palpation. (+) shifting dullness. Grade 4 (tense) ascites present.

▶ *Neurology*

Alert and oriented to Person only. To Place patient responded at "school" and to Date patient responded "1985" and unable to verbalize a month and date.

▶ *Extremities*

2+ Lower extremity edema

▶ *Genitourinary*

No oliguria

▶ *Rectal*

Deferred

Laboratory and Other Diagnostic Tests

Laboratory

	Conventional Units	SI Units
Na	135 mEq/L	135 mmol/L
K	3.9 mEq/L	3.9 mmol/L
Cl	91 mEq/L	91 mmol/L
CO_2	23 mEq/L	23 mmol/L
BUN	20 mg/dL	7.14 mmol/L
SCr	1.2 mg/dL	106.08 µmol/L
Glu	102 mg/dL	5.7 mmol/L
Ca	9.2 mg/dL	2.3 mmol/L
Mg	1.8 mEq/L	0.74 mmol/L
Phosphate	4.2 mg/dL	1.36 mmol/L
Hemoglobin	9.8 g/dL	98 g/L; 60.8 mmol/L
Hematocrit	29.2%	0.292
MCV	85 µm³	85 fL
WBC	12.5×10^3/mm³	12.5×10^9/L
WBC Differential % polymorphonu-clear neutrophils (PMN)/ eosinophils/ basophils/ lymphocytes/ monocytes	96.5/0.05/0.05/ 2.5/0.9	
WBC Differential % Bands	63	
Platelet	135×10^3/mm³	135×10^9/L
Albumin	2.4 g/dL	24 g/L
Bilirubin (Total)	1.2 mg/dL	20.52 µmol/L
Bilirubin (Direct)	0.3 mg/dL	5.13 µmol/L
AST	65 IU/L	1.08 µkat/L
ALT	51 IU/L	0.85 µkat/L
Alk Phos	124 IU/L	2.07 µkat/L
INR	1.6	
Prealbumin	10 mg/dL	100 mg/L
Ammonia	110 µ/dL	65 µmol/L

▶ *Imaging*

CT abdomen and pelvis showed cirrhotic liver, splenomegaly, and ascites. No ruptured viscus or obstruction.

▶ *Microbiologic Data*

Blood cultures pending

Ascitic fluid culture pending

▶ *Diagnostic Paracentesis*

Ascitic fluid analysis pending

Assessment

A 56-year-old male with signs and symptoms of a spontaneous bacterial peritonitis without hypovolemic shock at this time. An intra-abdominal source of infection has been ruled out with imaging and no surgical history.

Student Work-Up

Missing Information/Inadequate Data

Evaluate:	Patient database
	Drug therapy problems
	Care plan (by problem)

TARGETED QUESTIONS

1. What characteristics of the patient's case are consistent with a primary peritonitis or SBP?

   Hint: See p. 1147 in PPP

2. How does primary peritonitis management largely differ from secondary peritonitis?

   Hint: See p. 1149 in PPP

3. What are the likely pathogens given this patient's history and which antimicrobial would you choose to start empirically and why?

   Hint: See p. 1149 in PPP

4. When do most patients show clinical improvement after antimicrobials are started for intra-abdominal infections?

   Hint: See p. 1153 in PPP

5. In what circumstances would a typical course of 4-7 days of antibiotic therapy be inadequate?

   Hint: See p. 1154 in PPP

FOLLOW-UP

Patient JK was started on an IV antibiotic as soon as SBP was suspected and IV fluids were initiated. A large volume paracentesis was completed shortly after admission and 2 L of serosanguinous ascitic fliud were drained. Ascitic fluid cell count showed predominance in polymorphonuclear neutrophils (PMNs) with 265 PMNs/mm³. Albumin concentration in the fluid was <1 mg/dL. The calculated serum-ascites albumin gradient (SAAG) was >1.1 g/dL and the ascitic fluid total protein (AFTP) was <2.5 g/dL pointing to a cirrhotic cause of ascites. Forty-eight hours later the ascitic fluid culture grew *Klebsiella pneumoniae*, susceptibility and sensitivity report is still pending.

What is a common cause of early death in patients presenting with SBP and how can it be prevented?

Hint: See p. 1149 in PPP

☼ GLOBAL PERSPECTIVE

Gram-negative enteric organisms are the most common cause of SBP in cirrhotic patients, which is why empiric therapy with a third-generation cephalosporin (ceftriaxone, cefotaxime) is warranted. Gram-positive organisms however are rarely reported to cause SBP. Interestingly outside of the U.S. they are increasingly being implicated in the development of SBP in patients with underlying alcoholic liver disease or in liver cirrhosis. For example gram-positive organisms such as *Listeria monocytogenes*, *Bacillus cereus*, *Enterococcus cassiflavus* and *Enterococcus gallinarum*, which all rarely cause human disease, have been reported in case series and case reports of SBP. Infection with these organisms are documented in the scientific literature to increase awareness of their ability to cause disease in this patient population and to highlight the need to consider alternate or additional empiric antibiotic coverage as a third-generation cephalosporin would be inadequate therapy.

CASE SUMMARY

- The clinical presentation and past medical history of patient JK are typical and consistent with a primary peritonitis. Analysis of ascitic fluid following a paracentesis is key to confirm the diagnosis in which findings of PMNs ≥250/mm³ and isolation of a single organism are representative of an ascitic fluid infection caused by SBP in the absence of an intra-abdominal source of infection.

- In addition to patient JK's prior episode of SBP, his noncompliance with prescribed diuretics precipitates the development of ascites and also places him at higher risk of developing this infection.

- Early initiation of appropriate empiric antibiotic therapy is the mainstay of treatment in primary peritonitis and includes a third-generation cephalosporin. Initiation of antibiotics should not be delayed for the results of the ascitic fluid analysis.

For more information on the care plan and facilitator's guide please visit http://www.mhpharmacotherapy.com

86 Uncomplicated Urinary Tract Infection

Ronak Gandhi   Kathryn R. Matthias

PATIENT PRESENTATION

Chief Complaint
"It hurts when I pee."

History of Present Illness
Megan Ryder is a 25-year-old female who presents to your outpatient clinic for the first time complaining of painful urination and increased frequency for the past 3 days, which is completely new to her. The patient said her friend had similar symptoms and was treated by her primary care physician for something called a "urine infection" and wanted to know if she had the same problem. The patient also reports she took a course of antibiotics about 6 months ago when she had her wisdom teeth removed but cannot recall the name of the antibiotic.

Past Medical History
Exercise induced asthma

Keratoconjunctivitis sicca

Surgical History
Wisdom teeth removal 6 months ago

Family History
Mother and father are both alive. Father is 55 and has a history of diabetes and hypertension, and mother is 50 with a history of hyperlipidemia and psoriasis.

Social History
Patient is currently employed as a secretary at a law firm with health insurance. She is currently engaged and denies smoking, intravenous drug abuse, and drinks occasionally on the weekends.

Allergies
Penicillin (based on what her mother told her)

Medications
Albuterol inhaler, 2 puffs 30 minutes prior to exercise

Cyclosporine ophthalmic 0.05%, instill 1 drop in each eye every 12 hours

Review of System
Denies chest pain, shortness of breath, abdominal pain; (+) dysuria; (+) increase in urinary frequency (10-12 times per day for the past 3 days)

Physical Examination

▶ *General*

Well-appearing, 25-year-old Caucasian female in no acute distress

▶ *Vital Signs*

BP 118/72 mm Hg, P 98, RR 18, T 37.7°C

Weight 110 lb. (50 kg)

Height 64 in. (162.5 cm)

▶ *Skin*

Dry appearing skin; (–) rashes, (+) acne lesions

▶ *HEENT*

PERRLA with redness, EOMI; (–) sinus tenderness; TM appears normal

▶ *Neck and Lymph Nodes*

Thyroid gland symmetrical; (–) nodules; (–) lymphadenopathy

▶ *Chest*

Clear to auscultation

▶ *Cardiovascular*

Irregularly irregular rate, normal S_1, S_2, (–) S_3, (–) S_4

▶ *Abdomen*

Not tender; not distended; (–) organomegaly

▶ **Neurology**

Grossly Intact; DTRs normal

▶ **Extremities**

No swelling, redness, or pain

▶ **Genitourinary**

Normal external genitalia; (–) vaginal discharge; no costovertebral angle tenderness

▶ **Rectal**

No hemorrhoids

Laboratory Tests

	Conventional Units	SI Units
Na	135 mEq/L	135 mmol/L
K	5.0 mEq/L	5.0 mmol/L
Cl	106 mEq/L	106 mmol/L
CO_2	24 mEq/L	24 mmol/L
BUN	5 mg/dL	1.8 mmol/L
SCr	0.6 mg/dL	53 µmol/L
Glu	70 mg/dL	3.9 mmol/L
WBC	$12.1 \times 10^3/\mu L$	$12.1 \times 10^9/L$
HgB	12 g/dL	7.44 mmol/L
HcT	36%	0.36 (fraction)
Platelets	$250 \times 10^3/\mu L$	$250 \times 10^9/L$

▶ **Urinalysis**

pH	5.2	
Specific Gravity	1.023	
WBC	30 cells/mm³	$30 \times 10^6/L$
RBC	2 cells/mm³	$2 \times 10^6/L$
Proteins	Trace	
Glucose	(–)	
Ketones	(–)	
Blood	(–)	
Nitrite	(+)	
Leukocyte esterase	(+)	

Urine Cultures:

(+) 4+ Lactose fermenting Gram-negative rods (final results pending)

(+) 1+ yeast (final results pending)

Pregnancy Test Negative

Assessment

Twenty-five-year-old woman with symptoms and laboratory tests consistent with uncomplicated UTI.

Student Work-Up

Missing Information/Inadequate Data

Evaluate: Patient database

Drug therapy problems

Care plan (by problem)

TARGETED QUESTIONS

1. What signs and symptoms of an uncomplicated UTI does the patient have?

   Hint: See p. 1170 and Table 79-1 in PPP

2. What risk factors does the patient have for uncomplicated UTIs?

   Hint: See p. 1170 in PPP

3. If any, which antibiotic treatment options including duration of therapy should be considered in this patient?

   Hint: See pp. 1171-1173 and Tables 79-2 and 79-3 in PPP

4. If any, which antifungal treatment options including duration of therapy should be considered in this patient?

5. What risks and adverse effects of therapy should be discussed with the patient?

   Hint: See p. 1175 and Table 79-4 in PPP

FOLLOW-UP

One day later, the patient's urine culture and susceptibility results are reported:

Urine culture:

Escherichia coli

Candida albicans

>100,000 Escherichia coli

Drug	Interpretation	MIC (mcg/mL or mg/L)
Ampicillin/sulbactam	Susceptible	≤8/4
Amoxicillin-clavulanic acid	Susceptible	≤8/4
Cefazolin	Susceptible (urine)	8
Ceftriaxone	Susceptible	1
Ciprofloxacin	Susceptible	≤1
Gentamicin	Susceptible	1
Levofloxacin	Susceptible	1
Meropenem	Susceptible	≤0.25
Nitrofurantoin	Resistant	≥64
Tigecycline	Susceptible	≤4
Trimethoprim/ sulfamethoxazole	Susceptible	≤1/19

100-1000 Candida albicans

Drug	Interpretation	MIC (mcg/mL or mg/L)
Fluconazole	Susceptible	≤2
Caspofungin	Susceptible	≤0.25
Voriconazole	Susceptible	≤0.12

Based on the above cultures and susceptibility along with the patient's clinical status and past medical history, how would you change the patient's UTI therapy?

> *Hint: See pp. 1171-1173 in PPP*

⊘ GLOBAL PERSPECTIVE

Pivmecillinam is an oral Beta-lactam antibiotic that is considered a first line treatment per the 2011 International Clinical Practice Guidelines for the treatment of Acute Uncomplicated Cystitis. Per the guidelines Pivmecillinam 200-400 mg twice daily for 3-7 days provides adequate treatment for uncomplicated cystitis, however it is currently not available in the United States but the agent of choice in many European countries.

Pivmecillinam is the bioavailable form of mecillinam and is distinguished from other Beta-lactams because of its specificity for the urinary tract with minimal resistance or propensity for collateral damage. In a clinical study comparing 200 mg 3 times a day for 7 days, 200 mg twice a day for 7 days, and 400 mg twice a day for 4 days demonstrated clinical cure in 62%, 66%, and 55% respectively with bacteriologic cure rate of 93%, 94%, and 84% respectively. In a comparison to norfloxacin, pivmecillinam treatment resulted in lower bacterial and clinical cure. Overall efficacy rate is lower than many of the first line agents used in the United States, but *E. coli* resistance remains low.

REFERENCE

1. Gupta K, Hooton TM, et al. International Clinical Practice Guidelines for the Treatment of Acute Uncomplicated Cystitis an Pyelonephritis in Women: A 2010 update by the Infectious Diseases Society of America and the European Society of Microbiology and Infectious Diseases. Clin Infect Dis 2011 52:103-120.

CASE SUMMARY

- The patient's signs and symptoms are consistent with an uncomplicated urinary tract infection.

- Although there are several options for empiric treatment for uncomplicated urinary tract infection, patient-specific factors including allergies, renal function, drug-drug interactions, and teratogenicity potential should be evaluated prior to starting treatment.

- The patient should be counseled on potential adverse effects of antibiotics therapy.

For more information on the care plan and facilitator's guide please visit http://www.mhpharmacotherapy.com

87 Complicated Urinary Tract Infection

John J. Radosevich

PATIENT PRESENTATION

Chief Complaint

From patient's daughter: "She is not acting like herself… she seems really confused."

History of Present Illness

Erica Rhodes is a 64-year-old female that lives with her daughter who presents with confusion, fever, chills, nausea, and vomiting. Initial differential diagnosis includes sepsis with possible sources including meningitis, bacteremia, intra-abdominal, or urinary tract. On the basis of diagnostic studies including a chest x-ray and CT scan along with laboratory data, it is determined that the patient's altered mental status is due to a complicated UTI and dehydration from acute N/V. The patient is started on ciprofloxacin 200 mg IV q 12 h in the emergency department.

Past Medical History

Paraplegia s/p motor vehicle accident (MVA)

Neurogenic bladder s/p suprapubic catheter (changed every 3 months—last changed 1 week ago); history of *Klebsiella pneumoniae* extended spectrum β-lactamase (ESBL) urinary tract infections

Hypertension

Past Surgical History

History of spinal surgery s/p MVA (procedure unknown)

Suprapubic catheter placement

Cholecystectomy

Family History

Mother died at the age of 90 and had a past medical history significant for hypothyroidism and transient ischemic attack. Father died at the age of 75 and had a past medical history significant for type 2 diabetes mellitus and hypertension. Patient has 1 child and 2 grandchildren, none with any significant medical history.

Social History

Patient currently lives with her daughter and grandchildren in her daughter's home. As per the patient's daughter, she does not smoke or drink alcohol.

Allergies/Intolerances/Adverse Drug Events

Ciprofloxacin (severe pruritus)

Medications

Amlodipine 10 mg po daily

Lisinopril 20 mg po daily

Pantoprazole 40 mg po daily

Acetaminophen 500 mg po q 6 h prn pain

Multivitamin po daily

Review of Systems

(+) Fever; (+) vomiting; (−) eye changes; (−) neck pain

Physical Examination

▶ **General**

Acutely ill female with decreased level of consciousness who is sleepy but arousable and able to answer yes and no questions, but she is disoriented to time.

▶ **Vital Signs**

BP 111/51 mm Hg, P 105, RR 26, T 38.4° C, saturation 99% (0.99) on 2 liters/min of oxygen via nasal cannula

Weight 206.8 lb. (94 kg)

Height 59.8 in. (152 cm)

▶ **Skin**

Dry appearing skin; (−) rashes or lesions; (+) suprapubic catheter in place

▶ **HEENT**

PERRLA, EOMI, head normocephalic, mucous membranes dry, no thrush

► **Neck and Lymph Nodes**

(–) Nodules; (–) lymphadenopathy

► **Chest**

Clear to auscultation bilaterally

► **Cardiovascular**

RRR, normal S_1, S_2; no murmurs

► **Abdomen**

Not tender; not distended; (+) bowel sounds

► **Neurology**

Patient will open eyes to gentle stimulus; oriented to self; she is able to follow commands and move extremities

► **Genitourinary**

Normal external genitalia

► **Rectal**

No hemorrhoids

Laboratory Tests

	Conventional Units	SI Units
Na	140 mEq/L	140 mmol/L
K	4.1 mEq/L	4.1 mmol/L
Cl	108 mEq/L	108 mmol/L
CO_2	20 mEq/L	20 mmol/L
BUN	32 mg/dL	11.4 mmol/L
SCr	2.5 mg/dL	221 µmol/L
Glu	136 mg/dL	7.6 mmol/L
Ca	9.0 mg/dL	2.25 mmol/L
WBC	$16.4 \times 10^3/mm^3$	$16.4 \times 10^9/L$
Neutrophils	82%	0.82
Bands	9%	0.09
Hgb	13.1 g/dL	121 g/L; 7.51 mmol/L
HCT	39.6%	0.396
Platelets	$174 \times 10^3/mm^3$	$174 \times 10^9/L$
Urinalysis		Urine is yellow, cloudy
pH	5.50	
SG	1.012	
WBC	>150 cells/mm³	$>150 \times 10^6/L$
RBC	25 cells/mm³	$48 \times 10^6/L$
Protein	(+)	
Glucose	(–)	
Ketones	(–)	
Blood	Moderate	
Nitrite	(+)	
Casts	(+)	
Leukocyte Esterase	(+)	
Urine toxicology	(–)	

Urine cultures (from suprapubic catheter): results finalized on day 2 of admission

Escherichia coli (>100,000 colonies/mL [$>100 \times 10^6$/L])

Drug	Interpretation	MIC (mcg/mL or mg/L)
Ampicillin	Resistant	>16
Ampicillin/Sulbactam	Resistant	>16/8
Cefazolin	Susceptible	1
Ceftriaxone	Susceptible	1
Cefepime	Susceptible	1
Levofloxacin	Susceptible	≤1
Gentamicin	Susceptible	≤2
Meropenem	Susceptible	1
Nitrofurantoin	Susceptible	≤16
Piperacillin/tazobactam	Susceptible	≤2/4
Trimethoprim/ sulfamethoxazole	Susceptible	1/19

Blood Cultures:

(+) *Esherichia coli*—see above for susceptibility

Assessment

Sixty-four-year-old woman with a recent suprapubic catheter exchange who presents with s/s and laboratory tests consistent with a complicated UTI with associated bacteremia.

Student Work-Up

Missing Information/Inadequate Data

Evaluate: Patient database

Drug therapy problems

Care plan (by problem)

TARGETED QUESTIONS

1. What risk factors and characteristics does the patient have consistent with a complicated UTI?

   Hint: See p. 1170 and Table 79-1 in PPP

2. How does the patient's suprapubic catheter affect your decision to diagnose and treat a complicated UTI?

   Hint: See p. 1174 and Table 79-1 in PPP

3. On day 2, the patient's serum creatinine has decreased to 0.8 mg/dL (70.7 μmol/L), and urine culture results are reported as above. On the basis of the patient's urine culture and clinical factors, what changes do you recommend to the patient's UTI therapy?

   Hint: See pp. 1171-1173 and Table 79-2 in PPP

4. How should the patient be monitored for resolution of infection and ADEs?

   Hint: See p. 1175 in PPP

5. How long should the patient continue UTI therapy?

   Hint: See pp. 1171-1173 in PPP

FOLLOW-UP

The patient's UTI symptoms improved over the first 72 hours of her admission, repeat blood cultures are negative, and she is ready for discharge home on day 5 of the current admission. The patient's internal medicine team consults the clinical pharmacist to provide a recommendation for oral therapy to complete the course of antibiotics.

What would be an appropriate oral regimen for the patient?

   Hint: See pp. 1171-1175 and Tables 79-2 and 79-3 in PPP

⦿ GLOBAL PERSPECTIVE

Worldwide, the most common cause of nosocomial infection is associated with the use of urinary catheters that lead to UTIs.[1,2] Patients with an indwelling catheter have an estimated daily 5% incidence of UTIs. Therefore, the best way to avoid catheter-associated UTIs is to remove the catheter when no longer indicated as soon as possible based on the patient's clinical status. In addition, catheter associated UTI has been estimated to cost more than 4 times the cost of symptomatic UTI in a patient without a catheter.[3]

CASE SUMMARY

- The patient's signs and symptoms are consistent with a complicated UTI.
- Although the majority of UTIs are caused by *E. coli*, non-*E. coli* causes are more common in patients with complicated UTIs, patients with recurrent UTIs, and nosocomial UTIs.
- Recommended duration of therapy is usually longer for complicated UTIs and catheter-associated UTIs compared with uncomplicated UTIs.

REFERENCES

1. Hooton TM, Bradley SF, Cardenas DD, et al. Diagnosis, prevention, and treatment of catheter-associated urinary tract infection in adults: 2009 International Clinical Practice Guidelines from the Infectious Diseases Society of America. Clin Infect Dis 2010;50:625-663.
2. Gould CV, Umscheid CA, Agarwal RK, et al. Healthcare Infection Control Practices Advisory Committee: guideline for prevention of catheter associated urinary tract infections, 2009. www.cdc.gov/hicpac/cauti/001_ cauti. html. Accessed April 17, 2013.
3. Saint S. Clinical and economic consequences of nosocomial catheter-related bacteriuria. Am J Infect Control 2000;28:68-75.

For more information on the care plan and facilitator's guide please visit http://www.mhpharmacotherapy.com

88 Syphilis

Lawrence David York   Kathryn R. Matthias

PATIENT PRESENTATION

Chief Complaint

"I have a rash everywhere, my head hurts, and my neck feels swollen."

History of Present Illness

A 48-year-old Caucasian male presents to a free public clinic with complaints of a systemic rash, headache, and lymphadenopathy. He states the rash and lymphadenopathy have been present for "several months" and decided to come in due to his persistent headaches as the rash and swelling have not bothered him. He states these started 2 months ago and, while not significantly painful, have been occurring more frequently and range from 13 to 16 times monthly. He generally experiences them "on both sides" of his head and sometimes feel like he is carrying weight on his shoulders. He is also concerned that he is going bald as he has noted patches of hair missing in his beard and on his head.

Past Medical History

HIV (6 years)

HTN (15 years)

Family History

Has not had contact with family for several years. Recalls father having diabetes and "heart issues." Does not recall mother having any health issues. Reports being an only child.

Social History

The patient has been electively homeless for 4 years. He denies any children but endorses having multiple sexual partners in the past. He is currently monogamous with one partner he has been seeing for approximately 1.5 years.

Tobacco/Alcohol/Substance Abuse

Smokes 0.5 ppd × 32 years; 3-4 beers weekly; previously injected heroin × 11 years but has been abstinent × 1 year

Allergies/Intolerances/Adverse Drug Events

ACE-inhibitors (angioedema)

Medications (Current)

Emtricitabine/tenofovir disoproxil fumarate 200/300 mg po daily

Dolutegravir 50 mg po daily

Acetaminophen 1000 mg po q 6 h prn

Review of Systems

Headache (HA) with occasional relief from acetaminophen; (–) dizziness; (–) vertigo; (–) photo/phonophobia; (+) cervical lymphadenopathy; maculopapular rash on torso/palms/soles; (+) patchy alopecia; A&O × 3

Physical Examination

▶ **General**

Ill-appearing adult male in no acute distress

▶ **Vital Signs**

BP 149/84 mm Hg, P 75, RR 16, T 38°C

Weight 162.8 lb. (74 kg)

Height 71 in. (180.34 cm)

▶ **Skin**

Red maculopapular lesions on torso, palms, and soles; hair and beard appear patchy/moth-eaten

▶ **HEENT**

PERRLA, EOMI, mucous membranes moist

▶ **Neck**

Minimally tender, firm posterior cervical lymphadenopathy

▶ **Neurology**

Speech and thinking appropriate to situation, cranial nerves intact. Nonpulsating pain rated 4/10 bilaterally on temporal aspects of skull.

▶ **Chest**

Bilateral wheezes on inspiration and expiration

▶ **Cardiovascular**

RRR, normal S_1, S_2; no murmurs

▶ *Abdomen*

Soft, nontender, nondistended

▶ *Genitourinary*

Examination refused

▶ *Rectal*

Examination refused

Laboratory Tests

	Conventional Units	SI Units
Na	136 mEq/mL	136 mmol/L
K	4.8 mEq/L	4.8 mmol/L
Cl	100 mEq/L	100 mmol/L
BUN	15 mg/dL	5.4 mmol/L
SCr	1.1 mg/dL	97.2 umol/L
Glucose	130 mg/dL	7.15 mmol/L
Hgb	10.4 g/dL	6.46 pmol/L
Hct	30.1%	0.301
WBC	$10.0 \times 10^3/mm^3$	$10.0 \times 10^9/L$
Lymphocytes	18.4%	0.184
Monocytes	7.0%	0.07
Eosinophils	0.5%	0.005
Basophils	0.3%	0.003
Neutrophils	73.8%	0.738
ANC	$7.40 \times 10^3/mm^3$	$7.4 \times 10^9/L$
HIV RNA	<20 copies/mL	
Absolute CD_4	726 cells/mm³	$726 \times 10^6/L$
RPR	1:128	

▶ *Blood Cultures*

No growth in 2/2 cultures

▶ *CSF Findings*

	Conventional Units	SI Units
WBC	2 cells/mm³	$2 \times 10^6/L$
Protein	19 mg/dL	190 mg/L
Glucose	77 mg/dL	4.2 mmol/L
Gram stain	Negative	
VDRL	Nonreactive	
FTA-ABS	Negative	

Assessment

A 48-year-old male with signs and symptoms, and laboratory tests consistent with secondary syphilis and frequent episodic tension-type HAs.

Student Work-Up

Missing Information/Inadequate Data

Evaluate: Patient database

Drug therapy problems

Care plan (by problem)

TARGETED QUESTIONS

1. Which microbial organism is responsible for causing syphilis and how did this patient likely acquire it?

   Hint: See p. 1183 in PPP

2. What clinical features are associated with secondary syphilis? What additional lab values might be useful to obtain in evaluating additional systemic effects of the patient's disease?

   Hint: See p. 1183 in PPP

3. What is the preferred medication, dose, route of administration, and number of doses to treat the patient's condition? What reaction should you warn the patient about after starting therapy and what should you do if it occurs?

   Hint: See pp. 1184-1188 and Figure 80-1 in PPP

4. If the patient had documented anaphylaxis to penicillin in the past 3 years, what alternate medication regimens (drug/dose/route/duration) could be considered and what are some advantages/disadvantages to using them?

   Hint: See p. 1184 in PPP

5. What follow-up would you schedule for the patient and what monitoring parameters would you wish to continue evaluating? What would you do if the patient failed to meet your desired endpoints?

   Hint: See p. 1188 and Table 80-1 in PPP

6. How would your therapeutic recommendations change if the patient presented with a history of maculopapular rash that had since resolved and a predicted date of infection more than 1 year ago?

   Hint: See pp. 1184-1188 in PPP

FOLLOW-UP

At his 6-month follow-up, the patient presents with his girlfriend who complains of vision changes. The patient states she has also recently not been acting like herself. Work-up is performed and the patient is found to have a VDRL (venereal disease research laboratory) of 1:64 in her cerebrospinal fluid.

What is your preferred treatment regimen for the patient's girlfriend?

The patient's girlfriend is refusing hospital admission at this time but is willing to come to clinic daily for treatment if necessary. What regimen may be used in this setting if adherence can be assured?

If the patient's girlfriend reported that she had a severe anaphylactic reaction to penicillin in the recent past, how would this alter your therapeutic recommendations? What course of action would be pursued and how would it be done?

⊙ GLOBAL PERSPECTIVE

Syphilis persists as one of the leading sexually transmitted infections across the world with approximately 10-12 million new cases each year. Concerns for unforeseen morbidity and mortality exist given that a large population of patients infected with syphilis may present asymptomatically. In some parts of the world, syphilis remains a substantial cause of stillbirths and miscarriages in pregnant patients. Failure to identify the presence of this disease early enough may also lead to irreversible hepatic, renal, cardiac, and neurological damage and, in extreme cases, death. Health care providers should be cognizant of the potentially elusive presentation of this particular STD and evaluate the sexual history of a patient at risk for contraction of syphilis. Though simple and relatively affordable to treat, global access to health care is a limiting factor as patients must be able to receive their full course of treatment and receive adequate, timely follow-up to assess disease response and possible need for continued treatment. As young patients (age 15-24) make up approximately 20% of the American population newly infected with syphilis each year, early sexual education may be beneficial in reducing the rates of STD infections and decreasing overall health care costs.

CASE SUMMARY

- The patient presents with a history of high-risk sexual behavior and concomitant HIV.
- The clinical presentation is consistent with secondary/early syphilis and requires treatment.
- The patient's partner should also be evaluated for syphilis and treated appropriately.

For more information on the care plan and facilitator's guide please visit http://www.mhpharmacotherapy.com

89 Gonorrhea, Chlamydia, and Herpes Simplex Type 2

David E. Nix

PATIENT PRESENTATION

Chief Complaint

"I have been having pain when I urinate. I tried an over-the-counter drug, but it didn't help. I just can't take it anymore. And please don't forget to refill all of my narcotics. Last time, the nurse only called in one of them."

History of Present Illness

CR is a 47-year-old Latin American female who regularly visits the local community health center for myriad health reasons, with the latest visit revolving around complaints of a purulent, vaginal discharge and pain on urination. After self-testing with Azo Test Strips and detecting a positive result, she subsequently began orally taking phenazopyridine for 4 days with minimal relief. She admits that her dysuric symptoms commenced approximately 10 days prior and have worsened over the past 2 days. Additionally, she admits to observing a cluster of small, painful, itchy bumps in her vaginal area. When asked by the clinician to describe her recent sexual history, she acknowledged that she does not have a steady boyfriend and that she currently engages in frequent sexual activity with two men, one of which she traveled to Hawaii with last week for vacation. Finally, as she requested a refill on her narcotics and her cholesterol medications, she divulged that she has been constipated for 3 days although she has been taking docusate sodium for 2 consecutive days.

Past Medical History

Hyperlipidemia (diagnosed 1 year ago)

Back pain from car accident that occured 3 months ago

Family History

The patient's father had coronary artery disease and died of a myocardial infarction at age 70. Her mother is alive at age 64 with hypertension, diabetes, and osteoporosis. She has two sisters, one of which has been recently diagnosed with diabetes.

Social History

The patient migrated to the United States at age 16 from Mexico. She speaks fluent Spanish and English, and is a single mother, who lives alone with one son, age 20, from a previous marriage. As a result of the recession, her original job as a receptionist for a car dealership was terminated 4 months ago. She was recently hired (3 weeks prior to her visit) as a receptionist for a prominent law firm.

Tobacco/Alcohol/Substance Abuse

Social drinker; (−) tobacco or illicit drug use

Allergies/Intolerances/Adverse Drug Events

Tetracycline (rash as a child)

Propoxyphene (rash)

Medications

Atorvastatin 40 mg po q AM

Calcium carbonate one to two tablets po q 8-12 h prn

Docusate sodium 100 mg po q AM

Hydrocodone 7.5 mg/acetaminophen 325 mg one to two tablets po q 4-6 h prn pain

Oxycodone 5 mg/acetaminophen 325 mg two tablets po q 4-6 h prn severe pain

Acetaminophen 325 mg one to two capsules po q 4-6 h prn pain

Review of Systems

Occasional headaches relieved by acetaminophen; (−) fever; (−) tinnitus and vertigo; increased urinary frequency with pain; (+) bowel distention on palpation; (−) history of seizures, syncope, or loss of consciousness; reports "tingling" in the extremities; (−) rhabdomyolysis; dry mucus membranes; deep and rapid breathing.

Physical Examination

▶ **General**

Overweight, middle-aged, Latin American woman in no acute distress

▶ **Vital Signs**

BP 126/79 mm Hg, P 74, RR 22, T 37.2°C (99.0°F)

Weight 190.3 lb. (86.5 kg)

Height 66 in. (168 cm)

▶ **Skin**

Skin slightly dry; (–) rash or lesions

▶ **HEENT**

PERRLA; EOMI; TMs appear normal

▶ **Neck and Lymph Nodes**

Thyroid gland smooth and symmetrical; (–) thyroid nodules; (+) lymphadenopathy

▶ **Chest**

Clear to auscultation

▶ **Breasts**

Examination deferred

▶ **Cardiovascular**

RRR, normal S_1, S_2; (–) S_3 or S_4

▶ **Abdomen**

Nontender/distended; (–) organomegaly

▶ **Neurology**

Grossly intact; deep tendon reflexes normal

▶ **Genitourinary**

Cluster of vesicles; (+) vaginal discharge

▶ **Rectal**

Examination deferred

Laboratory Tests

Fasting, Obtained 3 months ago

	Conventional Units	SI Units
Na	139 mEq/L	139 mmol/L
K	4.4 mEq/L	4.4 mmol/L
Cl	103 mEq/L	103 mmol/L
CO_2	22 mEq/L	22 mmol/L
BUN	12 mg/dL	4.3 mmol/L
SCr	0.9 mg/dL	80 mmol/L
Glu	135 mg/dL	7.5 mmol/L
Ca	10.1 mg/dL	2.53 mmol/L
Mg	1.7 mEq/L	0.85 mmol/L
Phosphate	3.7 mg/dL	1.20 mmol/L
pH (arterial)	7.38	
Hgb	13 g/dL	130 g/L; 8.07 mmol/L
Hct	41%	0.41
WBC	$4.1 \times 10^3/mm^3$	$4.1 \times 10^9/L$
MCV	89 μm³	89 fL
Albumin	3.9 g/dL	39 g/L
Total cholesterol	183 mg/dL	4.73 mmol/L
LDL cholesterol	91 mg/dL	2.35 mmol/L
HDL cholesterol	36 mg/dL	0.93 mmol/L
AST	45 IU/L	0.75 μkat/L
ALT	51 IU/L	0.85 μkat/L
HbA1c	6.9%	0.069

Fasting, Obtained Yesterday

	Conventional Units	SI Units
Na	135 mEq/L	135 mmol/L
K	3.5 mEq/L	3.5 mmol/L
Cl	107 mEq/L	107 mmol/L
CO_2	23 mEq/L	23 mmol/L
BUN	40 mg/dL	14.3 mmol/L
SCr	1.3 mg/dL	115 mmol/L
Glu	180 mg/dL	10 mmol/L
Ca	10.1 mg/dL	2.53 mmol/L
Mg	1.8 mEq/L	0.90 mmol/L
Phosphate	3.8 mg/dL	1.23 mmol/L
pH (arterial)	7.41	
Urinalysis	(+) ketones	
Hgb	14 g/dL	140 g/L; 8.69 mmol/L
Hct	42%	0.42
WBC	$10.7 \times 10^3/mm^3$	$10.7 \times 10^9/L$
MCV	88 μm³	88 fL
Albumin	3.7 g/dL	37 g/L
Total cholesterol	185 mg/dL	4.78 mmol/L
LDL cholesterol	92 mg/dL	2.38 mmol/L
HDL cholesterol	34 mg/dL	0.88 mmol/L
AST	120 IU/L	2 μkat/L
ALT	130 IU/L	2.17 μkat/L

▶ **Urethral Exudate**

Gram stain shows many Gram negative diplococci (some intracellular). *C. trachomatis* and *N. gonorrheae* nucleic acid identification testing ordered for confirmation.

Assessment

A 47-year-old woman with signs and symptoms consistent with a gonococcal infection.

Further, the patient has constipation and hyperlipidemia.

Student Work-Up

Missing Information/Inadequate Data

Evaluate:	Patient database
	Drug therapy problems
	Care plan (by problem)

TARGETED QUESTIONS

1. What are the signs and symptoms of a gonococcal infection?

   Hint: See p. 1180 in PPP

2. Are there any other possible infections besides gonorrhea?

   Hint: See p. 1179 in PPP

3. When infected with gonorrhea, what is the probability of a coinfection?

   Hint: See pp. 1182 in PPP

4. What would be the recommended drug therapy for gonococcal infections in patients with anaphylaxis to cephalosporins?

   Hint: See the CDC 2015 Sexually Transmitted Diseases Treatment Guidelines: http://www.cdc.gov/std/tg2015/

5. Should treatment be provided for her partner?

   Hint: See pp. 1181 and 1182 in PPP

6. What is the etiology of the elevated hepatic enzymes?

   Hint: Liver enzymes may be elevated for a variety of reasons. Since the patient's past medical history is inconsistent with hepatic damage, a medication-induced elevation of liver enzymes is a reasonable suspicion

FOLLOW-UP

Twelve weeks later, the patient returns for a follow-up. Although re-evaluation of her infection is not required, it is vital to express the importance of altering her sexual behaviors and reiterate the importance of practicing preventive measures (i.e., condoms, spermicides) and to determine whether her partners have received treatment. Essential to this process is an interaction between the patient and a knowledgeable, yet patient-friendly, clinician.

How can this be accomplished?

Hint: See p. 1179 in PPP

Finally, the clinician and the patient must gain control of her chronic conditions promoting a healthy diet, exercise, and continuous self-monitoring.

🌐 GLOBAL PERSPECTIVE

Globally, new cases of sexually transmitted diseases (STDs) amenable to antimicrobial treatment amount to approximately 340 million per year. Evidence supports the need for better control of gonorrhea, especially with the emergence of fluoroquinolone-resistant strains of *Neisseria gonorrhoeae*. Such strains have been documented in several other countries, including Australia, China, India, Korea, and New Zealand. Another notable concern is the appearance of diminished gonococcal susceptibility to the third-generation cephalosporins, of which cefixime and ceftriaxone are commonly prescribed as effective options. Once 5% resistance or more to an antibiotic is recognized, the WHO recommends that the antibiotic be removed from the treatment recommendations for gonorrhea. Diminished susceptibility of *N. gonorrhoeae* to drugs of choice has been attributed to the overuse and misuse of antibiotics in a nonregulated environment. Although instituting change may be complex, global integration of treatment measures may be more feasible than continuing to rely on antibiotics as the primary mechanism of control.

CASE SUMMARY

- Her clinical picture is consistent with a gonococcal infection and with herpes simplex type 2. Patient counseling and effective treatment measures are necessary. In addition to covering the primary organisms, treatment should also cover *Chlamydia trachomatis* which is commonly present as a coinfection.

- Ceftriaxone 250 mg IM and azithromycin 1 g po as a one-time dose is recommended to cover the coverage of gonorrhea and chlamydia. Fluoroquinolones and oral cefixime are no longer recommended by the CDC guidelines for the treatment of gonococcal infections

- Valacyclovir 1 g orally twice daily for 7-10 days is appropriate for an initial episode of genital herpes simplex.

- Expedited partner treatment should be instituted in this case.

For more information on the care plan and facilitator's guide please visit http://www.mhpharmacotherapy.com

90 Acute Osteomyelitis

Melinda M. Neuhauser
Susan L. Pendland

PATIENT PRESENTATION

Chief Complaint

"I have horrible pain in my right hip and thigh. It hurts worse when I move my right leg. Please give me something to stop the pain. The pain meds that I am taking now are not working."

History of Present Illness

KJ is a 72-year-old African-American female who presented to the emergency department complaining of severe pain in her right hip and thigh. She had been transferred recently to the nursing home for rehabilitation after undergoing an ORIF (open reduction and internal fixation) to stabilize her proximal right femur which was fractured in a fall at her home. She had received preoperative vancomycin and was discharged to the nursing home on prn pain medications. At the time of discharge, the patient showed no signs of infection and required only occasional hydrocodone-acetaminophen for pain. The nursing home staff noted that she had been running a fever for several days and was being treated with clindamycin for cellulitis around the surgical site. They also noted that she had complained of increasing pain that was not relieved by hydrocodone/acetaminophen, even after her dose was increased to 2 tablets every 3 hours as needed.

Past Medical History

Cellulitis

Fractured proximal femur with subsequent ORIF

Non-insulin dependent diabetes mellitus (NIDDM)

Hypertension (HTN)

Dyslipidemia

Recurrent urinary tract infections (UTIs)

Family History

Both parents died of a myocardial infarction (MI). She has two sisters, both alive, who have HTN, NIDDM, and dyslipidemia. She is a widow and has no children.

Social History

The patient is a retired teacher. She was independent of daily activities prior to the fall and subsequent femur fracture.

Tobacco/Alcohol/Substance Use

Social drinker (occasional glass of wine); denies tobacco and illicit drug use

Allergies/Intolerance/Adverse Drug Events

Penicillin: anaphylaxis

Codeine: nausea

Medications (Current)

Metformin 500 mg 1 tablet po twice daily

Atorvastatin 80 mg 1 tablet po at bedtime

Amlodipine 5 mg 1 tablet po once daily

Hydrochlorothiazide 25 mg 1 tablet po once daily

Clindamycin 300 mg 1 tablet po 4 times daily

Docusate sodium 100 mg 1 tablet po once daily

Senna 8.6 mg 1-2 tablets po once daily prn constipation

Acetaminophen 325 mg 1-2 tablets po prn q 6 h mild to
 moderate pain

Hydrocodone-acetaminophen 5/325 mg 2 tablets po prn
 q 3 h severe pain

Review of Systems

(+) Pain (8/10) not relieved by hydrocodone-acetaminophen; (+) fever; (−) nausea, vomiting, diarrhea, constipation; (−) dysuria or change in urinary frequency

Physical Examination

▶ *General*

Ill-appearing 72-year-old African-American female in acute distress

▶ *Vital Signs*

BP 148/78 mm Hg, P 78, RR 20, T 38°C

Weight 147 lb (66.8 kg)

Height 5'7" (170.2 cm)

▶ *Skin*

Swelling and erythema around the surgical site

Laboratory Tests

Obtained Today in Emergency Department

	Conventional Units	SI Units
Na	140 mEq/L	140 mmol/L
K	3.6 mEq/L	3.6 mmol/L
Cl	103 mEq/L	103 mmol/L
CO_2	23 mEq/L	23 mmol/L
BUN	24 mg/dL	8.6 mmol/L
SCr	1.3 mg/dL	114.9 umol/L
Glu	183 mg/dL	10.2 mmol/L
Hgb	12.8 g/dL	128 g/L; 7.9 mmol/L
Hct	38.7%	0.387
WBC	$16.3 \times 10^3/mm^3$	$16.3 \times 10^9/L$
Neutrophils	76%	0.76
Bands	12%	0.12
Lymphocytes	8%	0.08
Monocytes	4%	0.04
Platelets	$246 \times 10^3/mm^3$	$246 \times 10^9/L$
ESR	76 mm/h	NA
CRP	25 mg/dL	250 mg/L

Microbiology

Blood culture (× 2): Pending

Bone Aspirate:

Gram stain: Gram positive cocci in clusters

Culture: Pending

Imaging

Plain Film Radiograph: Diffuse soft tissue swelling

Magnetic Resonance Imaging (MRI): Positive for increased uptake in right proximal femur

Assessment

A 72-year-old female with signs, symptoms, laboratory and imaging tests consistent with acute osteomyelitis.

Student Work-Up

Missing Information/Inadequate Data

Evaluate:	Patient database
	Drug therapy problems
	Care plan (by problem)

TARGETED QUESTIONS

1. What signs, symptoms, laboratory and imaging data support a diagnosis of acute osteomyelitis?

   Hint: See p. 1200 in PPP

2. How would you classify this patient's osteomyelitis?

   Hint: See pp. 1199 in PPP

3. What microorganism would be the most likely cause of infection in this patient?

   Hint: See p. 1199 in PPP

4. What empiric antimicrobial agent(s), dosage regimen and monitoring parameters would you recommend for this patient?

   Hint: See pp. 1201-1202, Table 81-1, and Table 81-2 in PPP

5. What duration of antimicrobial therapy do you anticipate for this patient?

   Hint: See pp. 1201 in PPP

FOLLOW-UP

The patient was started on Vancomycin 1 gram IV q 24 h at the hospital. The bone aspirate grew *S. aureus* (resistant to cefazolin, clindamycin, erythromycin, oxacillin, penicillin; susceptible to ceftaroline, daptomycin, linezolid, rifampin, tetracycline, trimethoprim-sulfamethoxazole (TMP-SMX), vancomycin). Blood cultures were negative with no growth × 5 days. The MIC (minimum inhibitory concentration) of vancomycin was 2 mcg/mL (1.4 μmol/L) and the steady-state trough concentration was 13.8 mcg/mL (9.5 μmol/L). After one week of IV vancomycin, the patient still requires frequent pain medication. WBC (white blood cell count), ESR (erythrocyte sedimentation rate) and CRP (c-reactive protein) have only declined minimally. She is returning to the nursing home to continue antimicrobial therapy and for physical therapy.

What modifications, if any, would you recommend regarding this patient's therapy?

Hint: See p. 1201 and Table 81-1 in PPP

The patient was changed to your recommendation and has received 6 weeks of IV therapy. She is ready to be discharged home and the physician is considering changing to po antibiotics to complete therapy. What po agent would you recommend?

Hint: See p. 1201 and Table 81-1 in PPP

⊙ GLOBAL PERSPECTIVE

Acute osteomyelitis affects patients, particularly pediatrics, throughout the world. In developing countries, the diagnosis of acute osteomyelitis may be more challenging with limited access to advanced imaging studies (e.g., MRI). Antimicrobial therapy may differ globally on the basis of local or regional susceptibility patterns, access to hospitals or infusion centers, drug availability and cost.

CASE SUMMARY

- The patient's clinical picture and diagnostic tests are consistent with acute osteomyelitis secondary to direct inoculation during surgery.

- IV antimicrobial therapy should be initiated on the basis of suspected etiologic organism(s) with definitive therapy per microbiology culture and susceptibility results.

- A dosage regimen should be utilized to obtain optimal drug concentrations at the site of infection.

- The patient should be routinely monitored for effectiveness as well as detection of potential adverse drug reactions.

For more information on the care plan and facilitator's guide please visit http://www.mhpharmacotherapy.com

The views expressed in this article are those of the authors and do not necessarily reflect the position or policy of the Department of Veterans Affairs or the United States government.

91 Sepsis

Sara A. Stahle   Brian L. Erstad

PATIENT PRESENTATION

Chief Complaint

"I don't feel right, and I'm in a lot of pain."

History of Present Illness

Gregory Parker is a 64-year-old male who was admitted to the hospital 4 days ago for a scheduled surgical resection of his colon secondary to colon cancer. Following his surgery, he was initially admitted to the intensive care unit for closer observation and received perioperative antibiotic prophylaxis for 24 hours after the operation. He transferred to the general surgical floor the following day and has been recovering well, working with physical therapy and progressing with his diet.

This morning during bedside report, the overnight nurse mentioned that the patient did not sleep well and that he was slightly confused this morning. She also mentioned that the patient complained of pain, and that the pain was not relieved by oxycodone. During her first assessment of the day, the day shift nurse noticed that the patient was still confused and was currently only oriented to person and place. He was also grimacing in pain. Upon taking his vital signs, she found that he was febrile, hypotensive, and tachycardic, which was significantly different from the patient's previous values.

She notified the surgeon on-call and activated the hospital's rapid response team for further evaluation. The patient was quickly administered one liter of normal saline, and stat labs and cultures were obtained. The patient was quickly transferred back to the intensive care unit.

Past Medical History

Colon cancer (diagnosed 1 month ago), with low anterior colonic resection
Chronic obstructive pulmonary disease (5 years)
Hyperlipidemia (11 years)
Hypertension (15 years)

Family History

Father died of lung cancer at age 68. Mother was diagnosed with colon cancer at age 59, and died due to complications following a hip fracture at age 82. He has one younger sister who is alive at age 58 with hypertension. He has one daughter, age 41, and two sons, ages 38 and 34, who are all alive and healthy.

Social History

Retired firefighter. Lives with his wife.

Tobacco/Alcohol/Substance Use

Former cigarette smoker (1 pack per day for 18 years), quit at age 44. Drinks 2-3 beers per day. No history of illicit substance use.

Allergies/Intolerances/Adverse Drug Events

Sulfa (hives)

Medications (Current)

Acetaminophen 650 mg po every 6 hours
Albuterol sulfate 2 puffs inhaled every 6 hours as needed
Alvimopan 12 mg po twice daily
Fluticasone 250 mcg/Salmeterol 50 mcg, 1 puff inhaled every 12 hours
Lisinopril 20 mg po daily
Omeprazole 40 mg po daily
Oxycodone 10 mg po every 4 hours as needed
Nifedipine ER 30 mg po daily
Simvastatin 10 mg po daily

Review of Systems

Distressed and confused male with hypotension, tachycardia, fever, and worsening abdominal pain.

Physical Examination

▶ *General*

Ill-appearing African-American male in acute distress.

▶ *Vital Signs*

BP 90/55 mm Hg, P 136, RR 26, T 38.6°C (101.5°F)
Weight 185 lb. (84 kg)
Height 68 in. (172.7 cm)
Pain rating 9 on a 10-point scale

▶ *Skin*

Cold; (–) erythema; (–) rash

► **HEENT**

Scleral icterus; dry mucus membranes; pinpoint pupils

► **Neck and Lymph Nodes**

(–) JVD; no nodules; minimal lymphadenopathy

► **Chest**

Decreased breath sounds; minimal wheezes and rales bilaterally

► **Cardiovascular**

Sinus tachycardia; (–) M/R/G; (–) bruits; (+) femoral and pedal pulses

► **Abdomen**

Tender, distended. Bowel sounds absent. Significant guarding.

► **Neurology**

A&O × 2 (place and person), (+) confusion

► **Genitourinary**

Deferred

► **Rectal**

Decreased tone; (+) bright red blood per rectum (BRBPR)

Laboratory Tests

	Conventional Units	SI Units
Na	139 mEq/L	139 mmol/L
K	4.7 mEq/L	4.7 mmol/L
Cl	104 mEq/L	104 mmol/L
CO_2	18 mEq/L	18 mmol/L
BUN	52 mg/dL	18.6 mmol/L
sCr	1.7 mg/dL	150 μmol/L
Glucose	193 mg/dL	10.7 mmol/L
Ca	7.9 mg/dL	1.98 mmol/L
Mg	2.1 mEq/L	1.05 mmol/L
Phosphate	4.7 mg/dL	1.52 mmol/L
ABG		
pH	7.28	
pCO_2	32 mm Hg	4.3 kPa
pO_2	82 mm Hg	10.9 kPa
Lactate	5.2 mEq/L; 46.8 mg/dL	5.2 mmol/L
Hgb	9.3 g/dL	93 g/dL; 5.77 mmol/L
Hct	27.9%	0.279
WBC	$17.4 \times 10^3/\mu L$	$17.4 \times 10^9/L$
Platelets	$175 \times 10^3/\mu L$	$175 \times 10^9/L$
Albumin	2.8 g/dL	28 g/L
AST	49 IU/L	0.82 μkat/L
ALT	58 IU/L	0.97 μkat/L
Alk Phos	132 IU/L	2.2 μkat/L
Bilirubin (total)	1.3 mg/dL	22.2 μmol/L

Assessment

A 68-year-old man with vital signs, physical examination, and laboratory tests consistent with sepsis in the setting of recent surgery.

Student Work-Up

Missing Information/Inadequate Data

Evaluate:
Patient database
Drug therapy problems
Care plan (by problem)

TARGETED QUESTIONS

1. What signs and symptoms of sepsis does this patient have?

   Hint: See Table 82-1, pp. 1208-1209 in PPP, and reference by Singer et al.

2. What monitoring parameters should be utilized to determine if this patient is responding to initial therapy?

   Hint: See pp. 1211-1212 in PPP

3. What approach should be taken with regard to IV fluid therapy in this patient?

   Hint: See p. 1211 in PPP

4. What factors should be considered when determining appropriate antimicrobial therapy for this patient?

   Hint: See pp. 1211-1212 in PPP

5. Which vasoactive agent(s) would be an appropriate initial choice in this patient and why?

   Hint: See pp. 1212-1213 in PPP

FOLLOW-UP

Eight hours later, the patient has received 3 liters of normal saline and is receiving vasopressor therapy with norepinephrine (current rate is 0.1 mcg/kg/min). Cultures are in progress in the laboratory, and broad-spectrum antibiotic therapy has been initiated. The patient has a central line in place; central venous pressure (CVP) has been maintained above 8 mm Hg and mean arterial pressure (MAP) has been maintained over 65 mm Hg on the current rate of norepinephrine for the past 3 hours. The surgery resident is considering initiating steroids out of concern for possible adrenal insufficiency.

Should corticosteroids be initiated for possible adrenal insufficiency in this patient? Why or why not?

   Hint: See p. 1213 in PPP

☉ GLOBAL PERSPECTIVE

Despite a landmark trial demonstrating a reduction in mortality with early goal-directed therapy (EGDT) in sepsis, use of EGDT has not been as widely adopted worldwide as expected. Potential factors affecting the implementation of EGDT include complexity of treatment, concerns regarding the external validity of the trial, and resource and infrastructure challenges, among others. To further examine the impact of EGDT compared to contemporary sepsis care, as well as examine the effect of individual protocol elements, multiple government-funded trials have been conducted and published recently to further examine the impact of EGDT. These trials, completed in the United States, Australasia and the United Kingdom, have provided valuable information regarding EGDT compared to usual care in sepsis patients.

The ProCESS trial, conducted in 31 emergency departments in the United States, randomized patients to one of three groups: protocol-based EGDT; protocol-based therapy that did not require placement of a central line, inotropes or blood transfusions; or usual care. There was no difference among the three groups with respect to the primary outcome of 60-day mortality. Both the ARISE trial, conducted at 51 centers primarily in Australia and New Zealand, and the ProMISe trial, conducted at 56 centers in the UK, randomized patients to receive EGDT or usual care. There was no difference between the two groups regarding the primary outcome of 90-day mortality in either trial. These newly published trials could potentially affect future published guidelines and clinical practice regarding early sepsis treatment going forward.

REFERENCES

1. The ARISE Investigators and the ANZICS Clinical Trials Group. Goal-directed resuscitation for patients with early septic shock. *NEJM* 2014;371:1496-1506.

2. Mouncey PR, Osborn TM, Power GS, et al. Trial of early, goal-directed resuscitation for septic shock. *NEJM* 2015;372:1301-1311.

3. The ProCESS Investigators. A randomized trial of protocol-based care for early septic shock. *NEJM* 2014;370:1683-1693.

4. Rivers E, Nguyen B, Havstad S, et al. Early goal-directed therapy in the treatment of severe sepsis and septic shock. *NEJM* 2001;345:1368-1377.

5. Singer M, Deutschman CS, Seymour CW, et al. The Third International Consensus Definitions for Sepsis and Septic Shock (Sepsis-3). *JAMA* 2016;315(8):801-810.

CASE SUMMARY

- The patient's acute clinical picture is consistent with septic shock, likely due to an infectious process in the setting of recent surgery.

- Initial treatment of sepsis should include aggressive IV fluid resuscitation with crystalloids and/or colloids, as well as broad-spectrum antibiotic therapy targeted toward suspected sources of infection.

- Vasoactive agents, with norepinephrine as the preferred agent, should be initiated if initial fluid resuscitation is inadequate to reach hemodynamic goals.

- Use of corticosteroids for stress-induced adrenal insufficiency is controversial, and should only be initiated in patients who remain hemodynamically unstable despite adequate fluid and vasopressor therapies.

For more information on the care plan and facilitator's guide please visit http://www.mhpharmacotherapy.com

92 Dermatophytosis

Lauren S. Schlesselman
Daniel J. Ventricelli

PATIENT PRESENTATION

Chief Complaint

"I have an itchy rash in my groin area. It looks like little red rings. By the way, I don't know if it is related but I also have been having itching and burning between my toes. Now the skin between my toes is peeling, too. I have been rubbing hydrocortisone cream on my feet and putting powder on my groin, but it does not seem to help."

History of Present Illness

Corey Samson is a 26-year-old man who presents to the physician's clinic complaining of severe inguinal itching and soreness, accompanied by a red ring-shaped rash. He has been applying powder to decrease the moisture around his groin. He also presents with itching and burning between his toes, accompanied by skin peeling. He has been applying hydrocortisone cream to his feet to reduce the redness. Other than powder, he has not tried any over-the-counter products for the inguinal rash. He has also not tried any other products on his feet than the hydrocortisone. He is an otherwise healthy male who has never been to the clinic before today.

Past Medical History

No significant medical history

Family History

Father is alive at age 55 with no significant medical history. Mother is alive at age 53 and has hypertension. He has one brother who is 30-years-old with no significant medical history.

Social History

Single and lives with a roommate and a cat; has no children. Employed as a wilderness survival instructor and regularly competes as a triathlete and ultra-marathoner.

Tobacco/Alcohol/Substance Use

Denies alcohol, tobacco, or illicit drug use

Allergies/Intolerances/Adverse Drug Events

Sulfa (rash)

Medications

No current oral medications

Talc powder to groin area prn

Hydrocortisone 1% cream to feet prn

Review of Systems

▶ **General**

Healthy and fit-appearing, Caucasian man in no acute distress

▶ **Vital Signs**

BP 100/60 mm Hg, P 48, RR 12, T 36.2°C

Weight 165 lb. (75 kg)

Height 72 in. (183 cm)

Denies pain

▶ **Skin**

Follicular papules and pustules on medial thigh and inguinal folds; fissures and maceration present between toes; thickening and yellowing of large toenail on right foot

▶ **HEENT**

PERRLA, EOMI; (–) sinus tenderness; TMs appear normal

▶ **Neck and Lymph Nodes**

Thyroid gland symmetrical; (–) nodules; (–) lymphadenopathy; (–) carotid bruits

▶ **Chest**

Clear to auscultation

▶ **Cardiovascular**

RRR, normal S_1, S_2; (–) S_3 or S_4

▶ **Abdomen**

Not tender; not distended; (–) organomegaly

▶ **Neurology**

Grossly intact; deep tendon reflexes normal

▶ **Genitourinary**

Follicular papules and pustules on medial thigh and inguinal folds

▶ *Rectal*

Examination deferred

Laboratory Tests

No labs

Assessment

A 26-year-old man with signs and symptoms consistent with tinea pedis, tinea cruris, and onychomycosis.

Student Work-Up

Missing Information/Inadequate Data

Evaluate: Patient database

                   Drug therapy problems

                   Care plan (by problem)

TARGETED QUESTIONS

1. What signs and symptoms of tinea pedis, tinea cruris, and onychomycosis does the patient have?

   Hint: See p. 1224 and Table 83-5 in PPP

2. What treatment options are available for treating tinea pedis, tinea cruris, and onychomycosis?

   Hint: See p. 1225 and Tables 83-6, 83-7, and 83-8 in PPP

3. What risk factors does the patient have for tinea pedis, tinea cruris, and onychomycosis?

   Hint: See p. 1225 and Table 83-5 in PPP

4. What adverse effects of therapy would you discuss with the patient?

   Hint: See p. 1227 in PPP

5. What nonpharmacologic treatment options should be recommended to the patient?

   Hint: See p. 1225 in PPP

FOLLOW-UP

Would the treatment plan change if the infection site were significantly inflamed and oozing by his groin?

Hint: See p. 1226 in PPP

🌐 GLOBAL PERSPECTIVE

Many cultures have strong beliefs related to feet and hands, which the practitioner must be aware of when treating patients with mycotic conditions. In Arab countries, showing the bottom of the foot is a grave insult therefore patients may be hesitant to show their feet to the practitioner. In other countries, the open palm "high five" gesture is considered insulting. When treating patients with infections on the hand, the practitioner should refrain from making such gestures while discussing the patient's hand infection.

CASE SUMMARY

- His current clinical picture is consistent with tinea pedis, tinea cruris, and onychomycosis. Anti-fungal therapy should be initiated.

- For the treatment of tinea pedis, clotrimazole, tolnaftate, or terbinafine cream applied 1-2 times daily for 4 weeks is recommended.

- For the treatment of tinea cruris, clotrimazole or terbinazine cream or solution applied 1-2 times daily for 2 weeks is recommended.

- Systemic therapy should be reserved for refractory cases or widespread lesions. Treatment should be continued at least 1 week after resolution of symptoms.

- For the treatment of onychomycosis, patients should be aware that resolution of infection will require treatments of multiple months.

For more information on the care plan and facilitator's guide please visit http://www.mhpharmacotherapy.com

93 Vaginal Candidiasis

Lauren S. Schlesselman

PATIENT PRESENTATION

Chief Complaint

"My vagina is really itchy and burns and has a thick discharge. I am fed up with these vaginal infections – I have already had 4 of them in the past 6 months!"

History of Present Illness

Erica Aspen is a 35-year-old woman who presents to the primary care office complaining of severe vaginal itching and burning, accompanied by a thick vaginal discharge. The patient reports a history of recurrent vaginal candidiasis, including four episodes in the last six months (excluding this episode) but no documentation or cultures from those episodes are available due to self-treatment. She expresses frustration with the repeated infections.

Patient also reports attempting to lose weight through low-impact swimming and convenience since her daughter's swim practice and meets occur at this pool. She reports not changing out of her bathing suit until after her daughter's swimming is complete, typically 2-4 hours.

Past Medical History

Type 2 diabetes mellitus (T2DM) (diagnosed 8 years ago)
Obesity
Nonadherence to therapy (patient reported)

Family History

Father is alive at age 61 with history of hypertension. Mother deceased at age 49 due to acute myocardial infarction; history of DM. No siblings.

Social History

Married; has one daughter (age 10). Occupation: homemaker

Tobacco/Alcohol/Substance Use

(–) alcohol use; (–) tobacco or illicit drug use

Allergies/Intolerances/Adverse Drug Events

Ciprofloxacin (rash)

Medications (Current)

Glipizide 5 mg po bid
Metformin 500 po tid

Review of Systems

► *General*

Well-appearing, obese Caucasian woman in no acute distress

► *Vital Signs*

BP 124/68 mm Hg, P 68, RR 13, T 36.5°C (97.7°F)
Weight 175 lb. (80 kg)
Height 60 in. (152 cm)
Denies pain

► *Skin*

Dry-appearing skin; (–) rashes or lesions

► *HEENT*

PERRLA, EOMI; (–) sinus tenderness; TMs appear normal

► *Neck and Lymph Nodes*

Thyroid gland symmetrical; (–) nodules; (–) lymphadenopathy; (–) carotid bruits

► *Chest*

Clear to auscultation

► *Breast*

Examination deferred

► *Cardiovascular*

RRR, normal S_1, S_2; (–) S_3 or S_4

► *Abdomen*

Not tender; not distended; (–) organomegaly

► *Neurology*

Grossly intact; deep tendon reflexes normal

► *Genitourinary*

White exudate; (+) thick, curd-like discharge; inflamed tissue

► *Rectal*

Examination deferred

Laboratory Tests

Vaginal smear (↑) *Candida albicans*

Assessment

A 35-year-old woman with signs, symptoms, and laboratory tests consistent with vulvovaginal candidiasis.

Student Work-Up

Missing Information/Inadequate Data

Evaluate:
- Patient database
- Drug therapy problems
- Care plan (by problem)
- Potential risk factors

Additional information:

Information on how closely the previous VVC episodes occurred could significantly impact therapy selection. If these episodes were not actually effectively treated with therapy, this could lead to concerns about resistant organisms, immune system concerns, or nonadherence. The lack of information on previous therapies utilized for VVC and the effectiveness of these therapies limits the ability to consider other treatment options. Patient preference on therapies is also not considered due to lack of information. For the treatment of VVC, patient preference can play a significant role, particularly for adherence to therapy. Patient has admitted to nonadherence therefore the causes of this need to evaluated to ensure adherence with VVC and DM therapies.

TARGETED QUESTIONS

1. What signs and symptoms of vaginal candidiasis does the patient have?

   Hint: See p. 1218 in PPP

2. What treatment options are available for treating vaginal candidiasis?

   Hint: See p. 1219 and Table 83-2 in PPP

3. What risk factors does the patient have for vaginal candidiasis?

   Hint: See p. 1217 and Table 83-1 in PPP

4. What risks and adverse effects of therapy would you discuss with the patient?

   Hint: See p. 1219 in PPP

5. Is the patient a candidate for suppressive therapy and why or why? What options are available if suppressive therapy is needed?

   Hint: See pp. 1219-1220 and Table 83-3 in PPP

6. What treatment options would be recommended if the patient was pregnant?

   Hint: See p. 1220 in PPP

⟲ GLOBAL PERSPECTIVE

Practitioners are treating an increased number of patients who have undergone female genital mutilation, the intentional alteration or injury of female genitalia undergone for cultural or religious reasons, particularly in Africa and the Middle East. Women who have undergone genital mutilation, more politically correctly called genital cutting, suffer acute and chronic complications. Patients with female genital mutilation may suffer from recurrent VVC due to inadequate drainage of vaginal fluids. Regardless of the practitioner's opinion on the practice, the practitioner must be sensitive to the patient's feeling and cultural values.

CASE SUMMARY

- Her current clinical picture is consistent with vaginal candidiasis and antifungal therapy should be initiated.
- A single dose of fluconazole 150 mg orally is recommended. The dose can be repeated in 3 days.
- Suppressive therapy of weekly fluconazole should be considered due to her history of recurrent candidiasis.

For more information on the care plan and facilitator's guide please visit http://www.mhpharmacotherapy.com

94 Invasive Fungal Infection

Russell E. Lewis   P. David Rogers

PATIENT PRESENTATION

Chief Complaint

Multiple postoperative complications and peritonitis following ruptured diverticulum.

History of Present Illness

Stephen Daedalus is a 39-year-old male who underwent exploratory laparotomy for peritonitis secondary to a ruptured diverticulum. He developed multiple postoperative complications, including small-bowel obstruction, enterocutaneous fistula, and hepatic and renal insufficiency. The patient required extensive surgical resection of the small bowel, and total parenteral nutrition (TPN). He developed an episode of catheter related bloodstream infection with positive blood cultures for Coagulase-negative *Staphylococcus*, *Escherichia coli* and *Candida albicans* that was managed with catheter exchange, broad-spectrum antibiotics, and fluconazole with good clinical response. However, on day 7 of piperacillin-tazobactam 3.375 grams every 6 hours plus vancomycin 1 g q 12 h, and fluconazole 400 mg IV q 24 h, he has developed a new fever (39.0°C) and his blood pressure has dropped to 90/66 mm Hg.

Past Medical History

Peptic ulcer disease

Merckel's diverticulum (diagnosed at age 32)

Family History

Father had coronary artery disease and died of an myocardial infarction at age 57. Mother is alive at age 68 with type 2 diabetes mellitus.

Social History

Real estate agent in Texas. No recent travel or unusual exposures. Unmarried and lives with girlfriend of 2 years, one pet dog.

Tobacco/Alcohol Substance Abuse

Social drinker; (–) illicit drug use

Allergies/Intolerances/Adverse Drug Events

None

Medications (Current)

Piperacillin/Tazobactam 3.375 g IV q 6 h

Vancomycin 1 g IV q 12 h

Fluconazole 400 mg IV q 24 h

Total parenteral nutrition, standard central vein formula with electrolytes, 1294 mL IV q 24 h:

(700 carbohydrate calories, 70 g protein, 200 fat calories, standard 3 in 1 fat emulsion, 100 mEq Na, 70 mEq K, cation-balanced with acetate, 100 mEq Cl, 10 mm phosphorous, 15 mEq Calcium, 16 mEq magnesium, plus multivitamins, plus trace elements)

Fentanyl 75 mcg/h IV

Lorazepam 0.05 mg/kg/h IV

Pantoprazole 40 mg IV daily

Acetaminophen 500 mg po q 6 h prn

Diphenhydramine 50 mg po q 4-6 h prn

Review of Systems

The patient is difficult to arouse and is possibly developing a nonconfluent rash on the chest and back.

Physical Examination

▶ *General*

Somewhat ill-appearing, difficult-to-arouse male in late 30's with extremities that are cool to touch. The patient is not intubated.

▶ *Vital Signs*

BP 90/60 mm Hg, P 90, RR 18, T 39.0°C

Weight 163 lb. (74 kg)

Height 67 in. (172 cm)

▶ *Skin*

Decreased skin turgor. Central venous catheter (CVC) site is not indurated or inflamed. A light diffuse morbilliform rash evident on the upper chest that is spreading on the arms, neck, and back. Surgical sites are clean and dressed without signs of erythema or pus.

▶ **HEENT**

PEERLA, EOMI; (–) sinus tenderness; TMs appear normal; mucus membranes dry

▶ **Neck and Lymph Nodes**

(–) Evidence of lymphadenopathy; thyroid nodules; (–) carotid bruits

▶ **Chest**

Dullness to percussion in lower right and left bases; (–) wheezes; (–) crackles during inspiration

▶ **Cardiovascular**

Tachycardia (90), S_1, S_2 normal; negative for for S_3 or S_4

▶ **Abdomen**

Tender, not distended.

▶ **Neurology**

The patient moderately sedated and not well oriented to person, place, or time

▶ **Genitourinary**

Foley catheter present

▶ **Rectal**

Examination deferred

Laboratory Tests

	Conventional Units	SI Units
Na	139 mEq/L	139 mmol/L
K	3.4 mEq/L	3.4 mmol/L
Cl	104 mEq/L	104 mmol/L
CO_2	25 mEq/L	25 mmol/L
BUN	23 mg/dL	8.2 mmol/L
SCr	1.1 mg/dL	97 μmol/L
Glu	122 mg/dL	6.8 mmol/L
Ca	9.2 mg/dL	2.30 mmol/L
Mg	1.2 mEq/L	0.60 mmol/L
Phos	3.3 mg/dL	1.07 mmol/L
Albumin	3.3 g/dL	33 g/L
AST	77 IU/L	1.28 μkat/L
ALT	92 IU/L	1.53 μkat/L
ALP	250 IU/L	4.17 μkat/L
Total bilirubin	2.1 mg/dL	36.0 μmol/L
Hgb	11 g/dL	110 g/L; 6.83 mmol/L
Hct	58%	0.58
WBC	$12.9 \times 10^3/mm^3$	12.9×10^9
Segs	49%	0.49
Bands	9%	0.09
Lymphocytes	28%	0.28
Monocytes	6%	0.06
Eosinophils	8%	0.08
Platelets	$290 \times 10^3/mm^3$	$290 \times 10^9/L$
Procalcitonin, serum	1.1 ng/mL	1.1 ng/mL

▶ **Culture Results**

Blood: (+) Coagulase negative *Staphylococcus* (vancomycin MIC 0.5 mg/L) and *Escherichia coli* (piperacillin-tazobactam MIC 2 mg/L), and *Candida albicans* (MIC testing not performed).

Urine: (+) yeast, species not reported

Wound swab: (–)

Urinalysis: Na 15 mEq/L (15 mmol/L); osmolality 500 mOsmol/kg (500 mmol/kg); hyaline casts; WBC (–); RBC (–); protein (–)

Assessment

A 39-year-old male s/p abdominal laparotomy with new-onset fever on broad-spectrum antibiotic therapy and fluconazole, hypotension and tachycardia, with a possible drug hypersensitivity reaction.

Student Work-Up

Missing Information/Inadequate Data

Evaluate: Patient database

Drug therapy problems

Care plan (by problem)

TARGETED QUESTIONS

1. What are the patient's risk factors for developing an opportunistic mycosis? Which fungal pathogen is most likely?

   Hint: See pp. 1235-1236 in PPP

2. In the absence of definitive microbiologic data, what antifungal therapy should be started in this patient?

   Hint: See pp. 1235-1236 and Table 84-2 in PPP

3. What is the most likely fungal pathogen in the setting of breakthrough infection on fluconazole therapy?

   Hint: See p. 1236 in PPP

4. Is the (+) yeast culture from the urine indicative of true infection or colonization in this patient?

   Hint: Review results of the urinalysis and see p. 1238 in PPP

5. What is the most likely explanation of this patient's rash?

   Hint: Review the CBC with differential

FOLLOW-UP

Fluconazole was discontinued and an alternative IV antifungal therapy was started. Three days later, a second yeast isolated from the blood (*Candida glabrata*). Susceptibility testing was performed and showed an MIC to fluconazole of 64 mcg/mL, which is considered resistant to fluconazole. The isolate was reported susceptible to echinocandins and amphotericin B. The patient has improved clinically since starting antifungal therapy and a second exchange of the catheter, and the patient has transitioned from TPN to enteral feeding. After 10 days of intravenous antifungal therapy for the *C. glabrata* bloodstream infections, you are asked if the patient can be switched to voriconazole oral solution to complete the treatment course for candidemia.

What is your recommendation?

Hint: See pp. 1236 and 1238 in PPP

☺ GLOBAL PERSPECTIVE

Candida species are the third to fourth most commonly isolated bloodstream pathogens in hospitalized patients associated with crude mortality rates approaching 40%. Like many opportunistic invasive fungal pathogens, invasive candidiasis can be difficult to diagnose early. Therefore, early suspicion of infection in patients with multiple risk factors for infection (e.g., central venous catheters, broad-spectrum antibiotic therapy, recent intra-abdominal surgery, colonization with *Candida* at multiple sites) should prompt empiric treatment during the diagnostic workup, as delays in the initiation of appropriate antifungal therapy have been associated with increased mortality. Selection of antifungal therapy is guided by local epidemiology (i.e., prevalence of *C. glabrata* and *C. krusei* in the institution), previous antifungal exposures, and underlying comorbidities of the host. For reasons not entirely understood, *C. glabrata* is more common in institutions in North America than South America or Europe, while *C. parapsilosis* is a more frequent pathogen in Latin America and Spain. For most patients, initial therapy with an echinocandin antifungal is recommended until pathogen identification and clinical response can be assessed.

CASE SUMMARY

- The patient's clinical picture is consistent with breakthrough invasive candidiasis and or bacterial bloodstream infection on fluconazole treatment, requiring immediate empiric changes in antibacterial and antifungal therapy.

- Because the patient is at relatively higher risk (possible early sepsis) and has failed prior fluconazole therapy initial therapy with an echinocandin would be appropriate. The patient should receive at least 2 weeks of therapy and have the PICC (peripherally inserted central catheter) line replaced.

- Because the patient has a fluconazole-resistant *C. glabrata*, he should not be considered as a candidate for step-down (oral) voriconazole therapy.

For more information on the care plan and facilitator's guide please visit http://www.mhpharmacotherapy.com

95 Pediatric Immunizations

Hanna Phan   Lynn C. Wardlow

PATIENT PRESENTATION

Date of clinic visit: October 25, 2015 at 10:00 a.m.

Chief Complaint

"We are here for a refill on my daughter's asthma medicine and wanted to ask if there were any other options. The nebulizer takes a while to do. Plus, since she has been diagnosed with asthma, we are ready to try out the flu vaccine."

History of Present Illness

Mary Jacobs is a 4-year-old African-American female who was brought into her pediatrician's office by her father. The father notes that it takes too long to give her budesonide and sometimes misses doses because of it (about 1-2 times per week). No current acute illness noted.

Past Medical History

Patient has had mild, persistent asthma 6 months ago with no history of asthma-related hospitalizations since diagnosis, received one course of systemic corticosteroids (3 months after diagnosis). During the first year of life, the patient was treated several times for respiratory tract infections, including one minor hospitalization at age 10 months. Diagnosed with sickle cell disease at birth (HbSS) of which she takes pencillin as prophylaxis against pneumococcal disease.

Social History

The patient lives at home with mother and father. Both parents smoke 1 pack per day. She attends day care during the weekdays as both parents work full-time. Siblings include a one-year-old presently healthy sister who also attends day care with no underlying comorbidities. Pet at home: 1 cat who sleeps wherever, including the children's bedroom.

Allergies/Intolerances/Adverse Drug Events

Latex (rash)

Medication History (Current)

Budesonide 0.25 mg via nebulizer twice daily

Albuterol HFA MDI 1-2 puffs with spacer every 4-6 hours as needed for shortness of breath

Pencilin VK 250 mg po bid

Immunizations

Per father, the patient has not experienced any adverse reactions with immunizations except for diarrhea following the third dose of rotavirus vaccine as an infant. Previously declined the influenza vaccine due to concern of "getting sick" from it.

Immunization Record

Name: Mary C. Jacobs
Birthdate: 1/1/2011

Vaccine	Product Name	Date Given	Route and Site	Vaccinator Signature/Initials
Hepatitis B	Recombivax HB	1/1/2011	IM RT	A.R.
	Pediarix	3/5/2011	IM RT	B.C.
	Pediarix	5/16/2011	IM LT	A.B.
	Pediarix	7/23/2011	IM LT	A.B.

(Continued)

Immunization Record (*Continued*)

Vaccine	Product Name	Date Given	Route and Site	Vaccinator Signature/Initials
Diptheria, tetanus, pertussis	Pediarix	3/5/2011	IM RT	*B.C.*
	Pediarix	5/16/2011	IM LT	*A.B.*
	Pediarix	7/23/2011	IM LT	*A.B.*
	Infanrix	4/15/2012	IM RDM	*P.T.*
Haemophilus influenzae type b	ActHIB	3/5/2011	IM LT	*B.C.*
	ActHIB	5/16/2011	IM RT	*A.B.*
	ActHIB	7/23/2011	IM RT	*A.B.*
	ActHIB	1/5/2012	IM LT	*P.T.*
Hepatitis A	Havrix	1/5/2012	IM RT	*P.T.*
Polio	Pediarix	3/5/2011	IM RT	*B.C.*
	Pediarix	5/16/2011	IM LT	*A.B.*
	Pediarix	7/23/2011	IM LT	*A.B.*
Pneumococcal	Prevnar	3/5/2011	IM LT	*B.C.*
	Prevnar	5/16/2011	IM LT	*A.B.*
	Prevnar	7/23/2011	IM RT	*A.B.*
Rotavirus	RotaTeq	3/5/2011	PO	*B.C.*
	RotaTeq	5/16/2011	PO	*A.B.*
	RotaTeq	7/23/2011	PO	*A.B.*
Measles, mumps, rubella	ProQuad	1/5/2012	SC LT	*P.T.*
Varicella	ProQuad	1/5/2012	SC LT	*P.T.*

Review of Systems

Negative for recent weight loss, rashes, bruising, heart murmur or palpitations, negative for fever, changes in respiratory status; negative for odynophagia, nausea/vomiting, diarrhea.

Physical Examination

▶ General

A well-nourished (54th percentile BMI for age), well-appearing 4-year-old female.

▶ Vital Signs

BP 100/60 mm Hg, HR 80, RR 20, T 37°C

Weight 36 lb. (16.4 kg)

Height 40 in. (102 cm)

▶ Skin

No abnormalities noted; normal skin turgor

▶ HEENT

PERRLA, EOMI; moist mucous membranes (mmm); No erythema, bulging or limitation in mobility of the tympanic membrane.

▶ Neck and Lymph Nodes

(–) lymphadenopathy

▶ Chest

No wheezes and crackles, bilaterally

▶ Cardiovascular

RRR, normal s_1, s_2; (–) s_3 or s_4

▶ Abdomen

Not tender/not distended; (–) organomegaly

▶ Neurology

Grossly intact; deep tendon reflexes normal

▶ Genitourinary

Examination deferred

▶ Rectal

Examination deferred

Laboratory Tests

August 2015 (Fasting)

	Conventional Units	SI Units
Na	140 mEq/L	140 mmol/L
K	4.1 mEq/L	4.1 mmol/L
Cl	105 mEq/L	105 mmol/L
CO_2	23 mEq/L	23 mmol/L
BUN	10 mg/dL	3.57 mmol/L
SCr	0.3 mg/dL	27 µmol/L
Glu	70 mg/dL	3.9 mmol/L
Ca	9.0 mg/dL	2.25 mmol/L
Mg	1.8 mEq/L	0.90 mmol/L
Phosphate	5 mg/dL	1.62 mmol/L
Hgb	12.2 g/dL	122 g/L; 7.57 mmol/L
Hct	36.7%	0.367
WBC	$5.2 \times 10^3/mm^3$	$5.2 \times 10^9/L$
MCV	$80\ \mu m^3$	80 fL
Albumin	4.2 g/dL	42 g/L
WBC	$5.5 \times 10^3/mm^3$	$5.5 \times 10^9/L$
Hgb	13.5 g/dL	135 g/L
Hct	37%	0.37
Platelet	$250 \times 10^3/mm^3$	$250 \times 10^9/L$

Assessment

A 4-year-old female child needing an asthma medication refill and inquiry about other less timely drug options. Pharmacist to review immunization record and recommend any necessary immunizations for today.

Student Work-Up

Missing Information/Inadequate Data

Evaluate: Patient database

Drug therapy problems

Care plan (by problem)

TARGETED QUESTIONS

1. What should be evaluated to determine if Mary should receive immunizations today?

   Hint: See guide to vaccine contraindications and precautions (by the CDC), http://www.cdc.gov/vaccines/recs/vac-admin/contraindications.htm -or- http://www.cdc.gov/vaccines/recs/vac-admin/contraindications-vacc.htm

2. What adverse effects should the patient's father be educated about regarding Mary's immunizations?

   Hint: See Table 86-1 in PPP

3. Is premedication (e.g., acetaminophen) before immunizations appropriate for Mary? Why or why not?

   Hint: See p. 1257 in PPP

4. What resource could the pediatrician access to find a list of commercially available latex-free vaccine products?

   Hint: See latex in vaccine packaging (by the cdc), http://www.cdc.gov/vaccines/pubs/pinkbook/downloads/appendices/b/latex-table.pdf

5. Which of Mary's missing vaccines is/are likely to cause body temperature elevation?

   Hint: See Table 86-1 in PPP

FOLLOW-UP

Mary and her father return to the clinic for a routine checkup in mid-January of the following year (2016), she has been to clinic since you last saw her in October. Mary is well nourished, not in distress, with mild upper respiratory infection. Rapid influenza A and B antigen (nasal aspirate) is negative and rapid respiratory syncytial virus (RSV) antigen (nasal aspirate) is positive. Her body temperature is 37.6°C. The pediatrician asks you if it is okay to give her immunizations today and which ones she will need today. Is it appropriate to administer immunizations today? If so, which ones?

   Hint: See Table 86-2 in PPP

🌐 GLOBAL PERSPECTIVE

Immunization of children remains a significant public health concern internationally. According to the WHO, immunizations do not reach every child worldwide, resulting in an estimated 1.5 million deaths from diseases preventable by vaccines recommended by the WHO. Up to 29% of deaths amongst infant and children worldwide are attributable to vaccine preventable diseases such as pneumococcal disease, rotovirus, and pertussis.[1] Due to growing immunization programs, improved access to clean water, improved nutrition, and sanitary living conditions by public health organizations, such as the WHO, the number of children dying every year has fallen from 9.6 million in 2000 to 7.6 million in 2010.[2] Optimal outreach of immunizations to the world's children is faced with challenges in financial support, logistics of organizing national and local public health groups, and support of caregivers regarding the importance of immunization for individual and community health.

KEY READINGS/REFERENCES

1. World Health Organization. Estimates of disease burden and cost-effectiveness. http://www.who.int/immunization/monitoring_surveillance/burden/estimates/en/ Accessed May 15, 2015.

2. World Health Organization. Global vaccine action plan 2011-2020. http://www.who.int/iris/bitstream/10665/78141/1/9789241504980_eng.pdf. Accessed May 15, 2015.

For more information on the care plan and facilitator's guide please visit http://www.mhpharmacotherapy.com

Joshua C. Caraccio   Kathryn R. Matthias

PATIENT PRESENTATION

Chief Complaint

"I was recently discharged from a hospital and they told me to ask about receiving a "pneumonia" vaccine. I am not sure if I really need this vaccine. Is it the flu shot since I had that a couple of months ago?"

History of Present Illness

GK is a 68-year-old female patient who was admitted to the hospital for confusion, abdominal pain, and word-finding issues. Her problems began 1 day prior to admission when her husband and sons noticed some confusion. She was brought to the emergency department and found to have altered mental status, fever, and flank pain due to pyelonephritis. On day 1 of hospitalization, she returned to normal mental status and was feeling much better. She had a 3-day hospitalization with no major problems and excellent recovery. During the hospitalization, the nurses and physician asked her if she wanted the "pneumonia" vaccine. She told them she would follow-up with the pharmacist at her medical clinic to see if she needs this vaccine. GK is discharged with antibiotics for pyelonephritis and a scheduled visit to her primary care clinic. GK comes to you 3 days after discharge with questions about this "pneumonia" vaccine and other inquiries.

Past Medical History

Pyelonephritis

Past Surgical History

Right knee replacement surgery (10 years ago)
Spleen removed (6 months ago after a motor vehicle crash)

Family History

Married. Father deceased from heart attack (age 76). Mother is 88 and has a history of chronic obstructive pulmonary disease, hyperlipidemia, and loves to gamble. Brother with no significant past medical history. She has two sons and one 1-month-old grandson.

Social History

She moved to the United States in 1998 from Italy. She is currently retired but travels frequently across the United States and has traveled to Europe a couple times in the past 5 years. No current or past smoking or illicit drug use. She drinks socially 2-3 drinks a week.

Allergies/Intolerances/Adverse Drug Events

NKDA

Medications

Ciprofloxacin 750 mg po bid × 10 days

Immunizations

A complete immunization record is missing and the patient only brought her discharge paperwork from the hospital. As per the patient's discharge paperwork from the hospital from the past week, no administered vaccinations were listed.

The patient states that she got her annual influenza vaccine a couple of months ago at a community pharmacy near her house. She does not remember the exact date and did not bring an immunization record with her to clinic today but thinks it was mid-November and tells you the name and location of the community pharmacy.

Review of Systems

No current issues.

Physical Examination

▶ *General*

Sixty-eight-year-old Caucasian female in no acute distress.

▶ *Vital Signs*

BP 118/70 mm Hg, P 76, RR 16, T 37.2°C
Weight 128 lb. (58 kg)
Height 65 in. (165 cm)

▶ *Skin*

Scar on right knee and on abdomen

► **HEENT**

PERRLA, EOMI

Head, ears, nose, throat—no apparent issues

► **Neck and Lymph Nodes**

(–) Lymphadenopathy

► **Chest**

Clear to auscultation

► **Cardiovascular**

RRR, normal S_1, S_2; (–) S_3 or S_4

► **Abdomen**

No apparent issues

► **Neurological**

Grossly intact; DTRs normal

► **Genitourinary**

Examination deferred

► **Rectal**

Examination deferred

Laboratory Tests

Per discharge paperwork: obtained 3 days ago on day of discharge from hospital

	Conventional Units	SI Units
Na	137 mEq/L	137 mmol/L
K	4.2 mEq/L	4.2 mmol/L
Cl	101 mEq/L	101 mmol/L
CO_2	27 mEq/L	27 mmol/L
BUN	5 mg/dL	1.8 mmol/L
SCr	0.6 mg/dL	54 μmol/L
Glu	105 mg/dL	5.9 mmol/L
Ca	9.7 mg/dL	2.43 mmol/L
Hgb	13.9 g/dL	139 g/L; 8.63 mmol/L
HCT	39.7%	0.397
MCV	95 μm³	95 fL
Platelets	294 × 10³/mm³	294 × 10⁹/L
WBC	5.4 × 10³/mm³	5.4 × 10⁹/L

Assessment

Sixty-eight-year-old Caucasian woman in no acute distress recently discharged from an acute care hospital with recommendation to obtain "pneumonia" vaccine. Pharmacist to review immunization record.

Student Work-Up

Missing Information/Inadequate Data

Evaluate: Patient database

Drug therapy problems

Care plan (by problem)

TARGETED QUESTIONS

1. GK comes to see you about this "pneumonia vaccine." Based on the most current CDC recommendations, what is the best treatment plan for GK in regard to her pneumococcal vaccination? Why did the nurses and physician recommend this vaccine for GK?

   Hint: See p. 1258 in PPP

   Hint: See guide to Vaccine-Preventable Adult Diseases (by the CDC), http://www.cdc.gov/vaccines/adults/vpd.html

2. Since you are missing a complete vaccination record for GK, which vaccinations do you recommend for GK at this time?

   Hint: See pp. 1255-1259 in PPP

   Hint: See Adult Immunization Schedule (by the CDC): http://www.cdc.gov/vaccines/schedules/hcp/adult.html

3. During your interview with GK, she says, "When I am watching TV, I notice they say I should ask a health care professional about the HPV vaccine. Is that something I should get?" Explain who should receive the human papillomavirus vaccination, and if GK should or should not receive this vaccine and why.

   Hint: See p. 1257 in PPP

   Hint: See Who Should Receive (by the CDC): http://www.cdc.gov/vaccines/schedules/hcp/adult.html

4. Upon review of the medical record, you discover GK had her spleen removed 6 months ago. You ask if she received any vaccinations after her surgery. She says she thinks they are unimportant. Explain why specific vaccines are important in asplenic patients, what are the vaccines recommended in GK since her spleen was removed, and when should they have been given?

   Hint: See Adult Immunization Schedule (by the CDC), http://www.cdc.gov/vaccines/schedules/hcp/adult.html

5. What are the common and serious potential adverse effects of recommended vaccines determined in questions 1, 2, and 4?

   Hint: See pp. 1259 and 1260 and Table 86-1 in PPP

   Hint: See Guide to Vaccine Contraindications and Precautions (by the CDC), http://www.cdc.gov/vaccines/recs/vac-admin/contraindications.htm

FOLLOW-UP

Two months later, GK comes back to the clinic and tells you she is planning a trip to Kenya in 4 months. What is the vaccination regimen for GK's trip to Kenya? Select three other countries to evaluate immunization recommendations where GK might travel.

> *Hint: See the Yellow Book (by the CDC), http://wwwnc.cdc.gov/travel/yellowbook/2016/table-of-contents specifically Appendix B: Travel Vaccine Summary Table*

🌐 GLOBAL PERSPECTIVE

The World Health Organization (WHO) and United Nations Children's Fund (UNICEF) conduct an annual review of immunizations reports from countries and territories from across the world.[1] Although global rates of certain immunizations have increased dramatically over the past 40 years, many vaccines on the United States' Immunization Schedule are not yet recommended in other countries' national immunization schedules. Although the United States and other industrialized countries have estimated vaccinated target populations (by antigen) above 90% based on childhood recommended immunization schedule, missed opportunities to vaccinate adult patients often occur. In a case-cohort study of two large tertiary medical centers in Australia only 2.3% of patients had their vaccination status for influenza or pneumococcal determined during a hospital visit.[2] In another study of adult patients who developed invasive pneumococcal disease, it was determined that 92% of these patients had at least one missed opportunity for vaccination such as a hospital, emergency department, or primary care visit in the 2 years prior to infection.[3] Due to high rates of missed opportunities to vaccinate, the Advisory Committee on Immunization Practices (ACIP) through the Centers for Disease Control (CDC) has recommended the use of institution protocols for standing order immunization programs for administration of vaccines by nurses or pharmacists to decrease rates of eligible, unvaccinated patients.[4]

REFERENCES

1. World Health Organization: Immunization surveillance, assessment and monitoring. http://www.who.int/immunization_monitoring/data/en/. Accessed January 3, 2016.
2. Skull SA, Andrews RM, Byrnes GB, et al. Missed opportunities to vaccinate a cohort of hospitalized elderly with pneumococcal and influenza vaccines. Vaccine 2007;25:5146-5154.
3. Kyaw MH, Greene CM, Schaffner W, et al. Adults with invasive pneumococcal disease: Missed opportunities for vaccination. Am J Prev Med 2006;31(4):286-292.
4. Centers for Disease Control and Prevention. Use of standing orders programs to increase adult vaccination rates. MMWR 2000;49(No. RR-1):15-26.

CASE SUMMARY

- GK presents to the clinic 3 days after discharge from the hospital due to pyelonephritis. She wanted to follow up with you to determine if this "pneumonia" vaccine is needed.

- GK has no acute problems but based on her medical record and interview GK's vaccination record is incomplete leaving her vulnerable to infection that a can be prevented.

- GK should receive missing immunization per the recommended adult immunization schedule provided be the CDC.

- GK should be counseled on potential adverse effects of recommended vaccines.

For more information on the care plan and facilitator's guide please visit http://www.mhpharmacotherapy.com

97 Human Immunodeficiency Virus

Emily L. Heil   Amanda H. Corbett

PATIENT PRESENTATION

Chief Complaint

"I am having trouble remembering to take my evening dose of medication."

History of Present Illness

Ronald Parker is a 55-year-old Caucasian male who has been infected with HIV since 2008. He has been stable on a regimen of raltegravir and Truvada (emtricitabine/tenofovir) for the past 7 years, and has recently changed jobs and is now working a night shift. He presents to the infectious disease (ID) clinic and states that he has been forgetting his evening dose of raltegravir prior to heading to work and is interested in a new regimen. Additionally, his routine lab work revealed an increase in his serum creatinine since his previous labs.

Past Medical History

HIV (7 years)
Depression (15 years)
Diabetes mellitus (3 years)
Hypertension (15 years)
GERD (2 years)

Family History

His father passed away after a STEMI (ST-elevation myocardial infarction) at the age of 65, and his mother passed away from breast cancer at the age of 78.

Social/Work History

He is currently employed as a toll-booth attendant and recently switched to a night shift.

Tobacco/Alcohol/Substance Use

Smokes 2 ppd; drinks about 10-12 drinks a week; former IV heroin use, but clean for 1 year

Allergy/Intolerance/Adverse Drug Events

NKDA

Medication (Current)

Atorvastatin 20 mg po q 24 h
Bupropion XL 150 mg po q 24 h
Emtricitabine/tenofovir 200/300 mg 1 tab po q 24 h
Raltegravir 400 mg po q 12 h
Hydrochlorothiazide 25 mg po q 24 h
Metformin 1000 mg po q 12 h
Pantoprazole 40 mg po q 24 h

Review of Systems

(–) Weight loss; decreased appetite; (+) insomnia; (–) SOB; chest pain

Physical Examination

▶ *General*

Well-appearing Caucasian man in no acute distress

▶ *Vital Signs*

BP 170/90 mm Hg, P 72, RR 13, T 36.4°C
Weight 198 lb. (90 kg)
Height 70 in. (177.8 cm)
No pain

▶ *Skin*

Supple; (–) rashes

▶ *HEENT*

PERRL; no evidence of retinopathy. Oropharynx, no evidence of thrush.

▶ *Neck and Lymph Nodes*

Neck supple; no lymphadenopathy

▶ **Chest**

Clear to auscultation bilaterally

▶ **Cardiovascular**

RRR, normal S_1, S_2; (–) murmurs, rubs, or gallops

▶ **Abdomen**

Not tender/not distended; (–) organomegaly

▶ **Neurology**

Grossly intact; deep tendon reflexes normal

▶ **Extremities**

Dry upper and lower extremities with no edema

▶ **Genitourinary**

Examination deferred

▶ **Rectal**

Examination deferred

Laboratory Tests

Fasting, Obtained 1 week ago Prior to Clinic Visit

	Conventional Units	SI Units
Na	137 mEq/L	137 mmol/L
K	4.2 mEq/L	4.2 mmol/L
Cl	101 mEq/L	101 mmol/L
CO_2	25 mEq/L	25 mmol/L
BUN	40 mg/dL	14.3 mmol/L
SCr	2.0 mg/dL	176.8 μmol/L
Glucose	135 mg/dL	7.4 mmol/L
Hg	14 g/dL	140 g/L; 8.69 mmol/L
Hct	38%	0.38
WBC	6.4×10^3/mm³	6.4×10^9/L
Platelets	425×10^3/mm³	425×10^9/L
AST	30 IU/L	0.50 μKat/L
ALT	40 IU/L	0.67 μKat/L
HgA1c (%)	6.5	0.065
HIV RNA	1300 copies/mL	
CD4+ T-cell count	235 cells/mm³	0.235×10^9/L

Assessment

A 55-year-old man with HIV previously well-controlled on his previous regimen now presents with concern of missing doses of raltegravir due a change in his job. Newly identified kidney disease necessitates a change in his antiretroviral regimen. His DM, depression, and GERD are under control.

TARGETED QUESTIONS

1. Given the new finding of chroic kidney disease, what medication(s) need to be dose adjusted and/or changed in the patient's medication regimen?

   Hint: See Table 87-4 in PPP

2. To construct a new regimen for the patient, what additional laboratory information should be ordered at this visit?

   Hint: See pp. 1269-1270 in PPP for potential laboratory assessments in treatment-experienced patients

FOLLOW-UP

The patient returns to clinic 2 weeks later to follow-up on repeat labs and start a new regimen. His HIV genotype revealed wild type virus. His HLA B*5701 was negative. A repeat chemistry panel had a SCr of 1.9. His BP is 139/85 mm Hg.

What would you recommend as a once-daily regimen for the patient based on his follow up laboratory information?

What monitoring parameters would you recommend for the new regimen?

Are there any potential drug interactions for the patient's current regimen with your chosen regimen?

Hint: See Table 87-4 in PPP

⚙ GLOBAL PERSPECTIVE

HIV is a global pandemic with broad reaching effects outside of the United States. Access to care and antiretroviral medications is much more limited in resource-poor countries compared to those treated in the United States and other industrialized countries. Criterion for when to treat is variable and typically delayed until CD4+ T-cell counts are lower compared to the recommendation to consider treatment regardless of CD4+ T-cell count in the United States Department of Health and Human Services (DHHS) guidelines. Additionally, what antiretroviral medication to use differs and depends on the country-specific recommendations from the WHO guidelines. Many countries rely on generic antiretrovirals that are still under the U.S. FDA patent, funding from countries, including the United States, through programs such as PEPFAR (U.S. President's Emergency Plan for AIDS Relief) or resources from pharmaceutical industry. Not only are therapies limited, but often only first-line therapy is available with second-line therapy less readily available.

CASE SUMMARY

- This is an HIV-infected patient presenting with difficulty taking his current antiretroviral regimen and newly identify renal dysfunction.

- Multiple options for once-daily antiretroviral therapy are available and selection for this patient should factor in his renal function and potential for drug-drug interactions.

- Continued adherence consultations with this patient should be reinforced by the pharmacist at each visit to the clinic.

For more information on the care plan and facilitator's guide please visit http://www.mhpharmacotherapy.com

PATIENT PRESENTATION

Chief Complaint

"But it was just a lump."

History of Present Illness

Hermione Braccaone is a 50-year-old Caucasian female who has presented to your clinic after recent diagnosis of breast cancer. In December 2014, the patient noticed a painful tender lump in her left breast with no other associated symptoms. She was referred for a bilateral mammogram and ultrasound performed in January 2015. A focal asymmetry at the 3 o'clock position corresponding to the palpable lump measuring 6.9 cm was confirmed with both modalities. A large abnormal lymph node was also present in the left axilla. The right breast was found to be negative for abnormalities. The patient underwent ultrasound-guided core needle biopsy of the breast mass with pathology returning infiltrating ductal carcinoma, grade 3, ER/PR positive, and HER2 positive by IHC. Biopsy of the left enlarged axillary lymph node demonstrated metastatic carcinoma consistent with breast primary. The patient reports feeling very stressed out and anxious about this recent diagnosis. Her depression is stable and she notes that she has attempted many other medications in the past but she has failed every antidepressant with the exception of duloxetine. She reports that she is uncomfortable with changing antidepressant at this time. Since the time of diagnosis, she has had diffuse pain in her left breast, overall she reports her pain is currently controlled. The patient is extremely adamant about being aggressive in treatment, though she is very much interested in breast conservation approaches if at all possible.

Past Medical History

Major depressive disorder (2 years)

S/p total abdominal hysterectomy and bilateral oophorectomy (in 2003 for a benign tumor)

Deep vein thrombosis (DVT) in popliteal vein (1 month with unidentified cause)

Family History

Her mother and 2 aunts have been diagnosed with early stage breast cancer in the past, her mother was diagnosed at 40 years of age. No other relevant history.

Social History

She is an elementary teacher.

Tobacco/Alcohol/Substance Use

She drinks socially maybe 2 times a month, otherwise negative for pertinent positives.

Allergy/Intolerance/Adverse Event History

No known medication allergies

Gynecologic History

Menarche at 13 years of age. She gave birth to her only child at the age of 25. Hysterectomy and oophorectomy at the age of 38.

Medication History

▶ *Current Medications*

Metoprolol tartrate 25 mg by mouth twice daily for hypertension

Enoxaparin 120 mg subcutaneously twice daily for DVT

Cymbalta 60 mg by mouth daily for depression

Oxycodone 5 mg by mouth every 6 hours as needed for pain

▶ *Past Medications*

Multiple SSRIs/SNRIs (discontinued for intolerance)

Hormone replacement therapy (6 years following oophorectomy)

Review of Systems

Cardiovascular: patient reports occasional dizziness on standing rapidly

Skin: pain associated with lump in left breast

Physical Exam

▶ *Vitals*

BP 125/85 (85/65 standing), P 85, RR 16, T 36.8°C

Weight 112 kg

Height 172 cm

Pain 2/10

▶ *Breast*

Right breast without palpable masses. Firm mass at the 3 o'clock position of left breast is very tender.

Laboratory and Other Diagnostic Tests

	Conventional Units	SI Units
Na	137 mEq/L	137 mmol/L
K	4.4 mEq/L	4.4 mmol/L
Cl	103 mEq/L	103 mmol/L
CO_2	32 mEq/L	32 mmol/L
Gluc	110 mg/dL	6.11 mmol/L
BUN	10 mg/dL	3.6 mmol/L urea
Creatinine	0.6 mg/dL	46 μmol/L
Ca	9.6 mg/dL	2.4 mmol/L
AST	20 units/L	0.33 μKat/L
ALT	23 units/L	0.4 μKat/L
Alk Phos	83 units/L	1.4 μKat/L
Tbili	0.3 mg/dL	5.1 μmol/L
Albumin	4.4 g/dL	44 g/L
WBC	$7.0 \times 10^3/\mu L$	$7.0 \times 10^9/L$
Hgb	14.0 g/dL	8.68 mmol/L
Hct	41 %	0.41
Plt	$350 \times 10^3/\mu L$	$350 \times 10^9/L$
ANC (absolute neutrophil count)	$2.93 \times 10^3/\mu L$	$2.93 \times 10^9/L$

Ultrasound-guided core needle biopsy (breast mass): 6.5 cm at greatest dimension infiltrating ductal carcinoma, grade 3 (High grade), ER (98%)/PR (95%) positive, and HER2 positive (3+) by IHC

Ultrasound-guided core needle biopsy (left axillary lymph node): metastatic carcinoma consistent with breast primary

Bilateral diagnostic mammogram: Focal asymmetry at the 3 o'clock position of left breast corresponding to the palpable lump and measuring 6.9 cm

Left breast ultrasound: Mass identified in the area of palpable concern at 3 o'clock in the left breast measuring approximately 7 cm

Bone scan: No osseous metastatic disease found

CT scan of chest/abdomen: no distant metastases identified

Assessment

Ms. Braccione is a 50-year-old female with recent diagnosis of Stage IIIA (T3N1M0) or locally advanced ER/PR and HER2 positive invasive ductal carcinoma. Her preference is for breast conservation, therefore a neoadjuvant approach

with AC-THP may be preferred in this case (T = Taxotere or Taxol). She is experiencing symptoms of orthostasis upon standing. She is currently stable on her SNRI duloxetine and continues taking her enoxaparin for recent DVT. Her pain is well controlled at this time.

Student Work-Up

Missing Information/Inadequate Data

Evaluate:
- Patient database
- Drug therapy problems
- Care plan (by problem)

Additional Information:
- Patient's cardiac status

  Transthoracic echocardiogram: Left ventricular ejection fraction = 65 %, no other abnormalities
- PET-CT scan for full staging

  PET-CT scan demonstrated no FDG avid sites beyond the primary site (left breast) and the enlarged axillary lymph node

TARGETED QUESTIONS

1. List the risk factors that increase a patient's risk for developing breast cancer. Which of these are exhibited by our patient?

   Hint: See pp. 1317-1319 in PPP

2. Distinguish and list the positive and negative prognostic factors associated with the current patient's diagnosis.

   Hint: See p. 1321 in PPP

3. What advantages does a neoadjuvant approach to this therapy hold over an adjuvant approach in this patient?

   Hint: See p. 1326 in PPP

4. What are the dose-limiting and common toxicities and counseling points for anthracyclines, alkylating agents, taxanes and HER2 targeted agents?

   Hint: See Table 89-6 PPP

5. Discuss some counselling points for patients taking anastrazole.

FOLLOW-UP

Two years after her initial presentation, Hermione is admitted to the emergency department following a serious fall in her home. Imaging demonstrates she sustained a significant hip fracture and MRI demonstrated multiple lytic bone lesions. Biopsy of one lesion has demonstrated recurrence of her breast cancer with an identical overall phenotype to the original cancer.

Discuss the theoretical advantages of the agent known as trastuzumab-DM1 as a future therapeutic option for this patient.

CASE SUMMARY

- Multiple extrinsic and intrinsic factors can significantly contribute to a patient's risk for developing breast cancer. In addition, multiple characteristics of each breast cancer case contribute to the overall prognosis of the patient.

- Patient preference can play an important role in the type of treatment that may be undertaken. Certain patients may even deny therapy, may opt for a less aggressive approach, or even choose a cosmetically appealing approach—these factors must be considered in the decision-making process.

- Neoadjuvant therapy in locally advance breast cancer is a viable option for many patients today, even in patients with more aggressive tumors such as HER2+ tumors.

- The management of a cancer patient relies on a coordinated effort between all parties including the patient. Emphasis should be placed on educating patients so they are prepared if confronted with chemotherapy cytotoxic side effects or other associated complications.

For more information on the care plan and facilitator's guide please visit http://www.mhpharmacotherapy.com

99 Colorectal Cancer

Patrick J. Medina   Emily B. Borders

PATIENT PRESENTATION

Chief Complaint

"I've been having irregular bowel movements for the past 2 months with some red color to it every once in a while. I've also been more tired then usual. In the last week, I've had only had one bowel that was very red. I'm not sure what is going on."

History of Present Illness

Phil Luisi is a 64-year-old Hispanic male who presented to his primary care physician with irregular bowel movements and generalized fatigue for 2 months. In the past week, he has significant constipation and large amounts of blood in his stool. Over-the-counter milk of magnesia had been recommended for the constipation and provided minimal relief. He also reports a loss of appetite due to "feeling bloated" and constipated. A complete blood count (CBC) revealed microcytic anemia thrombocytopenia. Fecal occult blood test was positive. Colonoscopy demonstrated a 5 cm (2-inch) frond-like, obstructing, villous lesion arising from the transverse colon. Biopsies were positive for high-grade, moderately differentiated adenocarcinoma. Tumor marker carcinoembryonic antigen (CEA) was 180 ng/mL (180 mcg/L) [normal 0–5 ng/mL (0–5 mcg/L)]. Metastatic disease was found on staging CT scans with 3 lesions ranging in size from 1-3-cm found in the liver. Final pathology revealed 4.5-cm (1.8-inch), high-grade, moderately differentiated adenocarcinoma invading into the muscularis propria. The tumor was found to be positive for *kras* mutations in codon 12. The final diagnosis was stage IV colon cancer. He underwent surgical resection to relieve pain from the obstruction and is being evaluated 4 weeks later in your clinic for metastatic treatment with the FOLFOX + bevacizumab regimen.

Past Medical History

Hypertension (HTN)

Hypercholesterolemia

Past Surgical History

Surgical debulking for the colon mass

Family History

Mother deceased at age 75 with colon cancer diagnosed at age 73. Father deceased at age 66 from a hemorrhagic stroke. Sister diagnosed with early stage breast cancer at the age of 52; no additional family history of cancer in family per the patient's report.

Social History

The patient is a lifelong resident of the state of New Jersey. He currently works as a school teacher. He is married and has two children.

Tobacco/Alcohol/Substance Use

The patient has 20-year pack history of smoking, but quit 10 years ago, drinks alcohol daily (3-5 drinks a day), and denies any drug use.

Allergies/Intolerances/Adverse Drug Events

No known drug allergies

Medications (Current)

Amlodipine 10 mg po q 24 h

Atorvastatin 10 mg po q 24 h

Milk of Magnesia 30 ml po prn constipation

Hydrocodone/acetaminophen 5/325 mg 1 tablet po prn pain

Review of Systems

Abdominal pain/constipation with minor relief with milk of magnesia; the patient has moderate postsurgical pain relieved with as-needed hydrocodone/acetaminophen. He denies any other symptoms, and additional review of symptoms is negative.

Physical Examination

▶ *General*

Thinly built, well-dressed, Hispanic male in mild acute distress

▶ *Vital Signs*

BP 114/79 mm Hg, P 67, RR 13, T 36.4°C

Weight 155 lb. (70.3 kg)

Height 68 in. (172.7 cm)

Mild abdominal and postsurgical pain

▶ *Skin*

Pale with good turgor; (–) lesions or pigments noted

▶ **HEENT**

PERRLA; (–) pallor, icterus; oropharynx clear

▶ **Neck**

Supple; no jugular venous distention; no significant lymphadenopathy

▶ **Respiratory**

Clear to auscultation

▶ **Cardiovascular**

RRR; no murmurs

▶ **Abdomen**

Soft; tender on palpation; normal BS; (+) hepatomegaly

▶ **Extremities**

(–) Edema, cyanosis, clubbing

▶ **Neurology**

AAO × 3; CNS grossly intact; no focal deficits noted

▶ **Rectal**

Stool is guaiac (+).

Laboratory and Other Diagnostic Tests

Fasting, Obtained 5 days ago. S/p Surgery 4 weeks ago

	Conventional Units	SI Units
Na	142 mEq/L	142 mmol/L
K	3.5 mEq/L	3.5 mmol/L
Cl	108 mEq/L	108 mmol/L
CO_2	22 mEq/L	22 mmol/L
BUN	18 mg/dL	6.7 mmol/L
SCr	0.8 mg/dL	70.7 µmol/L
Glu	88 mg/dL	4.9 mmol/L
Ca	8.8 mg/dL	2.20 mmol/L
Mg	1.9 mEq/L	0.95 mmol/L
WBC	$8.1 \times 10^3/mm^3$	$8.1 \times 10^9/L$
Hgb	11.4 g/dL	114 g/L; 7.1 mmol/L
Hct	35.2%	0.352
Platelets	$165 \times 10^3/mm^3$	$165 \times 10^9/L$
Albumin	2.9 g/dL	29 g/L
Total cholesterol	192 mg/dL	4.97 mmol/L
LDL cholesterol	140 mg/dL	3.62 mmol/L
HDL cholesterol	32 mg/dL	0.84 mmol/L
Total bilirubin	1.2 mg/dL	20.5 µmol/L
Alanine amino-transferase (ALT, SGPT)	173 U/L	2.9 µKat/L
Aspartate amino-transferase (AST, SGOT)	116 IU/L	1.9 µKat/L
Alkaline phosphatase	253 IU/L	4.2 µKat/L
CEA	18 ng/mL	18 mcg/L

▶ **CT Scans**

Liver positive for 3 lesions (1 cm; 1.8 cm; 3 cm). All other organs negative for metastatic disease.

▶ **Mutation Testing**

kras mutation positive – A G12D mutation was detected in the primary tumor biopsy. This results in an amino acid substitution at position 12 in *kras*, from a glycine (G) to an aspartic acid (D).

Assessment

A 64-year-old male with signs, symptoms, and pathology results diagnostic of stage IV colon cancer.

Student Work-Up

Missing Information/Inadequate Data

Evaluate: Patient database

Drug therapy problems

Care plan (by problem)

TARGETED QUESTIONS

1. What are the signs and symptoms this patient has for colon cancer?

   Hint: See p. 1350 in PPP

2. What risk factors did this patient have for the development of colon cancer?

   Hint: See Table 91-1 in PPP

3. What is the recommended therapy for this patient?

   Hint: See pp. 1350-1355 in PPP

4. Why are cetuximab and panitumumab not recommended to be added to this patient's regimen?

5. What risk factors and adverse effects of therapy would you discuss with this patient?

   Hint: See p. 1359 and Table 91-6 in PPP

FOLLOW-UP

The patient has been receiving the FOLFOX plus bevacizumab regimen for 4 months (eight cycles) with minimal adverse effects. During routine follow-up prior to his ninth cycle, he states he has noticed an increase in his daily blood pressure readings.

What is most likely causing this problem? What actions, if any, would you take?

🌐 GLOBAL PERSPECTIVE

Colon cancer is one of the most common cancers worldwide. The highest rate of colon cancer is in industrialized countries such as the United States as well as many countries in Europe. Industrialized countries tend to have diets high in fat, which partially explains the increased incidence, though other dietary and genetic factors play a role in its development. Early stage colon cancer (stages I–III) is curable with either surgery alone or surgery in combination with chemotherapy. Most patients receive 6 months of adjuvant chemotherapy following surgical resection of the tumor. Metastatic disease (stage IV) is currently incurable though patients can live 2 or more years. The initial treatment for most patients with metastatic disease consists of a combination chemotherapy backbone with targeted agents added as appropriate. Some of the chemotherapy agents (e.g., 5-fluorouracil, irinotecan) have pharmacogenomic factors, while others have tumor mutations (e.g., cetuximab and panitumumab) that determine their efficacy and toxicity.

CASE SUMMARY

- The patient is diagnosed with stage IV colon cancer requiring chemotherapy for metastatic disease.
- The initial regimen of FOLFOX plus bevacizumab is a reasonable choice, with therapy to progression of disease.
- *kras* mutations make therapies that target EGFR ineffective in colon cancer.
- Cumulative toxicities of the chemotherapy regimen should be evaluated at each clinic visit.

For more information on the care plan and facilitator's guide please visit http://www.mhpharmacotherapy.com

100 Acute Lymphocytic Leukemia

Shirley M. Abraham   Nancy H. Heideman
Richard L. Heideman

PATIENT PRESENTATION

Chief Complaint

Intermittent fevers, decreased appetite and weight loss.

History of Present Illness

JM is a 12-year-old Hispanic female who presented with a 3-week history of intermittent fevers, loss of appetite increased fatigue, headaches and weight loss. A few days prior, she also had a brief nose bleed, mild abdominal pain, followed by nausea and 1 episode of emesis. Patient's grandmother also noted a bruise on her right arm about 2 days prior.

Labs done at the outside hospital showed white blood cells of 129K/mm3, hemoglobin 8.7g/dl, hematocrit 27%, platelets 83K/mm3, and 96% blasts. Patient was transferred to the treating institution for further management of newly diagnosed acute leukemia.

Past Medical History

Full-term infant, uncomplicated birth and neonatal history. No prior hospital admissions or surgeries. Completely up-to-date on childhood immunizations for her age up to the time of diagnosis. Attained menarche 6 months prior.

Family History

Insulin dependent type I Diabetes Mellitus in several adult family members.

Social History

The patient is currently in seventh grade. She is a good student. She lives with both parents, 2 sisters and a brother.

Tobacco/Alcohol/Substance Use

Noncontributory

Allergies/Intolerance/Adverse Drug Events

None known

Prior to Admission Medications

None

Review of Systems

Patient has a 3-week history of fever and body pains. She also had a few days of abdominal pain, mild nausea and 1 episode of emesis. She had decreased oral intake and weight loss over the past 2 weeks. Patient also endorses malaise and headaches over the past 1 week. She attained menarche 6 months prior.

Physical Exam

▶ *General*

Obese, tired and pale appearing

▶ *Vital Signs*

BP 129/67 mmHg, P 104, RR 20, T 37.7°C

Weight 69.8 kg

Height 157.5 cm

Pain 5/10

▶ *Skin*

Warm, soft, acanthosis nigricans at nape of neck and axillae, few petechiae on back of neck

▶ *HEENT*

Within normal limits

▶ *Neck and Lymph Nodes*

Few shoddy cervical lymph nodes

▶ *Chest*

Clear to auscultation bilaterally

▶ *Cardiovascular*

Normal sinus rate and rhythm; good capillary refill; grade 2/5 systolic murmur at the apex

▶ *Abdomen*

Mildly tender in the right upper quadrant and epigastrium. Liver is a palpable 10 cm below the right costal margin and spleen is palpable 6 cm below the left costal margin.

▶ *Extremities*

Range of motion normal. No deformities noted. Some tenderness noted of both upper arms and legs.

▶ *Neurology*

Within normal limits

▶ *Genitourinary*

Tanner 4 female

Laboratory Tests

	Conventional Units	SI Units
Hgb	8.7 g/dL	87 g/L; 5.4 mmol/L
Hct	34%	0.34
WBC	$129 \times 10^3/mm^3$	$129 \times 10^9/L$
Blast count	96%	0.96
Platelets	$83 \times 10^3/mm^3$	$83 \times 10^9/L$
Uric acid	15 mg/dL	891 µmol/L
LDL cholesterol (calculated)	4762 mg/dL	123 mmol/L

Basic metabolic panel and liver function test results within normal limits.

Pathology: Peripheral blood and bone marrow evaluation showing 93% leukemic blasts that have CD19, CD10, CD34, HLA-DR, dim CD79a, TdT, CD22, dim CD45, minor subset with CD13, consistent with preB-acute lymphoblastic leukemia (ALL).

FISH: Positive for t(9;22) (q34;q11.2) in 87% (0.87) of the cells using Bcr/Abl1 dual fusion probe, negative for TEL/AML1 and MLL rearrangements.

Bcr-Abl transcript detected at ratio of 1.14 (>0.1 indicative of very high levels).

CNS status: CNS 2b (> 10 RBCs, <5 WBC, cytospin positive for blasts).

Assessment

A 12-year-old female with high risk acute preB-ALL, positive for Bcr-Abl (Philadelphia chromosome) who needs to be started on induction chemotherapy.

Student Work-Up

Missing Information/Inadequate Data

Evaluate:	Patient database
	Drug therapy problems
	Care plan (by problem)

TARGETED QUESTIONS

1. Identify the common presenting signs and symptoms of acute leukemia.

   Hint: See p. 1403 in PPP

2. Evaluate the prognostic factors for acute lymphoblastic leukemia (ALL) and evaluate the patient's potential risk for relapse.

   Hint: See pp. 1404-1405 and Table 95-5 in PPP

3. Recognize the immunophenotypic markers that help to make a diagnosis of preB ALL.

   Hint: See Table 95-4 in PPP

4. Identify the Philadelphia chromosome and its significance in ALL.

   Hint: See p. 1405 in PPP

5. What is the potential significance of acanthosis nigricans and obesity and family history of type 1 diabetes in this patient? How might her induction and subsequent treatment with dexamethasone present a problem?

   Hint: See 2015 American Diabetes Association Guidelines

FOLLOW UP

Patient had evidence of tumor lysis even before she started treatment as indicated by the high uric acid concentration. She received a dose of rasburicase and was placed on alkalinized fluids at twice maintenance. Patient started induction per high risk protocol and continued on this until day 15 when she was switched to the protocol specific for Philadelphia positive preB-ALL patients that includes Dasatinib, a tyrosine kinase inhibitor in addition to standard chemotherapy. Her day 29 MRD (minimal residual disease) was <0.01%, BCR-ABL transcript was negative by PCR and FISH.

As biologic agents like Dasatinib and others are introduced into treatment regimens, it is imperative that potential drug interactions and influences of diet be considered. What are some potential drug interactions with Dasatinib?

What are the signs of tumor lysis syndrome and how does rasburicase work?

What is the prognostic significance of MRD?

⟳ GLOBAL PERSPECTIVE

PreB-ALL is a heterogeneous disease characterized by multiple genetically defined subtypes. It is crucial that these genetic markers are identified early in treatment and the patient is appropriately risk stratified because these are important prognostic markers. The Philadelphia chromosome (Ph+) results from a reciprocal translocation between chromosomes 9 and 22, creating the BCR-ABL fusion protein, a constitutively activated form of ABL tyrosine kinase. The Philadelphia chromosome is found in 3-5% of pediatric ALL and 20-40% of adult ALL. The presence of this genetic change confers a significantly worse prognosis in both pediatric and adult ALL patients.

Until recently, hematopoietic stem cell transplant (HSCT), in first complete remission, offers the best chances for long-term survival in pediatric patients with Ph+ ALL. However, this was limited by the availability of a matched donor, and was also associated with significant post- transplant morbidity and mortality.

Currently the standard of treatment for this group of patients is the optimal integration of specific tyrosine kinase inhibitors such as imatinib or dasatinib into established multi-agent high-risk ALL backbone chemotherapy with the goal of improving overall survival.

CASE SUMMARY

- There are multiple other factors, such as potential comorbidities suggested by the physical exam and family history and social circumstances that should be considered as clues to problems that might develop during treatment.

- Think about the implications these issues for patient care, especially the impact of potential prediabetes in a patient who is starting a potent steroid.

For more information on the care plan and facilitator's guide please visit http://www.mhpharmacotherapy.com

101 Parenteral Nutrition

Michael D. Kraft   Melissa R. Pleva

PATIENT PRESENTATION

Chief Complaint

"I have fluid coming out of my surgery incision."

History of Present Illness

EF is a 58-year-old man who presented 7 days ago with a 2-month history of worsening abdominal pain and unintentional weight loss of ~20 kg (~44 lbs). Over the past month, the patient has also developed worsening nausea and vomiting, especially after eating, which has led to food avoidance. EF was admitted for further evaluation, including computed tomography (CT) scan that revealed a pancreatic mass. The patient was taken to the OR for an exploratory laparotomy and pancreaticoduodenectomy (i.e. Whipple procedure). Biopsies of the mass were positive for pancreatic adenocarcinoma. The team has attempted to advance oral intake, but so far this has been limited to clear liquids due to nausea and a few episodes of vomiting. Yesterday (post-operative day #5 (POD #5), hospital day #6 (HD #6)), the patient complained of a low-grade fever, and today (POD #6, HD #7), the patient was noted to have drainage at his surgical incision. The appearance of the fluid was consistent with intestinal fluid, so he was taken for a CT with oral contrast and a fistulogram. He was diagnosed with a high-output enterocutaneous (EC) fistula, likely originating from the mid-small bowel. He was made nil per os (NPO) status, his intravenous (IV) fluids increased to maintenance dose for hydration, a peripherally-inserted central catheter (PICC) was placed, and the team wants to initiate parenteral nutrition (PN).

Past Medical History

Depression

Alcoholism (25 years, quit in 2014)

Past Surgical History

Appendectomy in 1985

Family History

Remarkable for hypertension (mother and father) and hyperlipidemia (father)

Social History

Single, lives alone

Tobacco/Alcohol/Substance Abuse

History of alcoholism, abstinent since December 2014

Allergies/Intolerances/Adverse Drug Events

No known drug allergies

Medications (Current)

Heparin 5,000 units subcutaneous three times daily

Pantoprazole 40 mg IV daily

Morphine sulfate 2 to 4 mg IV q 4 h prn pain

Ondansetron 4 mg IV q 8 h prn nausea

Regular insulin (sliding-scale) q 6 h, dosage per capillary blood glucose measurements (chemsticks)

D5 ½ NS + 20 mEq/L KCL at 90 mL/hour

Medications Prior to Admission

Citalopram 20 mg po daily

Review of Systems

Subjectively reporting ongoing abdominal pain, nausea, no appetite, feels thirsty. Denies fever, chills, or other pain. (+) Dry mucus membranes.

Physical Examination

▶ *General*

Middle-aged African-American man, appears malnourished/cachectic

▶ *Vital Signs (Today – POD#6, HD#7)*

BP 110/68 mmHg, P 89, RR 14, T 38.3°C

Weight 56 kg (123 lbs)

Height 178 cm (70 in.)

Per patient, weight in December 2014 when he completed rehabilitation for alcoholism was 75 kg (165 lbs). Patient reports intermittent abdominal pain rated as 4–5 (on a scale of 1 – 10, 1 being no pain and 10 being the worst pain he has experienced), some relief with morphine; he also reports intermittent nausea and vomiting, relieved with ondansetron.

▶ **Skin**

Dry

▶ **HEENT**

PERRLA, EOMI, anicteric sclerae, mucus membranes dry

▶ **Chest**

Clear to auscultation bilaterally

▶ **Cardiovascular**

RRR; no murmurs, rubs, or gallops

▶ **Abdomen**

(+) Hypoactive/absent bowel sounds, mild tenderness around incision site, greenish drainage from surgical incision

▶ **Neurology**

A&O × 3; CNs II to XII intact

▶ **Extremities**

(−) Cyanosis, good pulse

▶ **Genitourinary**

Examination deferred

▶ **Rectum**

Examination deferred

Laboratory Tests

On Admission:

	Conventional Units	SI Units
Na	138 mEq/L	138 mmol/L
K	3.6 mEq/L	3.6 mmol/L
Cl	94 mEq/L	94 mmol/L
CO_2	28 mEq/L	28 mmol/L
BUN	12 mg/dL	4.3 mmol/L
SCr	0.5 mg/dL	44 μmol/L
Glu	152 mg/dL	8.4 mmol/L
Ca	7.6 mg/dL	1.9 mmol/L
Mg	1.5 mEq/L	0.75 mmol/L
Phosphate	3.1 mg/dL	1.0 mmol/L
Hgb	14.1 g/dL	141 g/L; 8.7 mmol/L
Hct	41.7%	0.417
WBC	$7.4 \times 10^3/mm^3$	$7.4 \times 10^9/L$
Platelets	$384 \times 10^3/mm^3$	$384 \times 10^9/L$
Albumin	2.4 g/dL	24 g/L
Total bilirubin	0.6 mg/dL	10.3 μmol/L
AST	17 IU/L	0.28 μkat/L

On Hospital Day 7 (Today):

	Conventional Units	SI Units
Na	135 mEq/L	135 mmol/L
K	3.3 mEq/L	3.3 mmol/L
Cl	92 mEq/L	92 mmol/L
CO_2	26 mEq/L	26 mmol/L
BUN	17 mg/dL	6.1 mmol/L
SCr	0.6 mg/dL	53 μmol/L
Glu	185 mg/dL	10.3 mmol/L
Ca	7.3 mg/dL	1.8 mmol/L
Mg	1.1 mEq/L	0.55 mmol/L
Phosphate	2.3 mg/dL	0.74 mmol/L
Hgb	13.2 g/dL	132 g/L; 8.2 mmol/L
Hct	38.4%	0.384
WBC	$8.9 \times 10^3/mm^3$	$8.9 \times 10^9/L$
Platelets	$297 \times 10^3/mm^3$	$297 \times 10^9/L$
Albumin	2.1 g/dL	21 g/L
Total bilirubin	0.9 mg/dL	15.4 μmol/L
AST	18 IU/L	0.30 μkat/L
ALT	19 IU/L	0.32 μkat/L
Alkaline phosphatase	34 IU/L	0.57 μkat/L

▶ **Radiology**

CT scan with oral contrast and fistulogram demonstrated enterocutaneous fistula, originating from the surgical site.

Assessment

This is a 58-year-old man who is status postexploratory laparotomy and Whipple's procedure for pancreatic adenocarcinoma, complicated by an EC fistula. He has a history of malnutrition and unintentional weight loss of 20 kg (~44 lbs) since December 2014. Given the apparent location of the fistula, the patient's ongoing nausea and vomiting, and his severe weight loss and severe malnutrition, the surgical team made the patient NPO, continued IV fluids for hydration, placed a PICC and wants to initiate PN therapy.

Student Work-Up

Missing Information/Inadequate Data

Evaluate: Patient database

Drug therapy problems

Care plan (by problem)

TARGETED QUESTIONS

1. Does this patient have an appropriate indication for PN therapy?

   Hint: See p. 1490, Table 100-1, and references 1 and 2 in Chapter 100 in PPP

2. Is this patient at risk of refeeding syndrome? If so, why?

   Hint: See p. 1502 and reference 42 in Chapter 100 in PPP

3. What signs, symptoms, and laboratory abnormalities are possible manifestations of refeeding syndrome?

   Hint: See p. 1502 and reference 42 in Chapter 100 in PPP

4. What steps would you take to prevent refeeding syndrome in this patient?

   Hint: See p. 1502 and reference 42 in Chapter 100 in PPP

5. What treatment would you recommend for his hyperglycemia? What target range for serum glucose concentrations would you recommend?

   Hint: See pp. 1500-1501 and references 31-33 in Chapter 100 in PPP

6. Is this patient receiving any medications that do not have an appropriate indication?

FOLLOW-UP

The surgical team takes your recommendations, and the patient's symptoms and electrolyte abnormalities have resolved, and his glucose control has improved. The team developed the following prescription for EF's goal PN formulation, with a plan to give 50% of this dose on day #1 (today) and then advance to goal on day #2 of PN (tomorrow):

Three-in-one PN formulation (all PN components admixed in the same container)

PN volume (dextrose/amino acid/micronutrient admixture) = 2,160 mL (90 mL/h)

Dextrose (70% stock solution) = 425 g/d

Amino acids (15% stock solution) = 110 g/d

IV fat emulsion (20% emulsion) = 50 g

Potassium chloride = 40 mEq/d (40 mmol/d)

Sodium chloride = 40 mEq/d (20 mmol/d)

Sodium acetate = 30 mEq/d (60 mmol/d)

Sodium phosphate = 15 mmol/d

Calcium gluconate = 10 mEq/d (5 mmol/d)

Magnesium sulfate = 10 mEq/d (5 mmol/d)

Parenteral adult multivitamin = 10 mL/d

Multi-trace element (concentrate) = 1 mL/d

What recommendations would you have about initiating PN in this patient? Develop a goal PN regimen, as well as a plan to initiate PN, advance PN to goal, and monitor PN therapy while in the hospital.

Hint: Calculate total calories and protein in the above PN prescription; note amounts of electrolytes (especially phosphate, potassium, magnesium, and sodium), total fluid, and any supplemental vitamins and trace elements, especially considering risk of refeeding syndrome; evaluate the patient's fluid needs and assess any abnormal fluid and electrolyte losses (e.g., GI losses); see p. 1499 and 1502, tables 100-3, 100-4, 100-5, 100-9, and references 1, 2, and 42 in Chapter 100 in PPP.

🌀 GLOBAL PERSPECTIVE

The refeeding syndrome is a constellation of metabolic derangements that can occur in patients who are malnourished or who have had a prolonged period of inadequate nutrition with significant weight loss. Refeeding syndrome can lead to serious complications, including death (although rare), and it can be one of the few true emergencies associated with nutrition therapy. In developing countries or areas where malnutrition is prevalent and nutrient and vitamin deficiencies are common, refeeding syndrome could be a significant concern if the person were to receive a more abundant source of nutrition (oral or parenteral). These individuals with severe protein and calorie malnutrition may be more likely to have underlying vitamin and trace element deficiencies that could complicate or worsen symptoms of refeeding syndrome (e.g., thiamine, folic acid, vitamin B_{12}, vitamin D, iron, selenium, zinc, copper).

This could be especially concerning in growing children with poor body protein and energy reserves and pregnant women who have added energy and nutrient demands. A good rule of thumb in individuals with moderate-to-severe malnutrition is to "start low and go slow" when initiating any type of nutrition whether PN, enteral nutrition, or oral diet. This slow-and-gradual approach is essential to avoid the complications of refeeding syndrome that may severely affect the cardiac, respiratory, neurologic, and neuromuscular systems. It is also important to provide aggressive supplementation of electrolytes, vitamins, and trace elements before initiating nutrition, and regularly as needed during nutrition advancement guided by serum electrolyte concentrations and clinical status.

CASE SUMMARY

- This Patient has an indication for PN given the presence (and location) of a high-output EC fistula, as well as evidence of severe malnutrition. Given these conditions, he is also at risk for refeeding syndrome when initiating PN therapy.

- Refeeding syndrome can lead to serious electrolyte abnormalities and associated complications, including death (although rare). A good approach in patients at risk for refeeding syndrome is to "start low and go slow" when initiating nutrition therapy (PN, enteral nutrition, or even an oral diet), aggressively correct serum electrolyte abnormalities (especially phosphorus, potassium, and magnesium) before initiating and while providing nutrition therapy, provide supplemental thiamine and folic acid for the first 5-7 days of therapy, evaluate for and develop a plan to correct other nutritional deficiencies, and monitor closely for abnormalities and complications. A specific prevention and treatment plan should be outlined.

- The patient also has depression and was taking citalopram which is currently on hold. Therefore, a plan must be developed to manage depression and potentially withdrawal effects from holding citalopram.

For more information on the care plan and facilitator's guide please visit http://www.mhpharmacotherapy.com

102 Obesity

Maqual R Graham

PATIENT PRESENTATION

Chief Complaint (CC)

"My wife thinks that I may feel better if I lost a few pounds. Can you recommend something to help me lose weight?"

History or Present Illness (HPI)

BT is a 57-year-old white male who reports to the pharmacist-managed Weight Loss Clinic for an initial evaluation. Patient states that his wife strongly feels that he might become more energetic and feel healthier overall if he could just lose a little weight. Complaints from patient include low energy and occasional lower back pain (rated as a 4 on a scale of 1-10). Upon further questioning, you determine that he has tried a variety of diets in the past but did not adhere to any of them. He prefers to eat whatever he pleases even though he knows which foods are considered healthy/unhealthy. He reports eating pancakes or biscuits with gravy for breakfast, a hamburger, fried chicken or pork tenderloin sandwich with French fries or onion rings for lunch and again for dinner. He typically eats ice cream or a chocolate candy bar before going to bed each night. Of note, patient presents with a large fountain drink from QuickTrip. Patient is not currently exercising. Patient claims that being an over-the-road truck driver impedes his ability to consume healthy food and adhere to an exercise regimen. Patient admits that he is "tired of making excuses and tired of feeling tired." Patient appears motivated to lose weight but would like something to help him achieve weight loss.

Past Medical History (PMH)

Hypertension (HTN) (diagnosed 6 years ago)
Depression (diagnosed 6 months ago) (first episode)
Occasional lower back pain (2 years)

Family History

Mother: Deceased, died at age 94, mother had HTN, diabetes, congestive heart failure
Father: Deceased, died at age 75 following "open heart surgery"

Social History

(+) alcohol, 2-4 beers during the weekend
(+) tobacco, ½ ppd for 40 years

Allergy/Intolerances

Amoxicillin causes a rash

Medication History

► **Current**

Hydrochlorothiazide 25 mg po q AM
Lisinopril 20 mg po q AM
Escitalopram 10 mg po q AM
Ibuprofen 600 mg po prn back pain

► **Prior Medication Use**

Sertraline 100 mg po daily (not effective for controlling depressive symptoms)

Review of Symptoms

(–) heartburn, dyspepsia; (–) dizziness, shortness of breath, chest pain

Physical Exam (PE)

► **Vital Signs**

BP 124/80 mm Hg, P 78 bpm, RR 15 rpm, T 98.0 (F Height 5′6″
Weight 217 pounds
WC 41 in.

► **HEENT**

Conjunctiva clear

► **Neck**

Supple

► **Cardiovascular**

Regular rhythm, no S_3 or S_4 noted

► **Chest**

Clear to auscultation (CTA) bilaterally

► **Abdomen**

Obese, soft, nontender, nondistended; (+) bowel sounds

► **Neurology**

Normal gait, normal speech

▶ *Extremeties*

(–) Edema

Laboratory Tests

	Conventional Units	*SI Units*
Na	142 mEq/L	142 mmol/L
K	4.3 mEu/L	4.6 mmol/L
Cl	107 mEq/L	107 mmol/L
CO_2	23 mEq/L	23 mmol/L
BUN	15 mg/dL	5.4 mmol/L
Creatinine	0.9 mg/dL	80 μmol/L
Glucose	76 mg/dL	4.2 mmol/L
TSH	1.4 μIU/mL	1.4 mIU/L

Assessment

A 57-year-old obese male patient presents to clinic requesting help to achieve weight loss.

Student Work-Up

Missing Information/Inadequate Data

Evaluate: Patient database

Drug therapy problems

Care plan (by problem)

TARGETED QUESTIONS

1. How would you classify this patient's BMI?

   Hint: See Table 102-1 in PPP

2. Does this patient have modifiable cardiovascular disease risk factors, and if so, which one(s)?

   Hint: See p. 1542 and Table 102-3 in PPP

3. Is this patient a candidate for weight loss, and if so, what is the initial weight loss goal?

   Hint: See p. 1542 (Key Concept #4) in PPP

4. Is nonpharmacologic therapy, pharmacologic therapy, or both recommended for this patient?

   Hint: See pp. 1525-1526 in PPP

5. How often should the patient return for follow-up and what patient parameters need assessed?

   Hint: See p. 1530 in PPP

FOLLOW-UP

The patient has returned for all scheduled follow-up assessment visits in the Obesity Management Clinic. At the 6-month follow-up visit, it was determined that the patient's weight decreased by 8 pounds (3.6 kg). His waist circumference is now 40 inches (102 cm). He appears compliant with the therapy previously recommended. He feels a little more energetic; however, he wishes that he was closer to his weight loss goal.

Should the initial therapeutic recommendations be altered, and if so, how?

Hint: See pp. 1530-1531 in PPP

⊙ GLOBAL PERSPECTIVE

Energy imbalance, or energy intake greater than energy expenditure, is a key factor in the development of obesity. The longer the imbalance occurs, the greater the extent of obesity. Height and weight can easily be assessed anytime a patient–provider interaction occurs. From these two parameters, BMI can be determined. Waist circumference should also be evaluated as well as presence of other comorbidities and cardiovascular disease risk factors. Weight reduction, maintaining weight loss, and preventing weight gain are the general therapeutic goals for obese patients. Controlling related risks is an additional goal in the management of obesity. Lifestyle changes (dietary modification, increased physical activity, and behavioral therapy), drug treatment, surgery, or a combination of strategies are necessary for meeting desired outcomes. Frequent follow-up is necessary to determine the success or failure of the treatment plan.

CASE SUMMARY

- BT is a Class 2 obese patient with a high-risk waist circumference and at least 2 modifiable cardiovascular disease risk factors that include hypertension and cigarette smoking.

- A comprehensive lifestyle intervention program is recommended to reduce his weight by 11-22 pounds (5-10 kg) in 6 months at a rate of 1–2 pounds (0.45–0.9 kg)/week.

- Aggressive management of related risks (blood pressure, cigarette smoking) is necessary for overall effective treatment of the obese patient.

For more information on the care plan and facilitator's guide please visit http://www.mhpharmacotherapy.com

Appendix A: Conversion Factors and Anthropometrics*

CONVERSION FACTORS

SI Units

SI (*le Systéme International d'Unités*) units are used in many countries to express clinical laboratory and serum drug concentration data. Instead of using units of mass (eg, micrograms), the SI system uses moles (mol) to represent the amount of a substance. A molar solution contains 1 mole (the molecular weight of the substance in grams) of the solute in 1 L of solution. The following formula is used to convert units of mass to moles (mcg/mL to μmol/L or, by substitution of terms, mg/mL to mmol/L or ng/mL to nmol/L).

▶ *Micromoles per Liter*

Micromoles per liter (μmol/L)

$$= \frac{\text{drug concentration (mcg/mL)} \times 1000}{\text{molecular weight of drug (g/mol)}}$$

▶ *Milliequivalents*

An equivalent weight of a substance is the weight that will combine with or replace 1 g of hydrogen; a milliequivalent is 1/1000 of an equivalent weight.

Milliequivalents per Liter

Milliequivalents per liter (mEq/L)

$$= \frac{\text{weight of salt (g)} \times \text{valence of ion} \times 1000}{\text{molecular weight of salt}}$$

$$\text{Weight of salt (g)} = \frac{\text{mEq/L} \times \text{molecular weight of salt}}{\text{valence of ion} \times 1000}$$

Approximate Milliequivalents: Weight Conversions for Selected Ions

Salt	mEq/g Salt	mg Salt/ mEq
Calcium carbonate ($CaCO_3$)	20.0	50.0
Calcium chloride ($CaCl_2 \cdot 2H_2O$)	13.6	73.5
Calcium gluceptate ($Ca[C_7H_{13}O_8]_2$)	4.1	245.2
Calcium gluconate ($Ca[C_6H_{11}O_7]_2 \cdot H_2O$)	4.5	224.1
Calcium lactate ($Ca[C_3H_5O_3]_2 \cdot 5H_2O$)	6.5	154.1
Magnesium gluconate ($Mg[C_6H_{11}O_7]_2 \cdot H_2O$)	4.6	216.3
Magnesium oxide (MgO)	49.6	20.2
Magnesium sulfate ($MgSO_4$)	16.6	60.2
Magnesium sulfate ($MgSO_4 \cdot 7H_2O$)	8.1	123.2
Potassium acetate ($K[C_2H_3O_2]$)	10.2	98.1
Potassium chloride (KCl)	13.4	74.6
Potassium citrate ($K_3[C_6H_5O_7] \cdot H_2O$)	9.2	108.1
Potassium iodide (KI)	6.0	166.0
Sodium acetate ($Na[C_2H_3O_2]$)	12.2	82.0
Sodium acetate ($Na[C_2H_3O_2] \cdot 3H_2O$)	7.3	136.1
Sodium bicarbonate ($NaHCO_3$)	11.9	84.0
Sodium chloride (NaCl)	17.1	58.4
Sodium citrate ($Na_3[C_6H_5O_7] \cdot 2H_2O$)	10.2	98.0
Sodium iodide (NaI)	6.7	149.9
Sodium lactate ($Na[C_3H_5O_3]$)	8.9	112.1
Zinc sulfate ($ZnSO_4 \cdot 7H_2O$)	7.0	143.8

Valences and Atomic/Molecular Weights of Selected Ions

Substance	Electrolyte	Valence	Atomic/ Molecular Weight
Calcium	Ca^{2+}	2	40.1
Chloride	Cl^-	1	35.5
Magnesium	Mg^{2+}	2	24.3
Phosphate	HPO_4^{2-}(80%)	1.8	96.0[a]
(pH = 7.4)	$H_2PO_4^-$(20%)		97.0
Potassium	K^+	1	39.1
Sodium	Na^+	1	23.0
Sulfate	SO_4^-	2	96.0[a]

[a]The atomic/molecular weight of phosphorus is only 31; that of sulfur is only 32.1.

*This appendix contains information from Appendices 1 and 2 of Smith KM, Riche DM, Henyan NN (eds.). Clinical Drug Data, 11th ed. New York: McGraw-Hill, 2010:1239–1246; With permission.

Anion Gap

The anion gap is the concentration of plasma anions not routinely measured by laboratory screening. It is useful in the evaluation of acid–base disorders. The anion gap is greater with increased plasma concentrations of endogenous species (eg, phosphate, sulfate, lactate, and ketoacids) or exogenous species (eg, salicylate, penicillin, ethylene glycol, ethanol, and methanol). The formulas for calculating the anion gap are as follows:

$$\text{Anion gap} = (Na^+ + K^+) - (Cl^- + HCO_3^-)$$

or

$$\text{Anion gap} = Na^+ - (Cl^- + HCO_3^-)$$

where the expected normal value for the first equation is 11 to 20 mmol/L and for the second equation is 7 to 16 mmol/L. Note that there is a variation in the upper and lower limits of the normal range.

Temperature

Fahrenheit to Centigrade: (°F − 32) × 5/9 = °C
Centigrade to Fahrenheit: (°C × 9/5) + 32 = °F
Centigrade to Kelvin: °C + 273 = °K

Weights and Measures

▶ Metric Weight Equivalents

1 kilogram (kg) = 1000 grams

1 gram (g) = 1000 milligrams

1 milligram (mg) = 0.001 gram

1 microgram (mcg, μg) = 0.001 milligram

1 nanogram (ng) = 0.001 microgram

1 picogram (pg) = 0.001 nanogram

1 femtogram (fg) = 0.001 picogram

▶ Metric Volume Equivalents

1 liter (L) = 1000 milliliters

1 deciliter (dL) = 100 milliliters

1 milliliter (mL) = 0.001 liter

1 microliter (μL) = 0.001 milliliter

1 nanoliter (nL) = 0.001 microliter

1 picoliter (pL) = 0.001 nanoliter

1 femtoliter (fL) = 0.001 picoliter

▶ Apothecary Weight Equivalents

1 scruple (℈) = 20 grains (gr)

60 grains (gr) = 1 dram (ʒ)

8 drams (ʒ) = 1 ounce (ℨ)

1 ounce (ℨ) = 480 grains (gr)

12 ounces (ℨ) = 1 pound (lb)

▶ Apothecary Volume Equivalents

60 minims (m) = 1 fluidram (fl ʒ)

8 fluidrams (fl ʒ) = 1 fluid ounce (fl ℨ)

1 fluid ounce (fl ℨ) = 480 minims (m)

16 fluid ounces (fl ℨ) = 1 pint (pt)

▶ Avoirdupois Equivalents

1 ounce (oz) = 437.5 grains

16 ounces (oz) = 1 pound (lb)

▶ Weight/Volume Equivalents

1 mg/dL = 10 mcg/mL

1 mg/dL = 1 mg%

1 ppm = 1 mg/L

▶ Conversion Equivalents

1 gram (g) = 15.43 grains (gr)

1 grain (gr) = 64.8 milligrams (mg)

1 ounce (ℨ) = 31.1 grams (g)

1 ounce (oz) = 28.35 grams (g)

1 pound (lb) = 453.6 grams (g)

1 kilogram (kg) = 2.2 pounds (lb)

1 milliliter (mL) = 16.23 minims (m)

1 minim (m) = 0.06 milliliter (mL)

1 fluid ounce (fl oz) = 29.57 milliliters (mL)

1 pint (pt) = 473.2 milliliters (mL)

1 US gallon = 3.78 liters (L)

1 Canadian gallon = 4.55 liters (L)

0.1 milligram = 1/650 grain

0.12 milligram = 1/540 grain

0.15 milligram = 1/430 grain

0.2 milligram = 1/320 grain

0.3 milligram = 1/220 grain

0.4 milligram = 1/160 grain

0.5 milligram = 1/130 grain

0.6 milligram = 1/110 grain

0.8 milligram = 1/80 grain

1 milligram = 1/65 grain

▶ Metric Length Conversion Equivalents

2.54 cm = 1 inch

30.48 cm = 1 foot

1 m = 3.28 feet

1.6 km = 1 mile

ANTHROPOMETRICS

Creatinine Clearance Formulas

▶ *Formulas for Estimating Creatinine Clearance in Patients with Stable Renal Function*

Cockcroft-Gault Formula

Adults (age 18 years and older)[1]:

$$CrCl\ (men) = \frac{(140 - age) \times weight}{SCr \times 72}$$

$$CrCl\ (women) = 0.85 \times above\ value^*$$

where CrCl is creatinine clearance (in mL/min), SCr is serum creatinine (in mg/dL [or μmol/L divided by 88.4]), age is in years, and weight is in kilograms.

Traub-Johnson Formula

Children (age 1–18 years)[2]:

$$CrCl = \frac{0.48 \times height \times BSA}{SCr \times 1.73}$$

where BSA is body surface area (in m²), CrCl is creatinine clearance (in mL/min), SCr is serum creatinine (in mg/dL [or μmol/L divided by 88.4]), and height is in centimeters.

▶ *Formula for Estimating Creatinine Clearance From a Measured Urine Collection*

$$CrCl\ (mL/min) = \frac{U \times V}{P \times T}$$

where U is the concentration of creatinine in a urine specimen in mg/dL, V is the volume of urine in mL, P is the concentration of creatinine in serum at the midpoint of the urine collection period in mg/dL, and T is the time of the urine collection period in minutes (eg, 6 hours = 360 minutes; 24 hours = 1440 minutes). Procedures for obtaining urine specimens should stress the importance of complete urine collection during the collection time period.

▶ *IDMS-Traceable MDRD Equation (Used for Creatinine Methods with Calibration Traceable to IDMS)*

For creatinine in mg/dL:

$$X = 175 \times creatinine^{-1.154} \times age^{-0.203} \times constant$$

For creatinine in μmol/L:

$$X = 175 \times (creatinine/88.4)^{-1.154} \times age^{-0.203} \times constant$$

where X is the glomerular filtration rate, constant for white men is 1 and for women is 0.742, and constant for African Americans is 1.212.

Ideal Body Weight

IBW is the weight expected for a non-obese person of a given height. The IBW formulas below and various life insurance tables can be used to estimate IBW. Dosing methods described in the literature may use IBW as a method in dosing obese patients.

Adults (age 18 years and older)[3]:

$$IBW\ (men) = 50 + (2.3 \times height\ in\ inches\ over\ 5\ ft)$$

$$IBW\ (women) = 45.5 + (2.3 \times height\ in\ inches\ over\ 5\ ft)$$

where IBW is in kilograms.

Children (age 1–18 years)[2] under 5 feet tall:

$$IBW = \frac{height^2 \times 1.65}{1000}$$

where IBW is in kilograms and height is in centimeters.

Children (age 1–18 years) 5 feet or taller:

$$IBW\ (males) = 39 + (2.27 \times height\ in\ inches\ over\ 5\ ft)$$

$$IBW\ (females) = 42.2 + (2.27 \times height\ in\ inches\ over\ 5\ ft)$$

where IBW is in kilograms.

REFERENCES

1. Cockcroft DW, Gault MH. Prediction of creatinine clearance from serum creatinine. Nephron. 1976;16:31-41.
2. Traub SI, Johnson CE. Comparison of methods of estimating creatinine clearance in children. Am J Hosp Pharm. 1980;37: 195-201.
3. Devine BJ. Gentamicin therapy. Drug Intell Clin Pharm. 1974; 8:650-655.

---

*Some studies suggest that the predictive accuracy of this formula for women is better *without* the correction factor of 0.85.

Appendix B: Common Laboratory Tests

The following table is an alphabetical listing of some common laboratory tests and their reference ranges for adults as measured in plasma or serum (unless otherwise indicated). Reference values differ among laboratories, so readers should refer to the published reference ranges used in each institution. For some tests, both the Système International Units and Conventional Units are reported.

Laboratory Test	Conventional Units	Conversion Factor	Système International Units
Acid phosphatase			
Male	2–12 U/L	16.7	33–200 nkat/L
Female	0.3–9.2 U/L	16.7	5–154 nkat/L
Activated partial thromboplastin time (aPTT)	25–40 seconds		
Adrenocorticotropic hormone (ACTH)	15–80 pg/mL or ng/L	0.2202	3.3–17.6 pmol/L
Alanine aminotransferase (ALT, SGPT)	7–53 U/L	0.01667	0.12–0.88 μkat/L
Albumin	3.5–5.0 g/dL	10	35–50 g/L
Albumin:creatinine ratio (urine)		0.113	
Normal	< 30 mg/g creatinine		< 3.4 mg/mmol creatinine
Microalbuminuria	30–300 mg/g creatinine		3.4–34 mg/mmol creatinine
Proteinuria	> 300 mg/g creatinine		> 34 mg/mmol creatinine
or	or		
Normal			
Male	< 18 mg/g creatinine	0.113	< 2.0 mg/mmol creatinine
Female	< 25 mg/g creatinine	0.113	< 2.8 mg/mmol creatinine
Microalbuminuria			
Male	18–180 mg/g creatinine	0.113	2.0–20 mg/mmol creatinine
Female	25–250 mg/g creatinine	0.113	2.8–28 mg/mmol creatinine
Proteinuria			
Male	> 180 mg/g creatinine	0.113	> 20 mg/mmol creatinine
Female	> 250 mg/mmol creatinine	0.113	> 28 mg/mmol creatinine
Alcohol			
See under Ethanol			
Aldosterone			
Supine	< 16 ng/dL	27.7	< 444 pmol/L
Upright	< 31 ng/dL	27.7	< 860 pmol/L
Alkaline phosphatase			
10–15 years	130–550 IU/L	0.01667	2.17–9.17 μkat/L
16–20 years	70–260 IU/L	0.01667	1.17–4.33 μkat/L
> 20 years	38–126 IU/L	0.01667	0.63–2.10 μkat/L
α-Fetoprotein (AFP)	< 15 ng/mL	1	< 15 mcg/L
α-1-Antitrypsin	80–200 mg/dL	0.01	0.8–2.0 g/L
Amikacin, therapeutic			
Peak	15–30 mg/L	1.71	25.6–51.3 μmol/L
Trough	≤ 8 mg/L	1.71	≤ 13.7 μmol/L
Amitriptyline	80–200 ng/mL or mcg/L	3.605	288–721 nmol/L
Ammonia (plasma)	15–56 mcg NH₃/dL	0.5872	9–33 μmol NH₃/L
Amylase	25–115 U/L	0.01667	0.42–1.92 μkat/L

(Continued)

Laboratory Test	Conventional Units	Conversion Factor	Système International Units
Androstenedione	50–250 ng/dL	0.0349	1.7–8.7 nmol/L
Angiotensin-converting enzyme	15–70 units/L	16.67	250–1167 nkat/L
Anion gap	7–16 mEq/L	1	7–16 mmol/L
Anti–double-stranded DNA (anti-ds DNA)	Negative		
Anti-HAV	Negative		
Anti-HBc	Negative		
Anti-HBs	Negative		
Anti-HCV	Negative		
Anti-Sm antibody	Negative		
Antinuclear antibody (ANA)	Negative		
Apolipoprotein A-1			
Male	95–175 mg/dL	0.01	0.95–1.75 g/L
Female	100–200 mg/dL	0.01	1.0–2.0 g/L
Apolipoprotein B			
Male	50–110 mg/dL	0.01	0.5–1.10 g/L
Female	50–105 mg/dL	0.01	0.5–1.05 g/L
Aspartate aminotransferase (AST, SGOT)	11–47 IU/L	0.01667	0.18–0.78 µkat/L
β_2-Microglobulin	< 0.2 mg/dL	10	< 2 mg/L
Bicarbonate	22–26 mEq/L	1	22–26 mmol/L
Bilirubin			
Total	0.3–1.1 mg/dL	17.1	5.1–18.8 µmol/L
Direct	0–0.3 mg/dL	17.1	0–5.1 µmol/L
Indirect	0.1–1.0 mg/dL	17.1	1.7–17.1 µmol/L
Bleeding time	3–7 minutes	60	180–420 seconds
Blood gases (arterial)			
pH	7.35–7.45	1	7.35–7.45
PO_2	80–105 mm Hg	0.133	10.6–14.0 kPa
PCO_2	35–45 mm Hg	0.133	4.7–6.0 kPa
HCO_3	22–26 mEq/L	1	22–26 mmol/L
O_2 saturation	≥ 95%	0.01	≥ 0.95
Blood urea nitrogen (BUN)	8–25 mg/dL	0.357	2.9–8.9 mmol/L
B-type natriuretic peptide (BNP)	0–99 pg/mL	1	0–99 ng/L
		0.289	0–29 pmol/L
B-type natriuretic peptide, N-terminal fragment (NT-proBNP)	0–299 pg/mL	1	0–299 ng/L
		0.118	0-35 pmol/L
BUN-to-creatinine ratio	10:1–20:1		40:1-100:1
C-peptide	0.51–2.70 ng/mL	331	170–894 pmol/L
		0.331	0.17–0.89 nmol/L
C-reactive protein	< 0.8 mg/dL	10	< 8 mg/L
CA-125	< 35 units/mL	1	< 35 kU/L
CA 15–3	< 30 units/mL	1	< 30 kU/L
CA 19–9	< 37 units/mL	1	< 37 kU/L
CA 27.29	< 38 units/mL	1	< 38 kU/L
Calcium			
Total	8.6–10.3 mg/dL	0.25	2.15–2.58 mmol/L
	4.3–5.16 mEq/L	0.50	2.15–2.58 mmol/L
Ionized	4.5–5.1 mg/dL	0.25	1.13–1.28 mmol/L
	2.26–2.56 mEq/L	0.50	1.13–1.28 mmol/L

(Continued)

Laboratory Test	Conventional Units	Conversion Factor	Système International Units
Carbamazepine, therapeutic	4–12 mg/L	4.23	17–51 µmol/L
Carboxyhemoglobin (nonsmoker)	< 2%	0.01	< 0.02
Carcinoembryonic antigen (CEA)			
Nonsmokers	< 2.5 ng/mL	1	< 2.5 mcg/L
Smokers	< 5 ng/mL	1	< 5 mcg/L
CD4 lymphocyte count	31%–61% of total lymphocytes	0.01	0.31–0.61 of total lymphocytes
CD8 lymphocyte count	18%–39% of total lymphocytes	0.01	0.18–0.39 of total lymphocytes
Cerebrospinal fluid (CSF)			
Pressure	75–175 mm H_2O	0.0098	0.74-1.72 kPa
Glucose	40–70 mg/dL	0.0555	2.2–3.9 mmol/L
Protein	15–45 mg/dL	0.01	0.15–0.45 g/L
White blood cell (WBC) count	< 10/mm³	1	< 10 × 10⁶/L
Ceruloplasmin	18–45 mg/dL	10	180–450 mg/L
Chloride	97–110 mEq/L	1	97–110 mmol/L
Cholesterol			
Desirable	< 200 mg/dL	0.0259	< 5.18 mmol/L
Borderline high	200–239 mg/dL	0.0259	5.18–6.19 mmol/L
High	≥ 240 mg/dL	0.0259	≥6.2 mmol/L
Chorionic gonadotropin (β-hCG)	< 5 mIU/mL	1	< 5 IU/L
Clozapine, minimum trough	300–350 ng/mL or mcg/L	3.06	918–1,071 nmol/L
		0.00306	0.92–1.07 µmol/L
CO_2 content	22–30 mEq/L	1	22–30 mmol/L
Complement component 3 (C3)	70–160 mg/dL	0.01	0.70–1.60 g/L
Complement component 4 (C4)	20–40 mg/dL	0.01	0.20–0.40 g/L
Copper	70–150 mcg/dL	0.157	11–24 µmol/L
Cortisol (fasting, morning)	5–25 mcg/dL	27.6	138–690 nmol/L
Creatine kinase			
Male	30–200 IU/L	0.01667	0.50–3.33 µkat/L
Female	20–170 IU/L	0.01667	0.33–2.83 µkat/L
MB fraction	0–7 IU/L	0.01667	0.0–0.12 µkat/L
Creatinine clearance (CrCl)	85–135 mL/min/1.73 m²	0.00963	0.82–1.30 mL/s/m²
		0.01667	85–135 mL/s/1.73 m²
Creatinine			
Male 4–20 years	0.2–1.0 mg/dL	88.4	18–88 µmol/L
Female 4–20 years	0.2–1.0 mg/dL	88.4	18–88 µmol/L
Male (adults)	0.7–1.3 mg/dL	88.4	62–115 µmol/L
Female (adults)	0.6–1.1 mg/dL	88.4	53–97 µmol/L
Cyclosporine			
Renal, cardiac, liver, or pancreatic transplant	100–400 ng/mL or mcg/L	0.832	83–333 nmol/L
Cryptococcal antigen	Negative		
D-dimers	< 250 ng/mL	1	< 250 mcg/L
Desipramine	75–300 ng/mL or mcg/L	3.75	281–1125 nmol/L
Dexamethasone suppression test (DST) (overnight), 8:00 am cortisol	< 5 mcg/dL	27.6	< 138 nmol/L

(Continued)

Laboratory Test	Conventional Units	Conversion Factor	Système International Units
DHEAS (dehydroepiandrosterone sulfate)			
Male	170–670 mcg/dL	0.0272	4.6–18.2 µmol/L
Female			
Premenopausal	50–540 mcg/dL	0.0272	1.4–14.7 µmol/L
Postmenopausal	30–260 mcg/dL	0.0272	0.8–7.1 µmol/L
Digoxin, therapeutic (heart failure)	0.5–0.8 ng/mL or mcg/L	1.28	0.6–1.0 nmol/L
Therapeutic (atrial fibrillation)	0.8–2.0 ng/mL or mcg/L	1.28	1.0–2.6 nmol/L
Erythrocyte count (blood)			
See under red blood cell (RBC) count			
Erythrocyte sedimentation rate (ESR)			
Westergren			
Male	0–20 mm/h		
Female	0–30 mm/h		
Wintrobe			
Male	0–9 mm/h		
Female	0–15 mm/h		
Erythropoietin	2–25 mIU/mL	1	2–25 IU/L
Estradiol			
Male	10–36 pg/mL	3.67	37–132 pmol/L
Female	34–170 pg/mL	3.67	125–624 pmol/L
Ethanol, legal intoxication (depends on location)	≥ 50–100 mg/dL	0.217	≥10.9–21.7 mmol/L
	≥ 0.05–0.1%	217	≥10.9–21.7 mmol/L
Ethosuximide, therapeutic	40–100 mg/L or mcg/mL	7.08	283–708 µmol/L
Factor VIII or factor IX			
Severe hemophilia	< 1 IU/dL	0.01	< 0.01 IU/mL
Moderate hemophilia	1–5 IU/dL	0.01	0.01–0.05 IU/mL
Mild hemophilia	> 5 IU/dL	0.01	> 0.05 IU/mL
Usual adult levels	60 to 140 IU/dL	0.01	0.60–1.40 IU/mL
Ferritin			
Male	20–250 ng/mL	1	20–250 mcg/L
		2.25	45-562 pmol/L
Female	10–150 ng/mL	1	10–150 mcg/L
		2.25	22-337 pmol/L
Fibrin degradation products (FDP)	2–10 mg/L		
Fibrinogen	200–400 mg/dL	0.01	2.0–4.0 g/L
Folate (plasma)	3.1–12.4 ng/mL	2.266	7.0–28.1 nmol/L
Folate (RBC)	125–600 ng/mL	2.266	283–1,360 nmol/L
Follicle-stimulating hormone (FSH)			
Male	1–7 mIU/mL	1	1–7 IU/L
Female			
Follicular phase	1–9 mIU/mL	1	1–9 IU/L
Midcycle	6–26 mIU/mL	1	6–26 IU/L
Luteal phase	1–9 mIU/mL	1	1–9 IU/L
Postmenopausal	30–118 mIU/mL	1	30–118 IU/L
Free thyroxine index (FT_4I)	6.5–12.5		
Gamma glutamyltransferase (GGT)	0–30 U/L	0.01667	0–0.50 µkat/L

(Continued)

Laboratory Test	Conventional Units	Conversion Factor	Système International Units
Gastrin (fasting)	0–130 pg/mL	1	0–130 ng/L
Gentamicin, therapeutic (traditional dosing)			
Peak	4–10 mg/L	2.09	8.4–21 µmol/L
Trough	≤ 2 mg/L	2.09	≤ 4.2 µmol/L
Globulin	2.3–3.5 g/dL	10	23–35 g/L
Glucose (fasting, plasma)	65–109 mg/dL	0.0555	3.6–6.0 mmol/L
Glucose, 2-hour postprandial blood (PPBG)	< 140 mg/dL	0.0555	< 7.8 mmol/L
Granulocyte count	$1.8–6.6 \times 10^3/mm^3$	10^6	$1.8–6.6 \times 10^9/L$
Growth hormone (fasting)			
Male	< 5 ng/mL	1	< 5 mcg/L
Female	< 10 ng/mL	1	< 10 mcg/L
Haptoglobin	60–270 mg/dL	0.01	0.6–2.7 g/L
Hepatitis B surface antigen, extracellular form (HBeAg)	Negative		
Hepatitis B surface antigen (HbsAg)	Negative		
Hepatitis B virus (HBV) DNA	Negative		
Hematocrit			
Male	40.7%–50.3%	0.01	0.407–0.503
Female	36.1%–44.3%	0.01	0.361–0.443
Hemoglobin (blood)			
Male	13.8–17.2 g/dL	10	138–172 g/L
		0.621	8.56–10.68 mmol/L
Female	12.1–15.1 g/dL	10	121–151 g/L
		0.621	7.51–9.36 mmol/L
Hemoglobin A1c	4.0%–6.0%	0.01	0.04–0.06
		[a]	20–42 mmol/mol hemoglobin
Heparin			
Via protamine titration method	0.2–0.4 units/mL		
Via antifactor Xa assay	0.3–0.7 units/mL		
High-density lipoprotein (HDL) cholesterol	> 35 mg/dL	0.0259	> 0.91 mmol/L
Homocysteine	3.3–10.4 µmol/L		
Ibuprofen			
Therapeutic	10–50 mcg/mL	4.85	49–243 µmol/L
Toxic	≥ 100 mcg/mL	4.85	≥ 485 µmol/L
Imipramine, therapeutic	100–300 ng/mL or mcg/L	3.57	357–1071 nmol/L
Immunoglobulin A (IgA)	85–385 mg/dL	0.01	0.85–3.85 g/L
Immunoglobulin G (IgG)	565–1765 mg/dL	0.01	5.65–17.65 g/L
Immunoglobulin M (IgM)	53–375 mg/dL	0.01	0.53–3.75 g/L
Insulin (fasting)	2–20 µU/mL or mU/L	7.175	14.35–143.5 pmol/L
International normalized ratio (INR), therapeutic	2.0–3.0 (2.5–3.5 for some indications)		
Iron			
Male	45–160 mcg/dL	0.179	8.1–28.6 µmol/L
Female	30–160 mcg/dL	0.179	5.4–28.6 µmol/L
Iron-binding capacity (total)	220–420 mcg/dL	0.179	39.4–75.2 µmol/L

(Continued)

Laboratory Test	Conventional Units	Conversion Factor	Système International Units
Iron saturation	15%–50%	0.01	0.15–0.50
Itraconazole			
Trough, therapeutic	0.5–1 mcg/mL or mg/L	1.42	0.7-1.4 µmol/L
Lactate (plasma)	0.7–2.1 mEq/L	1	0.7–2.1 mmol/L
	6.3–18.9 mg/dL	0.111	0.7–2.1 mmol/L
Lactate dehydrogenase (LDH)	100–250 IU/L	0.01667	1.67–4.17 µkat/L
Lead	< 25 mcg/dL	0.0483	< 1.21 µmol/L
Leukocyte count	$3.8–9.8 \times 10^3/mm^3$	10^6	$3.8–9.8 \times 10^9/L$
Lidocaine, therapeutic	1.5–6.0 mcg/mL or mg/L	4.27	6.4–25.6 µmol/L
Lipase	< 100 IU/L	0.01667	1.67 µkat/L
Lithium, therapeutic	0.5–1.25 mEq/L	1	0.5–1.25 mmol/L
Low-density lipoprotein (LDL) cholesterol			
Target for very high-risk patients	< 70 mg/dL	0.0259	< 1.81 mmol/L
Desirable LDL level and target for high-risk patients (optimal)	< 100 mg/dL	0.0259	< 2.59 mmol/L
Above desirable	100-129 mg/dL	0.0259	2.59-3.34 mmol/L
Borderline high risk	130–159 mg/dL	0.0259	3.36–4.11 mmol/L
High risk	160-189 mg/dL	0.0259	4.14-4.89 mmol/L
Very high risk	≥ 190 mg/dL	0.0259	≥ 4.91 mmol/L
Luteinizing hormone (LH)			
Male	1–8 mIU/mL	1	1–8 IU/L
Female			
Follicular phase	1–12 mIU/mL	1	1–12 IU/L
Midcycle	16–104 mIU/mL	1	16–104 IU/L
Luteal phase	1–12 mIU/mL	1	1–12 IU/L
Postmenopausal	16–66 mIU/mL	1	16–66 IU/L
Lymphocyte count	$1.2–3.3 \times 10^3/mm^3$	10^6	$1.2–3.3 \times 10^9/L$
Magnesium	1.3–2.2 mEq/L	0.5	0.65–1.10 mmol/L
	1.58–2.68 mg/dL	0.411	0.65–1.10 mmol/L
Mean corpuscular volume (MCV)	$80.0–97.6\ \mu m^3$	1	80.0–97.6 fL
Mononuclear cell count	$0.2–0.7 \times 10^3/mm^3$	10^6	$0.2–0.7 \times 10^9/L$
Nortriptyline, therapeutic	50–150 ng/mL or mcg/L	3.797	190–570 nmol/L
Osmolality (serum)	275–300 mOsm/kg	1	275–300 mmol/kg
Osmolality (urine)	250–900 mOsm/kg	1	250–900 mmol/kg
Parathyroid hormone (PTH), intact	10–60 pg/mL or ng/L	0.107	1.1–6.4 pmol/L
PTH, N-terminal	8–24 pg/mL or ng/L		
PTH, C-terminal	50–330 pg/mL or ng/L		
Phenobarbital, therapeutic	15–40 mcg/mL or mg/L	4.31	65–172 µmol/L
Phenytoin, therapeutic (total concentration)	10–20 mcg/mL or mg/L	3.96	40–79 µmol/L
Phosphate	2.5–4.5 mg/dL	0.323	0.81–1.45 mmol/L
Platelet count	$140–440 \times 10^3/mm^3$	10^6	$140–440 \times 10^9/L$
Potassium (plasma)	3.3–4.9 mEq/L	1	3.3–4.9 mmol/L
Prealbumin (adult)	19.5–35.8 mg/dL	10	195–358 mg/L
Primidone, therapeutic	5–12 mcg/mL or mg/L	4.58	23–55 µmol/L
Procainamide, therapeutic	4–10 mcg/mL or mg/L	4.25	17–42 µmol/L

(Continued)

Laboratory Test	Conventional Units	Conversion Factor	Système International Units
Progesterone			
Male	13–97 ng/dL	0.0318	0.4–3.1 nmol/L
Female			
Follicular phase	15–70 ng/dL	0.0318	0.5–2.2 nmol/L
Luteal phase	200–2500 ng/dL	0.0318	6.4–79.5 nmol/L
Prolactin	< 20 ng/mL	1	< 20 mcg/L
		43.5	< 870 pmol/L
Prostate-specific antigen (PSA)	< 4 ng/mL	1	< 4 mcg/L
Protein, total	6.0–8.0 g/dL	10	60–80 g/L
Prothrombin time (PT)	10–12 seconds		
Quinidine, therapeutic	2–5 mcg/mL or mg/L	3.08	6.2–15.4 µmol/L
Radioactive iodine uptake (RAIU)	< 6% in 2 hours		
Red blood cell (RBC) count (blood)			
Male	$4–6.2 \times 10^6/mm^3$	10^6	$4–6.2 \times 10^{12}/L$
Female	$4–6.2 \times 10^6/mm^3$	10^6	$4–6.2 \times 10^{12}/L$
Pregnant			
Trimester 1	$4–5 \times 10^6/mm^3$	10^6	$4–5 \times 10^{12}/L$
Trimester 2	$3.2–4.5 \times 10^6/mm^3$	10^6	$3.2–4.5 \times 10^{12}/L$
Trimester 3	$3–4.9 \times 10^6/mm^3$	10^6	$3–4.9 \times 10^{12}/L$
Postpartum	$3.2–5 \times 10^6/mm^3$	10^6	$3.2–5 \times 10^{12}/L$
Red blood cell distribution width (RDW)	11.5%–14.5%	0.01	0.115–0.145
Reticulocyte count			
Male	0.5%–1.5% of total RBC count	0.01	0.005–0.015
Female	0.5%–2.5% of total RBC count	0.01	0.005–0.025
Retinol-binding protein (RBP)	2.7–7.6 mg/dL	10	27–76 mg/L
Rheumatoid factor (RF) titer	Negative		
Salicylate, therapeutic	150–300 mcg/mL or mg/L	0.00724	1.09–2.17 mmol/L
	15–30 mg/dL	0.0724	1.09–2.17 mmol/L
Sirolimus (renal transplant)	4–20 ng/mL	1	4–20 mcg/L
		1.094	4–22 nmol/L
Sodium	135–145 mEq/L	1	135–145 mmol/L
Tacrolimus			
Renal, cardiac, liver, or pancreatic transplant	5–20 ng/mL	1	5–20 mcg/L
		1.24	6.2-24.8 nmol/L
Testosterone (total)			
Men	300–950 ng/dL	0.0347	10.4–33.0 nmol/L
Women	20–80 ng/dL	0.0347	0.7–2.8 nmol/L
Testosterone (free)			
Men	9–30 ng/dL	0.0347	0.31–1.04 nmol/L
Women	0.3–1.9 ng/dL	0.0347	0.01–0.07 nmol/L
Theophylline			
Therapeutic	5–15 mcg/mL or mg/L	5.55	28–83 µmol/L
Toxic	20 mcg/mL or mg/L or more	5.55	111 µmol/L or more
Thiocyanate	Toxic level unclear; units are mcg/mL or mg/L	17.2	µmol/L

(Continued)

Laboratory Test	Conventional Units	Conversion Factor	Système International Units
Thrombin time	20–24 seconds		
Thyroglobulin	< 42 ng/mL	1	< 42 mcg/L
Thyroglobulin antibodies	Negative		
Thyroxine-binding globulin (TBG)	1.2–2.5 mg/dL	10	12–25 mcg/L
Thyroid-stimulating hormone (TSH)	0.35–6.20 μIU/mL	1	0.35–6.20 mIU/L
TSH receptor antibodies (TSHRab)	0–1 units/mL		0–1 kU/L
Thyroxine (T_4)			
Total	4.5–12.0 mcg/dL	12.87	58–154 nmol/L
Free	0.7–1.9 ng/dL	12.87	9.0–24.5 pmol/L
Thyroxine index, free (FT_4I)	6.5–12.5		
TIBC—see Iron binding capacity (total)			
Tobramycin, therapeutic			
Peak	4–10 mcg/mL or mg/L	2.14	8.6–21.4 μmol/L
Trough	≤ 2 mcg/mL or mg/L	2.14	≤ 4.3 μmol/L
Transferrin	200–430 mg/dL	0.01	2.0–4.3 g/L
Transferrin saturation	30–50%	0.01	0.30–0.50
Triglycerides (fasting)	< 160 mg/dL	0.0113	< 1.81 mmol/L
Triiodothyronine (T_3)	45–132 ng/dL	0.0154	0.69–2.03 nmol/L
Triiodothyronine (T_3) resin uptake	25–35%		
Uric acid	3–8 mg/dL	59.48	178–476 μmol/L
Urinalysis (urine)			
pH	4.8–8.0		
Specific gravity	1.005–1.030		
Protein	Negative		
Glucose	Negative		
Ketones	Negative		
RBC	1–2 per low-power field		
WBC	< 5 per low-power field		
Valproic acid, therapeutic	50–100 mcg/mL or mg/L	6.93	346–693 μmol/L
Vancomycin, therapeutic			
Peak	20–40 mcg/mL or mg/L	0.690	14–28 μmol/L
Trough	10–20 mcg/mL or mg/L	0.690	7–14 μmol/L
Trough for central nervous system infections	15–20 mcg/mL or mg/L	0.690	10–14 μmol/L
Vitamin A (retinol)	30–95 mcg/dL	0.0349	1.05–3.32 μmol/L
Vitamin B_{12}	180–1000 pg/mL	0.738	133–738 pmol/L
Vitamin D_3, 1,25-dihydroxy	20–76 pg/mL	2.4	48–182 pmol/L
Vitamin D_3, 25-hydroxy	10–50 ng/mL	2.496	25–125 nmol/L
Vitamin E (a-tocopherol)	0.5–2.0 mg/dL	23.22	12–46 μmol/L
WBC count	$4–10 \times 10^3/mm^3$	10^6	$4–10 \times 10^9/L$
WBC differential (peripheral blood)			
Polymorphonuclear neutrophils (PMNs)	50%–65%	0.01	0.50–0.65
Bands	0%–5%	0.01	0–0.05
Eosinophils	0%–3%	0.01	0–0.03
Basophils	1%–3%	0.01	0.01–0.03
Lymphocytes	25%–35%	0.01	0.25–0.35
Monocytes	2%–6%	0.01	0.02–0.06

(Continued)

Laboratory Test	Conventional Units	Conversion Factor	Système International Units
WBC differential (bone marrow)			
PMNs	3%–11%	0.01	0.03–0.11
Bands	9%–15%	0.01	0.09–0.15
Metamyelocytes	9%–25%	0.01	0.09–0.25
Myelocytes	8%–16%	0.01	0.08–0.16
Promyelocytes	1%–8%	0.01	0.01–0.08
Myeloblasts	0%–5%	0.01	0–0.05
Eosinophils	1%–5%	0.01	0.01–0.05
Basophils	0%–1%	0.01	0–0.01
Lymphocytes	11%–23%	0.01	0.11–0.23
Monocytes	0%–1%	0.01	0–0.01
Zinc	60–150 mcg/dL	0.153	9.2–23.0 µmol/L

[a]Hemoglobin A1c (mmol/mol hemoglobin) = (Hemoglobin A1c (%) − 2.15) × 10.929.

REFERENCES

1. Medscape. Brain-Type Natriuretic Peptide (BNP). http://emedicine.medscape.com/article/2087425-overview. Accessed October 26, 2014.
2. Jacobs DS, Oxley DK, DeMott WR (eds.). (2001) Laboratory Test Handbook (5th ed.). Hudson OH: Lexi-Comp, Inc.
3. Young DS, Huth EJ (eds.). (1998) SI Units for Clinical Measurement. Philadelphia, PA: American College of Physicians. Reviewed and updated by Edward W. Randell.

Appendix C: Example Care Plans

Two pharmacotherapy care plans based on cases in the book have been provided so the student will have a better understanding of the structure and content of typical care plans. Note that some information has been left out of these examples so you will not have all the 'answers' for your own workup of these cases. As discussed in Chapter 1, the care plan forms are meant to be a guide in structuring your thoughts and information, and there is no single correct way to do it. As you gain more experience, developing the elements of the care plan will become more intuitive. Remember, your most important job is to provide the best possible drug therapy for the patient.

17 Peptic Ulcer Disease: Example Care Plan With Missing Data

Michael D. Katz

PATIENT DATABASE FORM

Patient Name: CC	Weight: 106 (48.1)	Location:	Completed by:
Patient MRN:	Height: 65 in (165 cm)	Physician:	
Age (or date of birth): 28	Race: Chinese	Pharmacy:	Pharmacist:
Date of Admission/Initial Visit: 9/15/15		Patient Occupation: Pharmacy resident	

Allergies/ Intolerances/ ADRs		HPI, FH, SH, and Additional Information
☐ No known drug allergies/ADRs		**HPI:** Increasing epigastric pain, nausea, decreased intake X 1 week, although she had similar sx in the past. Self-described as type A and a workaholic. Takes ibuprofen for HA. Hx hypothyroidism, on LT_4 replacemen t
☐ Not known/inadequate information		
Drug	**Reaction**	
Penicillin	Unknown reaction as child	
Alcohol	Flushing, nausea	**FH / SH:** FH noncontributory. Engaged and planning wedding. No tobacco, EtOH, illicit drugs
		Additional Information:

	Prioritized Medical Problem List	Medication Profile
1	Peptic ulcer disease, *H. pylori* +	
2	Hypothyroidism × 4 yrs	Levothyroxine 25 mcg PO q/d
3	HA, stress related?	Ibuprofen 200–400 mg PO PRN
4		
5		
6		

Health Maintenance:	vaccine status not known; need for contraception	Calcium carbonate 500 mg PO q/d
PMH with no therapy needed:		
Inadequate Database:	How much ibuprofen does she use?	

Vital Signs, Laboratory Data, and Diagnostic Test Results				
	Normal Range or Units			
Date		9/15/15		
Weight	lb (kg)	106 (48.1)		
Temperature	°C	37.2		
Blood Pressure	mmHg	110/68/104/62		
Pulse		64/78		
Respiratory Rate		12		
Na	135–145 mEq/L (135–145 mmol/L)	136 (136)		
K	3.3–4.9 mEq/L (3.3–4.9 mmol/L)	3.9 (3.9)		
Cl	97–110 mEq/L (97–110 mmol/L)	100 (100)		
CO_2/HCO_3	22–26 mEq/L (22–26 mmol/L)	24 (24)		
BUN	8–25 mg/dL (2.9–8.9 mmol/L)	18 (6.43)		
Serum Creatinine (adult)	male 0.7–1.3 mg/dL; female 0.6–1.1 mg/dL (male 62–115 μmol/L; female 53–97 μmol/L)	0.5 (44.2)		
Creatinine Clearance (adult)	85–135 mL/min (1.42–2.25 mL/s)	126 (1.21)		
Glucose (fasting)	65–109 mg/dL (3.6–6.0 mmol/L)	89 (4.9)		
Total Ca	8.6–10.3 mg/dL (2.15–2.58 mmol/L)	9.4 (2.35)		
Mg	1.3–2.2 mEq/L (0.65–1.10 mmol/L)	1.8 (0.9)		
PO_4	2.5–4.5 mg/dL (0.81–1.45 mmol/L)	3.8 (1.23)		
Hemoglobin	male 13.8–17.2 g/dL; female 12.1–15.1 g/dL (male 138–172 g/L; female 121–151 g/L)	12.1 (121, 7.51)		
Hematocrit	male 40.7–50.3%; female 36.1–44.3% (male 0.407–0.503; female 0.361–0.443)	36.2 (0.362)		
MCV	80.0–97.6 μm³ (80.0–97.6 fl)	79 (79)		
WBC	$4–10 \times 10^3/mm^3$ ($4–10 \times 10^9/L$)	8.2 (8.2)		
WBC Differential	% polymorphonuclear neutrophils (PMN)/ eosinophils/basophils/lymphocytes/monocytes	/ / / /	/ / / /	/ / / /
Platelets	$140–440 \times 10^3/mm^3$ ($140–440 \times 10^9/L$)	247 (247)		
Albumin	3.5–5 g/dL (35–50 g/L)			
Bilirubin (total)	0.3–1.1 mg/dL (5.13–18.80 μmol/L)			
Bilirubin (direct)	0–0.3 mg/dL (0–5.1 μmol/L)			
AST	11–47 IU/L (0.18–0.78 μkat/L)			
ALT	7–53 IU/L (0.12–0.88 μkat/L)			
Alk phos (adult)	38–126 IU/L (0.13–2.10 μkat/L)			
TSH	4.2 (4.2)			
H. pylori serology	positive			

Additional Notes: Stool occult blood neg; EGD biopsy *H. pylori* +

DRUG THERAPY PROBLEM WORKSHEET

Type of Problem	Possible Causes	Problem List	Notes
Correlation between drug therapy and medical problems	Drugs without obvious medical indications	PUD, *H. pylori*	
	Medication(s) unidentified		
	Untreated medical conditions		
Need for additional drug therapy	New medical condition requiring new drug therapy	PUD, *H. pylori*	
	Chronic disorder requiring continued drug therapy	Hypothyroidism	
	Condition best treated with combination drug therapy	*H. pylori*	
	May develop new medical condition without prophylactic or preventative therapy or premedication		
Unnecessary drug therapy	Medication with no valid indication or condition is better treated with nondrug therapy		
	Condition caused by accidental or intentional ingestion of toxic amount of drug(s) or chemical(s)		
	Medical problem(s) associated with use of or withdrawal from alcohol, drug(s), or tobacco		
	Taking multiple drugs when single agent is as effective		
	Taking drug(s) to treat an avoidable adverse reaction from another medication		
Appropriate drug selection	Current regimen not usually as effective or safe as other choices	Ibuprofen	
	Therapy not individualized to patient		
Wrong drug	Medical problem for which drug is not effective	Ibuprofen and PUD	
	Patient has risk factors that contraindicate use of drug		
	Patient has infection with organisms resistant to drug		
	Patient refractory to current drug therapy		
	Taking combination product when single agent appropriate		
	Dosage form inappropriate or medication error		
Drug regimen	PRN use not appropriate for condition		
	Route of administration/dosage form/mode of administration not appropriate for current condition		
	Length or course of therapy not appropriate		
	Drug therapy altered without adequate therapeutic trial		
	Dose or interval flexibility not appropriate		
Dose too low	Dose or frequency too low to produce desired response in this patient	Levothyroxine dose based on high TSH	
	Serum drug concentration below desired goal range for indication		
	Timing of antimicrobial prophylaxis not appropriate		
	Medication not stored properly or medication error		

DRUG THERAPY PROBLEM WORKSHEET

Type of Problem	Possible Causes	Problem List	Notes
Dose too high	Dose or frequency too high for this patient		
	Serum drug concentration above the desired goal range for indication		
	Dose escalated too quickly		
	Dose or interval flexibility not appropriate for this patient		
	Medication error		
Therapeutic duplication	Receiving multiple agents without added benefit		
Drug allergy/ adverse drug events	History of allergy or ADE to current (or chemically related) agents	Ibuprofen could worsen her PUD	
	Allergy or ADE history not in medical records		
	Patient not using alert for severe allergy or ADE		
	Symptoms or medical problems that may be drug induced		
	Drug administered too rapidly		
	Medication error, actual or potential		
Interactions (drug-drug, drug-disease, drug-nutrient, drug-laboratory test)	Effect of drug altered due to enzyme induction/inhibition, protein binding alterations, or pharmacodynamic change from another drug patient is taking	LT_4 absorption decreased with calcium	
	Bioavailability of drug altered due to interaction with another drug or food		
	Effect of drug altered due to substance in food		
	Patient's laboratory test altered due to interference from drug(s) the patient is taking		
Failure to receive therapy	Patient did not adhere with the drug regimen		
	Drug not given due to medication error		
	Patient did not take due to high drug cost/lack of insurance		
	Patient unable to take oral medication		
	Patient has no IV access for IV medication		
	Drug product not available		
Financial impact	The current regimen is not the most cost effective		
	Patient unable to purchase medications/no insurance		
Patient knowledge of drug therapy	Patient does not understand the purpose, directions, or potential side effects of the drug regimen		
	Current regimen not consistent with the patient's health beliefs		

PHARMACOTHERAPY CARE PLAN

	Medical Problems	Current Drug Regimen	Therapy Goals, Desired Endpoints	Therapeutic Recommendations	Therapeutic Alternatives	Rationale
1	PUD, *H. pylori* +		Eradicate H. pylori, no GI S/S	Clarithromycin 500 mg; metronidazole 500 mg; omeprazole 20 mg; each bid × 14 days. Continue PPI for total 4 weeks NS 500 ml IV over 30 min. Reassess ECF volume status. If able to take po, continue rehydration orally. Stress reduction	Bismuth subsalicylate 525 mg; metronidazole 500 mg; tetracycline 500 mg; lansoprazole 30 mg. Each bid × 14 day See Table 1 (page 9) for treatment regimens	First-line regimen with highest eradication rate × 14 days of therapy. Amoxicillin-containing regimen avoided due to hx penicillin reaction in past.
2	Hypothyroidism	Levothyroxine 25 mcg po q/d	TSH 1–1.5 uIU/ml (mIU/L), no S/S	Assess adherence; use with calcium. If adherent and not taking with calcium, increase dose to 50 mcg po q/d	If taking with calcium, space out administration and continue same LT_4 dose.	TSH above target and pt C/O cold intolerance.
3	HA	Ibuprofen 200–400 mg po prn	No HA	D/C ibuprofen. Obtain more detailed hx about HA. If tension HA, try nondrug therapy (e.g. stress reduction, relaxation) first. Acetaminophen 325 mg prn	If chronic or severe tension HA, consider TCA or other prophylactic therapy.	NSAID contraindicated with active PUD.
4						
5						
6						

Medical Problems	Planned Monitoring and Follow-Up	Patient Education Summary Points
1 PUD, *H. pylori* +	F/U in 14 days for resolution of S/S. Confirm eradication with stool antigen or breath test	The reason for taking these medications is to treat the *H. pylori* infection that is causing ulcers in your duodenum and causing your symptoms. To have the highest chance of success, several antibiotics along with medications that decrease stomach acid production must be used.
		It is vitally important to take these medications exactly as directed. This will require you to take these medications twice daily. It will be easy to forget taking these medications because of this and you should work with your pharmacist to develop a reminder plan to ensure you take your medications as directed. Pill calendars, e-mail reminders, or other devices can help you remember to take your medication. You must take all the medication(s)—even if you feel better.
		After you complete the antibiotic section of your treatment, you will continue the medication that decreases stomach acid production for another 2 weeks.
		If you miss a dose of any of these medications, take it as soon as you remember, unless it is within 2 hours of your next dose. If it is too close to your next dose, forget about the dose you missed and continue with your regular regimen. Do not take double doses.
		You should begin to feel better within 4–5 days of starting this regimen. Your nausea should improve first, followed by a decrease in the stomach pain.
		Remember to return to your primary care provider for follow-up.
		Adverse effects from this regimen are generally mild and may include discoloration of tongue or stools (both of which are harmless), metallic taste, diarrhea, nausea, and rarely, numbness in your fingers or toes. If any of these occur, contact your pharmacist or primary care physician. If diarrhea occurs and is severe, contact your primary care physician immediately.
		You should avoid consuming alcohol during the time you take this regimen. Not only can alcohol irritate the stomach lining, but it may interact with one of the medications in your regimen, causing flushing, nausea, or worse reactions.
2 Hypothyroidism	TSH is 6 weeks	Since your TSH is above the desired target level and you have some symptoms of hypothyroidism, we have increased your levothyroxine dose. Make sure you take it at the same time every day, and do not take it within 2 hours before or 4 hours after taking calcium.
3 HA	Patient will self-monitor S/S	NSAIDs like ibuprofen cannot be taken with peptic ulcer disease. If your headaches are due to stress or tension, then finding ways to reduce stress may help as much as medication. If you do need to take a medication, acetaminophen 325 mg would be the safest treatment.
4		
5		
6		

KEY INFORMATION FOR FACILITATOR

Question 1	What signs and symptoms of PUD does this patient have?
	Epigastric and postprandial pain, nausea, weight loss, decreased oral intake
Question 2	What treatment regimen for *H. pylori* infection would you select for this patient? What specific parts of the patient database would guide your decision?
	There are many regimens (see Table 1, page 9). In the United States, 14-day regimens containing clarithromycin, metronidazole, and a PPI have the highest eradication rates. Since this patient has an unspecified history of penicillin reaction, the amoxicillin-containing regimen is best avoided. Twice daily regimens are more likely to have full adherence versus three or four times daily regimens. The PPI should be continued for a total of 4 weeks. H_2RA-containing regimens are less effective than those containing a PPI.
Question 3	What medications should be *avoided* in this patient to treat her HA?
	NSAIDs
Question 4	What risks and adverse effects of therapy would you discuss with this patient?
	Eradication therapy usually is well tolerated. Adverse effects from this regimen are generally mild and may include discoloration of tongue or stools (both of which are harmless), metallic taste, diarrhea, nausea, and rarely, numbness in your fingers or toes. *Clostridium difficile*-associated diarrhea is possible though unlikely with a metronidazole-containing regimen.
Question 5	Would you make any changes in her hypothyroid therapy?
	Since her TSH is above the desired target and she has some symptoms of hypothyroidism, her current dose is not adequate. If she is adherent and not taking her levothyroxine at the same time as the calcium, increasing the dose to 50 mcg/d is reasonable. The TSH can then be rechecked in 6–8 weeks
Follow-up	The patient is referred to a new primary care physician to establish care and for follow-up. The patient is seen 5 days after completing *H. pylori* eradication therapy, even though she is still taking the PPI. Although she feels somewhat better, she still complains of epigastric pain after meals. However, this pain is diminished and the nausea she felt before has abated. She is eating and drinking normally at this time. Urea breath test is + for *H. pylori*. The patient confirms that she was adherent to the original *H. pylori* eradication regimen. She mentions that she has traveled to China every 1–2 years since she was in junior high school. What actions would you take?
	Since she was adherent to her eradication therapy, this is a true treatment failure, likely due to *H. pylori* resistance to clarithromycin and/or metronidazole. Metronidazole- and clarithromycin-resistant strains of *H. pylori* are more prevalent in Asia, and she may have acquired *H. pylori* in China. Several "rescue" or "salvage" regimens are available for those who fail first-line therapy (see Table 1). In areas with high levels of clarithromycin resistance, fluoroquinolone-containing regimens have been effective with 85–90% eradication rates.
Additional Information	

TABLE 1. Drug Regimens to Eradicate *Helicobacter Pylori*[a,b]	
Treatment Regimen	**Cure Rates[b]**
First Line: Three Drugs	
Clarithromycin 500 mg + metronidazole 500 mg + omeprazole 20 mg, each given twice daily	Good to excellent
Clarithromycin 500 mg + amoxicilin 1 g + lansoprazole 30 mg, each given twice daily	Good to excellent
First Line: Four Drugs	
Helidac (bismuth subsalicytate 525 mg + metronidazole 250 mg + tetracycline 500 mg, each given four times a day) + ranitidine 150 mg twice daily[c]	Good
Bismuth subsalicylate 525 mg four times a day + metronidazole 250 mg four times a day + tetracycline 500 mg four times a day + PPI twice daity OR ranitidine 150 mg twice daity[c]	Good
Py1era (bismuth subcitrate potassium 140 mg + metronidazole 125 mg + tetracycline 125 mg) three capsules twice daity + omeprazole 20 mg twice daity × 10 days	Good to excellent
Rescue/Salvage Therapy	
Bismuth subsalicylate 525 mg + tinidazole + tetracycline 500 mg, each given four times a day + omeprazole 20 mg twice daily[d]	Good to excellent
Amoxicillin 1 g + PPI (each given two times daily) + levoftoxacin 500 mg daity	Good
Other Proposed Regimens for Rescue/Salvage Therapy[f]	
• Sequential Therapy	
Days 1-5: Amoxicillin 1 g + esomeprazole 40 mg, each given twice daily	Good to excellent
Days 6-10: Oarithromycin 500 mg + metronidazole 500 mg + Esomeprazole 40 mg, each given twice daily	
• Modified Regimen	
Amoxicillin 1 g + standard dose PPI + levofloxacin 250 mg (each given twice daily)	Good
• Concomitant Regimen	
Esomeprazole 40 mg + amoxicillin 1 g + darithromycin 500 mg + metronidazole 500 mg, each given twice daity × 10 days	Good to excellent

[a]Regimens are based on efficacy for a 14-day treatment duration unless otherwise noted.

[b]Based on cure rates of 80% to 90% = Good; greater than 90% = Excellent.

[c]Although commercially available, regimens containing H_2RAs are not preferred.

[d]Duration of therapy is 7 to 10 days.

[e]Given for 10 to 14 days.

[f]Proposed for patients failing previous therapy.

H_2RA, histamine-2 receptor antagonist; PPI, proton pump inhibitor.

From Bourg C.A., May D., *Peptic ulcer disease*, in Chisholm-Burns et al Pharmacotherapy Principles and Practice, 4th edition, p. 299

88 Syphilis: Example Care Plan With Missing Data

Lawrence David York   Kathryn R. Matthias

Patient Name: PG	Weight: 162.8 lbs (74 kg)	Location: Free Public Health Clinic	Completed by:
Patient MRN: 5428465	Height: 71 in (180.34 cm)	Physician: Dr. Harry Lee	
Age (or date of birth): 48	Race: Caucasian	Pharmacy:	Pharmacist:
Date of Admission/Initial Visit: 2/3/16		Patient Occupation:	

Allergies/ Intolerances/ ADRs		HPI, FH, SH, and Additional Information
☐ No known drug allergies/ADRs		**HPI:** C/O systemic rash and lymphadenopathy ("several months") and persistent headaches for 2 months (13–16 times per month). He generally experiences them "on both sides" of his head and sometimes feels like he is carrying a weight on his shoulders. He is also concerned that he is going bald as he has noted patches of hair missing in his beard and on his head.
☐ Not known/inadequate information		
Drug	**Reaction**	
ACE-inhibitors	Angioedema	
		FH / SH:
		Father: diabetes and "heart issues."
		The patient has been electively homeless for four years. He denies any children but endorses having had multiple sexual partners in the past. He is currently monogamous with one partner he has been seeing for approximately $1\frac{1}{2}$ years.
		Additional Information: Smokes 0.5 ppd × 32 years; 3–4 beers weekly; previously injected heroin × 11 years but has been abstinent × 1 year

	Prioritized Medical Problem List	Medication Profile
1	Syphilis, secondary	None
2	Headaches, frequent episodic tension-type	Acetaminophen 1000 mg po q6h prn
3	Hypertension (× 15 years)	None
4	HIV (× 6 years)	Emtricitabine 200 mg/tenofovir disoproxil fumarate 300 mg po daily Dolutegravir 50 mg po daily
5	Smoking cessation	None
6		

Health Maintenance:	Smoking cessation	
PMH with no therapy needed:		
Inadequate Database:	Reason for acetaminophen use (headaches)? Liver function test results?	

Vital Signs, Laboratory Data, and Diagnostic Test Results				
	Normal Range or Units	Yesterday		
Date				
Weight	lb (kg)	162.8 (74)		
Temperature	°C	38		
Blood Pressure	mmHg	149/84		
Pulse		75		
Respiratory Rate		16		
Na	135–145 mEq/L (135–145 mmol/L)	136		
K	3.3–4.9 mEq/L (3.3–4.9 mmol/L)	4.8		
Cl	97–110 mEq/L (97–110 mmol/L)	100		
CO_2/HCO_3	22–26 mEq/L (22–26 mmol/L)			
BUN	8–25 mg/dL (2.9–8.9 mmol/L)	15 (5.4)		
Serum Creatinine (adult)	male 0.7–1.3 mg/dL; female 0.6–1.1 mg/dL (male 62–115 µmol/L; female 53–97 µmol/L)	1.1 (97.2)		
Creatinine Clearance (adult)	85–135 mL/min (1.42–2.25 mL/s)			
Glucose (fasting)	65–109 mg/dL (3.6–6.0 mmol/L)	130 (7.15)		
Total Ca	8.6–10.3 mg/dL (2.15–2.58 mmol/L)			
Mg	1.3–2.2 mEq/L (0.65–1.10 mmol/L)			
PO_4	2.5–4.5 mg/dL (0.81–1.45 mmol/L)			
Hemoglobin	male 13.8–17.2 g/dL; female 12.1–15.1 g/dL (male 138–172 g/L; female 121–151 g/L)	10.4 (6.46)		
Hematocrit	male 40.7–50.3%; female 36.1–44.3% (male 0.407–0.503; female 0.361–0.443)	30.1 (0.301)		
MCV	80.0–97.6 µm³ (80.0–97.6 fl)			
WBC	4–10 × 10³/mm³ (4–10 × 10⁹/L)	10		
WBC Differential	% polymorphonuclear neutrophils (PMN)/ eosinophils/basophils/lymphocytes/monocytes	73.8/0.5/0.3/18.47	////	////
Platelets	140–440 × 10³/mm³ (140–440 × 10⁹/L)			
Albumin	3.5–5 g/dL (35–50 g/L)			
Bilirubin (total)	0.3–1.1 mg/dL (5.13–18.80 µmol/L)			
Bilirubin (direct)	0–0.3 mg/dL (0–5.1 µmol/L)			
AST	11–47 IU/L (0.18–0.78 µkat/L)			
ALT	7–53 IU/L (0.12–0.88 µkat/L)			
Alk phos (adult)	38–126 IU/L (0.13–2.10 µkat/L)			
HIV RNA	copies/mL	<20		
Absolute CD4	cells/mL (10⁶/L)	726		

Additional Notes: RPR result: 1:128

Blood cultures: no growth in 2/2 cultures

CSF: WBC 2 cells/mm³ (2 × 10⁶/L)

CSF: Protein 19 mg/dL (190 mg/L)

CSF: Glucose 77 mg/dL (4.2 mmol/L)

CSF: Gram stain Negative

CSF: VDRL Nonreactive

CSF: FTA-ABS Negative

DRUG THERAPY PROBLEM WORKSHEET

Type of Problem	Possible Causes	Problem List	Notes
Correlation between drug therapy and medical problems	Drugs without obvious medical indications		
	Medication(s) unidentified		
	Untreated medical conditions		
Need for additional drug therapy	New medical condition requiring new drug therapy	Secondary syphilis	
	Chronic disorder requiring continued drug therapy	Headaches	
	Condition best treated with combination drug therapy		
	May develop new medical condition without prophylactic or preventative therapy or premedication		
Unnecessary drug therapy	Medication with no valid indication or condition is better treated with nondrug therapy		
	Condition caused by accidental or intentional ingestion of toxic amount of drug(s) or chemical(s)		
	Medical problem(s) associated with use of or withdrawal from alcohol, drug(s), or tobacco		
	Taking multiple drugs when single agent is as effective		
	Taking drug(s) to treat an avoidable adverse reaction from another medication		
Appropriate drug selection	Current regimen not usually as effective or safe as other choices		
	Therapy not individualized to patient		
Wrong drug	Medical problem for which drug is not effective		
	Patient has risk factors that contraindicate use of drug		
	Patient has infection with organisms resistant to drug		
	Patient refractory to current drug therapy		
	Taking combination product when single agent appropriate		
	Dosage form inappropriate or medication error		
Drug regimen	PRN use not appropriate for condition		
	Route of administration/dosage form/mode of administration not appropriate for current condition		
	Length or course of therapy not appropriate		
	Drug therapy altered without adequate therapeutic trial		
	Dose or interval flexibility not appropriate		
Dose too low	Dose or frequency too low to produce desired response in this patient		
	Serum drug concentration below desired goal range for indication		
	Timing of antimicrobial prophylaxis not appropriate		
	Medication not stored properly or medication error		
Dose too high	Dose or frequency too high for this patient		
	Serum drug concentration above the desired goal range for indication		
	Dose escalated too quickly		
	Dose or interval flexibility not appropriate for this patient		
	Medication error		

DRUG THERAPY PROBLEM WORKSHEET

Type of Problem	Possible Causes	Problem List	Notes
Therapeutic duplication	Receiving multiple agents without added benefit		
Drug allergy/ adverse drug events	History of allergy or ADE to current (or chemically related) agents		
	Allergy or ADE history not in medical records		
	Patient not using alert for severe allergy or ADE		
	Symptoms or medical problems that may be drug induced		
	Drug administered too rapidly		
	Medication error, actual or potential		
Interactions (drug-drug, drug-disease, drug-nutrient, drug-laboratory test)	Effect of drug altered due to enzyme induction/inhibition, protein binding alterations, or pharmacodynamic change from another drug patient is taking		
	Bioavailability of drug altered due to interaction with another drug or food		
	Effect of drug altered due to substance in food		
	Patient's laboratory test altered due to interference from a drug the patient is taking		
Failure to receive therapy	Patient did not adhere to the drug regimen		
	Drug not given due to medication error		
	Patient did not take due to high drug cost/lack of insurance		
	Patient unable to take oral medication		
	Patient has no IV access for IV medication		
	Drug product not available		
Financial impact	The current regimen is not the most cost effective		
	Patient unable to purchase medications/no insurance		
Patient knowledge of drug therapy	Patient does not understand the purpose, directions, or potential side effects of the drug regimen		Assess the patient's understanding regarding the importance of adherence to his HIV medications
	Current regimen not consistent with the patient's health beliefs		

PHARMACOTHERAPY CARE PLAN

	Medical Problems	Current Drug Regimen	Therapy Goals, Desired Endpoints	Therapeutic Recommendations	Therapeutic Alternatives	Rationale
1	Syphilis, secondary	None	Eradicate causative organism *Treponema pallidum*	Penicillin G benzathine 2.4 mill units IM one time	Alternative therapy options not recommended since patient does not have a documented penicillin allergy. Alternative therapy options include: Doxycycline 100 mg po bid × 14 days Azithromycin 2 g po × 1 dose Ceftriaxone 1 g IM/IV × 14 days	Drug of choice for this infection.
2	Headaches	Acetaminophen 1000 mg po q6h prn	Reduce incidence of headaches	No treatment at this time. Evaluate headache triggers and use of acetaminophen	If headache reported while patient in clinic: acetaminophen 500 mg po × once	Unknown use of acetaminophen prn and headache triggers.
3	Hypertension	None	BP <140/80 mmHg Reduction in CV and renal morbidity and mortality	No therapy recommended at this time. Recommend repeating BP measurement.	HCTZ 12.5 mg daily Institute diet and exercise modifications per current hypertension guidelines	BP may not be at goal. Recommend repeat BP readings to evaluate trend.
4	HIV	Emtricitabine 200 mg/tenofovir disoproxil fumarate 300 mg po daily Dolutegravir 50 mg po daily	Increase CD4 count annually Undetectable viral load	Continue current therapy	If the patient's CD4 count declines, viral load rises, or he becomes intolerant to current therapy, consider the use of combination emtricitabine/tenofovir disoproxil fumarate/ elvitegravir/cobicistat or emtricitabine/tenofovir disoproxil fumarate plus darunavir/cobicistat (or darunavir/ritonavir) if deemed adherent to current regimen	Current therapy is recommended per 2015 HIV AIDS treatment guidelines

PHARMACOTHERAPY CARE PLAN

Medical Problems	Current Drug Regimen	Therapy Goals, Desired Endpoints	Therapeutic Recommendations	Therapeutic Alternatives	Rationale
5 Smoking cessation	None	Stop smoking Improve CV health and prevent MI	Smoking cessation counseling: Nonpharmacologic therapy: • Brief physician/ practitioner advice • Telephone counselling • Self-help material Pharmacologic therapy: Bupropion SR 150 mg q24h for 3 d and then 150 mg po q12h Nicotine patch 21 mg/d for 4 wk, then 14 mg/d for 2 wk, and then 7 mg/d for 2 wk	Varenicline 0.5 mg q24h for 3 d, then 0.5 mg q12h for 4–7 d, and then 1 mg q 12 h for 2–12 wk	Combination therapy in addition to nonpharmacologic therapy improves a patient's chance of remaining abstinent.

	Medical Problems	Planned Monitoring and Follow-Up	Patient Education Summary Points
1	Syphilis, Secondary	• S/S of Jarisch-Herxheimer reaction • Repeat serologic titers at 6 and 12 months	• This infection is curable; however, your partner(s) will also require treatment. Using protection may reduce your chances of reinfection. • Symptoms of a serious allergic reaction may include rash, itching, swelling, severe dizziness, and trouble breathing. If you notice other effects not listed above, alert your nurse immediately.
2	Headaches	• Check baseline LFT • Monitor frequency of headaches	• Headaches can be triggered by factors such as environmental exposures, medication use, and food intake. • Evaluation and avoidance of triggers can be used to decrease rate of headaches.
3	Hypertension	BP q2–4 w	• Control of your blood pressure is extremely important and may decrease your chances of future health complications (i.e., heart disease, kidney disease). • Hydrochlorothiazide is a water pill that aids in the reduction of blood pressure. Since it may increase your glucose concentrations, monitoring your glucose is important.
4	HIV	CD4 count q3–4mo Viral load q3–4mo	• Emtricitabine/tenofovir disoproxil fumarate and dolutegravir are used to treat human immunodeficiency virus (HIV) infection. HIV causes acquired-immunodeficiency syndrome (AIDS). These medications do not cure HIV or AIDS, but they may slow the progress of the disease. It is important that you do not miss any doses of these medications, so do not allow yourself to run out of them. If you miss a lot of doses, or forget to take the drug, the virus can become stronger. When your supply of this medicine becomes low, contact your physician or pharmacy ahead of time. • Ask your physician or pharmacist before using any over-the-counter products, vitamins, or herbal products because they may affect how these medications work.
5	Smoking cessation	• Smoking cessation • Decrease in the number of cigarettes per day until cessation is achieved • Withdrawal symptoms • Adverse effects of medications (i.e., tachycardia, insomnia, dizziness, application site reaction, rash)	Your physician has prescribed bupropion SR to assist you in your quit attempt. He has also recommended that you use nicotine patches. • Swallow the bupropion SR tablet whole. Do not crush, chew, or break it. • Apply the nicotine patch once daily after removing the patch applied the previous day. Do not put the patch on the same place where you have worn a patch in the past week. • Do not cut the wrapper or patch.
6			

SIGNIFICANT REFERENCES RELATED TO THERAPY RECOMMENDATIONS

Panel on Antiretroviral Guidelines for Adults and Adolescents. Guidelines for the use of antiretroviral agents in HIV-1-infected adults and adolescents. Department of Health and Human Services. Available at <http://aidsinfo.nih.gov/contentfiles/lvguidelines/AdultandAdolescentGL.pdf>.

Centers for Disease Control and Prevention. Sexually Transmitted Diseases Treatment Guidelines, 2015. *MMWR.* 2015;64:3.

KEY INFORMATION FOR FACILITATOR

Question 1	Which microbial organism is responsible for causing syphilis and how did this patient likely acquire it?
	The responsible organism is *Treponema pallidum*, a spirochete that cannot be grown in culture and can only be directly identified when using darkfield microscopy. Though there are known cases of vertical transmission, this patient likely acquired the infection through sexual contact.
Question 2	What clinical features are associated with secondary syphilis? What additional lab values might be useful to obtain in evaluating additional systemic effects of the patient's disease?
	A rash is a trademark of secondary syphilis with the lesions appearing around the trunk and spreading to the extremities. Involvement of the hands and soles raises the suspicion for syphilis in the appropriate context. Lymphadenopathy may be present though it is not limited to only the cervical region. A "moth-eaten" alopecia of the scalp, beard, and eyebrows may also indicate secondary syphilis.
	Renal dysfunction and hepatitis may also manifest as a result of infection, making the availability of liver function tests useful. While neurologic and/or ocular symptoms such as altered mental status or uveitis may be present, these findings might be more suggestive of neurosyphilis.
Question 3	What is the preferred medication, dose, route of administration, and number of doses to treat the patient's condition? What reaction should you warn the patient about after starting therapy and what should you do if it occurs?
	For secondary syphilis (or early latent syphilis) the treatment of choice is penicillin G benzathine, 2.4 million units, intramuscularly, one time.
	After receiving the dose, the patient is at risk for the Jarisch-Herxheimer reaction, a febrile state that may result from dead *Treponema* cellular products stimulating cytokines throughout the body. Acetaminophen or other antipyretics may be considered purely for symptomatic management.
Question 4	If the patient had documented anaphylaxis to penicillin in the past three years, what alternate medication regimens (drug/dose/route/duration) could be considered and what are some advantages/disadvantages to using them?
	Alternate medications: • Doxycycline 100 mg po bid × 14 days • Azithromycin 2 g po × 1 dose • Ceftriaxone 1 g IM/IV × 14 days Some advantages include avoiding desensitization protocols in patients with anaphylactic penicillin allergies (for all regimens) and offering oral alternatives (for azithromycin, a one-time oral alternative). Disadvantages to these regimens include a concern for resistance (particularly with azithromycin) and repeated IM/IV injections with ceftriaxone.

KEY INFORMATION FOR FACILITATOR

Question 5	What follow-up would you schedule for the patient and what monitoring parameters would you wish to continue evaluating? What would you do if the patient failed to meet your desired endpoints?
	At a minimum, follow-up should be schedule for 6 and 12 months following treatment. Repeat serologic titers should be checked with the goal of therapy being a fourfold reduction from the original titer 1 year after treatment. If this is not achieved, treatment is generally repeated with penicillin G benzathine 2.4 million units IM given weekly × 3 weeks. Though there is data indicating some patients may be less likely to achieve a fourfold reduction based on initial titers and duration of disease, one should also consider the possibility of neurosyphilis based on disease presentation and acquire CSF studies if desired.
Question 6	How would your therapeutic recommendations be changed had the patient presented with a history of maculopapular rash that had since resolved and a predicted date of infection more than one year ago?
	In the case of late latent syphilis as described in the question, treatment recommendations would change from a one-time dose of penicillin G benzathine to a three-time dosing schedule, each administered one week apart.
Follow-up Question 7	At his six-month follow-up, the patient presents with his girlfriend who complains of vision changes. The patient states she has also recently not been acting like herself. Workup is performed and the patient is found to have a VDRL of 1:64 in her CSF. What is your preferred treatment regimen for the patient's girlfriend?
	The preferred treatment regimen for neurosyphilis is aqueous crystalline penicillin G 18–24 million units administered IV as either a continuous infusion or as 3–4 million units every 4 hours. Duration of therapy is approximately 10–14 days.
Question 8	The patient's girlfriend is refusing hospital admission at this time but is willing to the come to clinic daily for treatment if necessary. What regimen may be used in this setting if adherence can be assured?
	An alternate treatment regimen for neurosyphilis includes procaine penicillin G 2.4 million units IM daily for 10–14 days in combination with probenecid 500 mg po 4× daily for the total treatment duration.
Question 9	If the patient's girlfriend reported that she had a severe anaphylactic reaction to penicillin in the recent past, how would this alter your therapeutic recommendations? What course of action would be pursued and how would it be done?
	Penicillin is the only recommended drug for the treatment of neurosyphilis. In the event of an anaphylactic penicillin reaction, the patient would be desensitized using one of a number of different protocols. For one possible desensitization protocol please refer to the CDC STD guidelines under "Management of Persons Who Have a History of Penicillin Allergy."
	While ceftriaxone 2 g IV daily × 10–14 days has been used to some success, it should be noted that this regimen has a potential failure rate of approximately 25% and should be avoided if at all possible.
Additional Information	